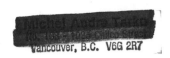

D0426837

The Relationship of
Theory and Research

The Relationship of Theory and Research

Third Edition

Jacqueline Fawcett, PhD, FAAN
University of Pennsylvania
School of Nursing
Philadelphia, Pennsylvania

F. A. Davis Company • Philadelphia

F. A. Davis Company
1915 Arch Street
Philadelphia, PA 19103

Printed in the United States of America

Last digit indicates print number: 10 9 8 7 6 5 4 3 2 1

Publisher: Lisa A. Biello
Acquisitions Editor: Joanne DaCunha, RN, MSN
Cover Designer: Louis J. Forgione

As new scientific information becomes available through basic and clinical research, recommended treatments and drug therapies undergo changes. The author and publisher have done everything possible to make this book accurate, up to date, and in accord with accepted standards at the time of publication. The author, editors, and publisher are not responsible for errors or omissions or for consequences from application of the book, and make no warranty, expressed or implied, in regard to the contents of the book. Any practice described in this book should be applied by the reader in accordance with professional standards of care used in regard to the unique circumstances that may apply in each situation. The reader is advised always to check product information (package inserts) for changes and new information regarding dose and contraindications before administering any drug. Caution is especially urged when using new or infrequently ordered drugs.

Library of Congress Cataloging-in-Publication Data

Fawcett, Jacqueline.
   The relationship of theory and research / Jacqueline Fawcett. —
3rd ed.
     p. cm.
   Includes bibliographical references and index.
   ISBN 0-8036-0406-8
   1. Research. 2. Theory (Philosophy) I. Title.
Q180.A1F39   1998   98-31324
001.4—dc21   CIP

This book is meant to fill a major gap in the literature of most disciplines by presenting a detailed discussion of the relationship between conceptual models, middle-range theories, and empirical research methods. Emphasis in this edition continues to be placed on information needed by both novice and accomplished scholars for the analysis and evaluation of research documents, including proposals for new studies and reports of completed studies.

The book is based on three philosophical premises. First, in keeping with a postpositivist perspective, I believe that all observation is theory-laden; that is, all theory development is based on implicit or explicit sets of assumptions that are derived from or are an inherent part of a conceptual model. Second, I believe that both conceptual models and theories without research and research without conceptual models and theories do little to advance knowledge in any meaningful way. Third, I believe that although it is true that the conceptual and theoretical aspects of research have been neglected by many investigators in favor of an emphasis on research methods, it is not true that there is no basis for conceptual models and theories in research documents. Rather, I believe that the paucity of explicit conceptual models and theories in research documents is due to the failure of investigators to articulate the conceptual and theoretical components of their studies.

This book goes beyond the many fine existing texts that concern conceptual models, theories, or research methods in its focus on the relations between conceptual models, theories, and empirical research methods. This edition includes the basic content of the first and second editions, inasmuch as the analytic techniques discussed are fundamental and have not changed over time. The third edition of the book presents a refinement and reorganization of the content of the previous editions. These modifications are the result of the author's experience in using the book as a text for a doctoral program course and of conversations with doctoral students and colleagues throughout the country. The major modification is the integration of content from Chapter 5 of the second edition into the relevant sections of Chapters 1, 2, 3, and 4 of the third edition. This modification reflects current thinking about the influence of conceptual models on research methods and should help readers to understand that the conceptual elements of research are not an afterthought, but rather are an integral aspect of any study.

Chapter 1 presents an overview of the relations between conceptual models, theories, and research and introduces the notion of the conceptual-theoretical-empirical structure for research. Accordingly, the discussion focuses on the definition and functions of conceptual models; the definitions, functions, and types of theories (descriptive, explanatory, predictive) and research designs (descriptive, correlational, experimental); and the selection of appropriate research designs for development of different types of theories. This edition includes updated definitions of conceptual models, theories, and research drawn from the latest editions of relevant textbooks from nursing and other disciplines. Chapter 1 also includes discussion of the most recent thinking about the distinctions between abstract conceptual models and more concrete theories, as well as the contributions of conceptual models and theories to theory-generating and theory-testing research designs. In addition, the chapter includes discussion of the issues surrounding the progression of theory development.

Chapter 2 presents a comprehensive format for analysis of conceptual-theoretical-empirical structures for theory-generating and theory-testing research. Emphasis is placed on analysis of the concepts and propositions that make up conceptual models and middle-range theories.

The close connection between conceptual models, theories, and research methods mandates evaluation of the conceptual and theoretical elements of a research document, as well as the empirical research methods used to generate or test the theory. Chapter 3, therefore, presents criteria for the evaluation of conceptual-theoretical-empirical structures for theory-generating and theory-testing research. In addition, the influence of research findings on the empirical adequacy of middle-range theories and the credibility of conceptual models is discussed in detail.

The credibility of a conceptual model and the empirical adequacy of a middle-range theory ultimately should be determined by evaluating the findings of the research that generated or tested the theory. Accordingly, Chapter 4 extends the discussion of the empirical adequacy of theories and the credibility of conceptual models, begun in Chapter 3, by describing formal procedures that can be used to prepare integrative reviews of the findings of related studies. Both qualitative and quantitative approaches to the integration of research findings are discussed.

Chapter 5 presents guidelines for the preparation of research documents that clearly describe how to write the conceptual-theoretical-empirical structure for theory-generating or theory-testing research. Examples drawn from existing research documents are to illustrate each guideline.

Numerous diagrams and tables are used to illustrate and summarize the narrative in each chapter. The reference list for each chapter is augmented by additional readings about conceptual models, theories, and research methods. The vast majority of examples given in Chapters 1, 2, 3, 4, and 5 are taken from published research reports and funded research proposals that present at least some aspect of conceptual models and middle-range theories in an explicit manner.

Complete formalization of the conceptual-theoretical-empirical structures for seven published reports, representing descriptive, correlational, and experimental research, are presented in the Appendices. This edition includes entirely new reports, all of which include the description of an explicit conceptual model that was used to guide the theory-generating or theory-testing research.

The book is intended for neophyte and mature scholars in all academic and professional disciplines. Theorists and researchers should find the chapters on analysis on conceptual-theoretical-empirical structures and integration of research findings particularly helpful. Researchers seeking funding for their proposals and journal publication of their findings will find the chapter on writing proposals and reports particularly helpful. Consumers of research, including clinicians, should find that the chapter on evaluation of conceptual-theoretical-empirical structures facilitates their understanding of the content of research documents and provides a systematic approach to judgments about the applicability of research findings in practical situations. Educators should find that the book as a whole assists students to comprehend the essential connections between conceptual models, middle-range theories, and research methods and improves their ability to analyze and evaluate existing research reports and prepare coherent research proposals. The book is most appropriate as a required text in graduate courses in theory development and research. It is also appropriate as a recommended text for undergraduate research courses to enhance students' understanding of the connections between conceptual models, middle-range theories, and research methods.

No words can adequately express my debt to Florence S. Downs, Professor Emeritus, University of Pennsylvania, who was my co-author for the previous two editions of the book. Florence is a mentor beyond compare. Her wisdom and insight into the relation of theory and research was the impetus for the first edition. Our many conversations over the years have contributed greatly to my ideas about the relations between conceptual models, middle-range theories, and research, and my ability to convey those ideas to the readers of this book.

I am continually stimulated by the questions from students and colleagues about conceptual models, theories, and research. These questions have challenged me to continue to refine and clarify my ideas and strive to write about those ideas as clearly as possible. In addition, I would like to acknowledge the helpful comments of the reviewers of the draft manuscript for this edition of the book. Their ideas stimulated refinements that I hope have enhanced the clarity of my ideas.

I am, as always, very grateful to my husband, John S. Fawcett, for the love and support he has steadfastly provided, no matter how distracted I have been by writing and teaching. I would be remiss if I did not mention that our move to Maine has provided a marvelous new environment in which to live and write with joy.

I continue to acknowledge the encouragement given by the editor of the first edition of the book, Charles Bollinger. And, I gratefully acknowledge the encouragement provided by my editors at F. A. Davis Company, Robert G. Martone and Joanne DaCunha. I also acknowledge the essential contributions of all the people who facilitated the production of this edition.

Jacqueline Fawcett

Reviewers

John R. Phillips, RN, PhD
Associate Professor, Nursing
Division of Nursing
School of Education
New York University
New York

Ruth M. Tappen, EdD, RN, FAAN
Christine E. Lynn Eminent Scholar and Professor
College of Nursing
Florida Atlantic University
Boca Raton, FL

Company from Broome, M.E. Integrative literature reviews in the development of concepts. In B.L. Rodgers & K.A. Knafl (Eds.), *Concept development in nursing: Foundations, techniques, and applications.* Copyright ©1993 W.B. Saunders.

Quotations in Chapter 5 were reprinted with the permission of: Sigma Theta Tau International Center Nursing Press from Sherman, D.W. (1996). Nurses' willingness to care to AIDS patients and spirituality, social support, and death anxiety. *Image: Journal of Nursing Scholarship, 28,* 205–213; and John Wiley & Sons, Inc. from Villarruel, A.M. (1995), Mexican-American cultural meanings, expressions, self-care and dependent-care actions associated with experiences of pain. *Research in Nursing and Health, 18,* 427–436.

Figure 5-1 and Table 5-3 were reprinted with the permission of Chestnut House Publications from Calvillo, E.R., & Flaskerud, J.H. (1993). The adequacy and scope of Roy's adaptation model to guide cross-cultural pain research. *Nursing Science Quarterly, 6,* 118–129.

Figure 5-2 and 5-3 and Tables 5-11 and 5-12 were reprinted with the permission of Sigma Theta Tau International Center Nursing Press from Hamner, J.B. (1996). Preliminary testing of a proposition from the Roy adaptation model. *Image: Journal of Nursing Scholarship, 28,* 215–220.

Tables 5-6 and 5-7 were reprinted with the permission of Sigma Theta Tau International Center Nursing Press from Dzurec, L.C. (1994). Schizophrenic clients' experiences of power: Using hermeneutic analysis. *Image: Journal of Nursing Scholarship, 26,* 155–159.

Tables 5-8 and 5-9 were reprinted with the permission of the Oncology Nursing Press, Inc. from Moore, J.B., & Mosher, R.B. (1997). Adjustment responses of children and their mothers to cancer: Self-care and anxiety. *Oncology Nursing Forum, 24,* 519–525.

Table 5-10 was reprinted with the permission of Sage Publications, Inc. from Yarcheski, A., & Mahon, N.E. Rogers's pattern manifestations and health in adolescents. *Western Journal of Nursing Research 17,* 383–397. Copyright ©1995 Sage Publications.

Artinian, N.T. (1991). Stress experience of spouses of patients having coronary artery bypass during hospitalization and 6 weeks after discharge. *Heart and Lung, 20,* 52–59, was reprinted with the permission of Mosby Year Book, Inc.

Bournaki, M-C. (1997). Correlates of pain-related responses to venipunctures in school-age children. *Nursing Research, 46,* 147–154, was reprinted with the permission of Lippincott-Raven Publishers. Copyright ©1997 Lippincott-Raven Publishers, Philadelphia, PA.

Breckenridge, D.M. (1997). Patients' perceptions of why, how, and by whom dialysis treatment modality was chosen. *American Nephrology Nurses Association Journal, 24,* 313–319, was reprinted with the permission of Anthony J. Jannetti, Inc.

Janelli, L.M., Kanski, G.W., Jones, H.M., & Kennedy, M.C. (1995). Exploring music intervention with restrained patients. *Nursing Forum, 30*(4), 12–18, was reprinted with the permission of NurseCom, Inc.

Newman, D.M.L. (1997). The Inventory of Functional Status-Caregiver of a

Child in Body Cast. *Journal of Pediatric Nursing*, *12*, 142–147, was reprinted with the permission of W.B. Saunders. Copyright ©1997 W.B. Saunders.

Roberts, K.L., Brittin, M., Cook, M-A., & deClifford, J. (1994). Boomerang pillows and respiratory capacity. *Clinical Nursing Research*, *3*, 157–165, was reprinted with the permission of Sage Publications, Inc. Copyright ©1994 Sage Publications.

Rosenthal-Dichter, C.H. (1996). The pediatric physiologic stress response: A concept analysis. *Scholarly Inquiry for Nursing Practice*, *10*, 211–234, was reprinted with the permission of Springer Publications Company, Inc., New York 10012.

Contents

1 An Overview of Conceptual Models, Theories, and Research

■ Many disciplines exist to generate, test, and apply theories that will improve the quality of people's lives. Every such theory-development effort is based on a particular frame of reference that provides an intellectual and sociohistorical context for theoretical thinking, for research, and ultimately, for practice. That context is provided by the conceptual model that guides theory development by means of empirical research. This chapter presents an overview of the components of conceptual-theoretical-empirical structures. The chapter begins with a presentation of the definitions and functions of conceptual models, theories, and research, continues with a discussion of appropriate research designs for development of different kinds of empirical theories, and concludes with a discussion of issues involved in the progression of theory development.

CONCEPTUAL-THEORETICAL-EMPIRICAL STRUCTURES

The components of any *conceptual-theoretical-empirical structure* include a conceptual model, a theory, and empirical research methods. Each conceptual model and theory is made up of concepts and propositions. A *concept* is a word or phrase that summarizes the essential characteristics or properties of a phenomenon. A *proposition* is a statement about a concept or the relation between concepts.

The components of conceptual-theoretical-empirical structures form a hierarchy that is based on levels of abstraction (Feigl, 1970; Gibbs, 1972; Margenau, 1972). The conceptual model that provides the context or frame of reference for theory-generating and theory-testing research is at the most abstract level of the structure. The theory that was generated or tested is at the intermediate level, and the empirical research methods used to collect and analyze the data are at the most concrete level (Fig. 1–1).

CONCEPTUAL MODEL

Definitions of Conceptual Model

Definitions assign meaning to terms. Inasmuch as scholars frequently attach different meanings to the same term or use different terms to mean the same thing, one author's use of a term cannot be assumed to be the same as another author's or the reader's. One of the best ways to be sure about the meaning of any term is to determine how each author has used it. Here are some typical definitions of the term *conceptual model*:

■ A conceptual model is a network of concepts, in relation, that accounts for broad nursing phenomena; synonymous with conceptual framework. (Kramer, 1997, p. 67)

■ A conceptual model is a set of abstract and general concepts and propositions that integrate those concepts into a meaningful configuration; synonymous with conceptual framework, conceptual system, paradigm, and disciplinary matrix. (Fawcett, 1997, pp. 13–14)

■ A conceptual framework is a general perspective of organizing and classifying concepts into a relevant structure. (Kim, 1997, p. 32)

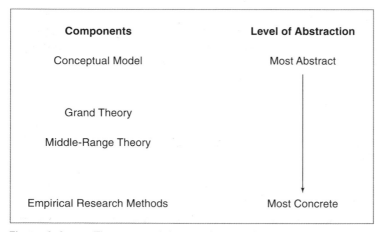

Figure I–I ■ The conceptual-theoretical-empirical structure: components and levels of abstraction.

Kramer, Fawcett, and Kim all agree that a conceptual model is made up of concepts that are organized in some way. Furthermore, all three authors agree that a conceptual model deals with relatively global phenomena. The following definition, which reflects the global and set-of-concepts notions of all three definitions, will be used in this book:

■ A conceptual model is a set of relatively abstract and general concepts and the propositions that describe or link those concepts.

The Function of a Conceptual Model

A conceptual model provides a distinctive frame of reference—"a horizon of expectations" (Popper, 1965, p. 47)—and "a coherent, internally unified way of thinking about . . . events and processes" (Frank, 1968, p. 45). Thus, each conceptual model provides a different lens or perspective for viewing the phenomena that are within the domain of inquiry of a particular discipline.

Furthermore, each conceptual model reflects the philosophical stance, cognitive orientation, research tradition, and practice tradition of a particular group of scholars within a discipline, rather than those of all members of the discipline. Most disciplines, therefore, have more than one conceptual model. Nursing, for example, has at least seven major conceptual models. Johnson's Behavioral System Model (1990) emphasizes the efficiency and effectiveness of the person's behavior. King's General Systems Framework (Frey and Sieloff, 1995) focuses on attainment of goals. Levine's Conservation Model (Schaefer and Pond, 1991) requires consideration of conservation of the individual's energy and structural, personal, and social integrity. Neuman's Systems Model (1995) highlights client system stability. Orem's Self-Care Framework (1995) emphasizes self-care capabilities. Rogers' Science of Unitary Human Beings (Barrett, 1990) draws attention to the unity of human life. Roy's Adaptation Model (Roy and Andrews, 1991) focuses on the individual's ability to adapt to a constantly changing environment.

Each conceptual model, then, focuses on certain phenomena that are regarded as relevant. Other phenomena are ignored because they are less important. For example, Johnson's Behavioral System Model declares that people are behavioral systems that perform specialized tasks to maintain their integrity. In contrast, Roy's Adaptation Model asserts that people are adaptive systems that respond to environmental stimuli. Note that Johnson mentions nothing about stimuli, and Roy does not mention specialized tasks. Thus, when a phenomenon is not mentioned, it is, in effect, ruled out of the domain of interest.

THEORY

Definitions of Theory

A theory, like a conceptual model, is made up of concepts and propositions and has many meanings. Here are some definitions of *theory* that are typical of the variability in the scope of the term's meaning:

■ A theory is a construct that accounts for or organizes some phenomenon. (Barnum, 1998, p. 1)

■ A theory is a set of interrelated concepts, definitions, and propositions that present a systematic view of essential elements in a field of inquiry by specifying relations among variables. (King, 1997, p. 23)

■ Theories comprise, first of all, a set of concepts. . . . Second, theories comprise a set of statements or propositions, each of which indicates a relationship among the concepts. . . . Third, the propositions must form a logically interrelated deductive system. (Polit and Hungler, 1995, p. 97)

These definitions place various restrictions on what is considered to be theory. Barnum's definition is the least restrictive, because it does not require that a theory state a relation, nor does it preclude statements of relations. Also, her definition is the only one that does not require a theory to take more than one concept into account, nor does it limit the theory to just one concept. This lack of restriction permits a description of one concept to be considered a theory.

King's definition is more restrictive, in that it requires a theory to state a relation between two or more concepts. A description of just one concept would not be considered a theory, according to her definition.

Polit and Hungler's definition, which is similar to Homans' (1964) and Kerlinger's (1986) frequently cited definitions, is the most restrictive, because it requires not only that relations be stated, but also that a deductive system of propositions be evident. Thus, theories that are developed by means of induction would not be considered legitimate theories. The restrictions imposed by Polit and Hungler would, therefore, preclude all but the most elaborate, deductively developed formulations from being considered theories.

The following definition, which draws primarily from Barnum's definition, is used in this book:

■ A theory is a set of relatively concrete and specific concepts and the propositions that describe or link those concepts.

The lack of restrictions imposed by this definition is advantageous, in that descriptions, explanations, and predictions all may be considered theories. Moreover, this definition reflects the difference in the level of abstraction of a conceptual model and a theory by requiring the concepts of a theory to be relatively concrete and specific, whereas those of a conceptual model are relatively abstract and general.

Theories themselves do, however, vary in their levels of abstraction and scope. The more abstract and broader type of theory is called a *grand theory*. The more concrete and narrower type of theory is called a *middle-range theory*.

More specifically, grand theories are rather broad in scope; they are made up of concepts and propositions that are less abstract and general than the concepts and propositions of a conceptual model but are not as concrete and specific as the concepts and propositions of a middle-range theory. Grand theories are developed by thoughtful and insightful appraisal of existing ideas or creative intellectual leaps beyond existing knowledge rather than by means of empirical research. Newman's

(1994) theory of health as expanding consciousness is an example of a grand theory. Her theory was derived from Rogers' Science of Unitary Human Beings and is made up of five rather abstract concepts—time, space, movement, consciousness, and pattern—and the rather general propositions that describe and link those concepts.

Middle-range theories are narrower in scope than grand theories. They are made up of a limited number of concepts and propositions that are written at a relatively concrete and specific level. Middle-range theories are generated and tested by means of empirical research. Examples are found in virtually all proposals for and reports of empirical research.

In summary, grand theories are less abstract and general than conceptual models but not as concrete and specific as middle-range theories. This book focuses on the analysis and evaluation of middle-range theories and their parent conceptual models.

The Function of a Theory

Middle-range theories represent intelligible and systematic schemata for observations. The value of those schemata lies in their ability to "unite phenomena which, without the theor[ies], are either surprising, anomalous, or wholly unnoticed" (Hanson, 1958, p. 121). Middle-range theories, then, provide structures for the interpretation of initially puzzling behavior, situations, and events. Moreover, they unify what is known by common sense (Collin, 1992).

Many middle-range theories are required to account for the vast array of experiences encountered by human beings. Each middle-range theory addresses a relatively concrete and specific phenomenon by stating what the phenomenon is, why it occurs, or how it occurs. The function of a middle-range theory, therefore, is to describe, explain, or predict phenomena.

CONCEPTUAL MODELS AND THEORIES

A conceptual model, whether implicit or explicit, is always the precursor to a grand theory or a middle-range theory. Indeed, the belief that theory development proceeds outside the context of a conceptual frame of reference is "absurd" (Popper, 1965, p. 46). As Slife and Williams (1995) explained:

> ■ All theories have implied understandings about the world that are crucial to their formulation and use. . . . [In other words,] all theories have assumptions and implications embedded in them [and] stem from cultural and historic contexts that lend them meaning and influence how they are understood and implemented. (pp. 2, 9)

More specifically, every theory is shaped by an a priori frame of reference, that is, a conceptual model that guides theory generation and theory testing by directing the questions that are asked and how they are asked (Babbie, 1998; Nagel, 1961). In particular, each conceptual model functions as a "canopy" of ideas and statements that guide theory-generating and theory-testing research (Downs, 1994,

p. 195). Hempel (1970) explained, "The specification of the model determines in part what consequences may be derived from the theory and, hence, what the theory can [describe,] explain or predict" (p. 157).

Many grand and middle-range theories are needed to fully describe, explain, and predict all the phenomena encompassed by a conceptual model. That is because each theory is more circumscribed than its parent conceptual model, and, therefore, deals only with a portion of the domain of inquiry identified by the conceptual model. Consequently, each theory may address one or a few of the many concepts and propositions that make up a conceptual model.

Some theories are derived directly from conceptual models. For example, Rogers (1986) derived three grand theories from the Science of Unitary Human Beings. Each one emphasizes a different aspect of the more abstract conceptual model. The theory of accelerating evolution posits that evolutionary change is speeding up and that the range of diversity of life processes is widening. The theory of rhythmical correlates of change, which focuses on human and environmental energy field rhythms, proposes that the accelerating evolution and increasing diversity of human field patterns are integral with the accelerating evolution and increasing diversity of environmental field patterns. The theory of paranormal phenomena provides explanations for various paranormal experiences, such as precognition, clairvoyance, and telepathy.

When grand theories are derived from conceptual models, they can serve as the starting points for middle-range theory development. Alligood (1991), for example, derived a middle-range theory of creativity, actualization, and empathy from Rogers' (1986) grand theory of accelerating evolution.

Alternatively, middle-range theories can be derived directly from the conceptual model. For example, Orem (1995) derived three middle-range theories from the Self-Care Framework. Each theory focuses on a different component of the more abstract conceptual model. The theory of self-care proposes that self-care is a learned behavior that intentionally regulates human structural integrity, functioning, and human development. The theory of self-care deficit proposes that people can benefit from nursing because they are subject to health-related or health-derived limitations that render them incapable of continuous self-care or care of others or result in ineffective or incomplete care. The theory of nursing systems proposes that nursing systems are formed when nurses use their abilities to prescribe, design, and provide nursing care.

Furthermore, existing middle-range theories can be linked with a conceptual model when the existing theory provides the necessary specificity of conceptual model concepts and propositions needed for a particular situation. In that case, there is no need to duplicate knowledge by deriving a new theory from the conceptual model. Care must be taken, however, to ensure that the conceptual model and the theory are logically congruent, that is, the model and the theory must reflect compatible views about the nature of the phenomena to be studied (Fawcett, 1993; Whall, 1986).

Suppose, for example, that a conceptual model includes the proposition that the person actively engages in interactions with the surrounding environment rather than being a passive reactor to external forces. Behavior modification theory is not compatible with the conceptual model because it proposes that the person's behavior is shaped by external conditioning stimuli. In contrast, the client-centered theory of personality is compatible with the conceptual model because it proposes that the individual is actively responsible for his or her behavior (Burton, 1974).

For example, the middle-range theory of planned behavior (Ajzen, 1991) has been linked to Neuman's Systems Model because it is logically congruent with Neuman's model. Moreover, the theory provided the requisite level of specificity for propositions that were tested in studies of behavioral intentions regarding smoking (Hanson, 1995) and cervical cancer screening (Jennings, 1997).

A conceptual model also may suggest ways to extend an existing middle-range theory. For example, the theory of planned behavior identifies several factors that influence the individual's intention to behave in a certain way, in terms of beliefs, attitudes, subjective norms, and perceived behavioral control. The theory also asserts that intention to behave in a certain way is highly correlated with actual behavior. The theory does not, however, identify clinical interventions or educational programs that might modify the factors that influence behavioral intentions. But linking the theory to Neuman's Systems Model guides the addition of particular primary, secondary, and tertiary prevention interventions that could be used to modify relevant factors (Hanson, 1995; Jennings, 1997).

It is important to point out that conceptual models and theories are not real or tangible entities. Rather, they are tentative formulations that represent scholars' best efforts to understand phenomena (Payton, 1994; Polit and Hungler, 1995). Their tentative nature means that the knowledge contained in conceptual models and theories carries with it a degree of uncertainty.

RESEARCH

Definitions of Research

The term "research," like "conceptual model" and "theory," has several meanings. Here are some representative definitions of the term *research*:

■ Research is the formal process of seeking knowledge and understanding through use of rigorous methodologies. (Parse, 1997, p. 74)

■ Research may be defined as systematic investigations that are rooted in objective reality and that aim to develop general knowledge about natural phenomena (Polit and Hungler, 1995, p. 9)

■ Research is systematic, controlled, empirical, and critical investigation of natural phenomena guided by theory and hypotheses about the presumed relations among such phenomena. (Kerlinger, 1986, p. 10)

These definitions, like those of theory, vary in their restrictiveness. Parse's definition is the least restrictive, because it does not require, and does not preclude, that the study be empirical. Thus, her definition does not call for a single mode of inquiry for the development of knowledge. Yet it is a strong definition that, like the others, requires the process of research to be formal and rigorous.

Polit and Hungler's definition is more restrictive than Parse's, in that it requires research to be objective. That requirement could be interpreted to mean that subjective methods of inquiry, such as phenomenology, are not considered research.

Kerlinger's definition is distinctive in that it emphasizes the connection between theory and research. It is, however, also the most restrictive definition; it requires study of relations, and thereby excludes investigation of single concepts. Furthermore, it requires direct experience or observation of data; that is, the empirical method. This requirement implies that nonempirical works, such as some philosophical inquiries, are not considered research. Finally, it requires the testing of existing theories and hypotheses. This requirement implies that inquiry directed toward the generation of theories would not be considered research.

The following definition, which reflects the least restrictive elements of the three definitions, is used in this book:

> ■ Research is a formal, systematic, and rigorous process of inquiry used to generate and test the concepts and propositions that comprise middle-range theories, which are derived from or linked with a conceptual model.

This definition reflects the levels of abstraction of conceptual-theoretical-empirical structures. In addition, although the focus of this book is on empirical research, the definition does not rule out other forms of inquiry.

The Function of Research

Research frequently is viewed as a systematic process employed to answer questions and solve problems. The process often is regarded as sterile—a linear series of steps to be surmounted in the search for solutions to problems. Research, however, is much more than a method of problem solving. In fact, as stipulated in its definition, the function of research is to generate or test the concepts and propositions of middle-range theories. More specifically, research is the vehicle for the development of middle-range theories and the refinement of conceptual models. In particular, research is one part of a cycle: the part that supplies the data. The other parts of the cycle—the conceptual model and the theory—give meaning to the data. That is true whether the purpose of the research is to generate a theory or to test one (Cook and Shadish, 1986; Lavee and Dollahite, 1991; Polit and Hungler, 1995; Schumacher and Gortner, 1992). The cycle is completed when the meanings ascribed to the data are used to draw conclusions regarding the adequacy and utility of the theory and the credibility of the conceptual model.

CONCEPTUAL MODELS, THEORIES, AND RESEARCH

Research *always* starts with a conceptual model. The influence of a conceptual model on research was explained by Batey (1971/1997), who pointed out that although two investigators may observe the same situation or event, "their notions of why it occurs, their conceptual organization about the problem, [and] the knowledge base they select for studying that problem, may differ" (p. 686). In other words, each investigator views situations and events through a particular lens or frame of reference, which is encapsulated in a conceptual model.

Although research always starts with a conceptual model, its global nature precludes direct empirical observation and testing of its concepts and propositions. Rather, each conceptual model contributes to theory development by guiding the generation and testing of theories through research. More specifically, conceptual models act as global research traditions for the generation and testing of middle-range theories. Laudan (1981) explained:

> ■ Research traditions are not directly testable, both because their ontologies are too general to yield specific predictions and because their methodological components, being rules or norms, are not straightforwardly testable assertions about matters of fact. Associated with any active research tradition is a family of theories. . . . The theories . . . share the ontology of the parent research tradition and can be tested and evaluated using its methodological norms. (p. 151)

A fully developed conceptual model reflects a particular research tradition that includes the following six rules that guide middle-range theory generation and testing (Laudan, 1981; Schlotfeldt, 1975):

- The first rule identifies the phenomena that are to be studied.
- The second rule identifies the distinctive nature of the problems to be studied and the purposes to be fulfilled by the research.
- The third rule identifies the source (individuals, groups, animals, documents) of the data and the settings in which data are to be gathered.
- The fourth rule identifies the research designs, instruments, and procedures that are to be employed.
- The fifth rule identifies the methods to be employed in reducing and analyzing the data.
- The sixth rule identifies the nature of contributions that the research will make to the advancement of knowledge.

Each rule is derived from the distinctive substantive content and focus of the conceptual model and the model author's view of research. The research rules of Orem's Self-Care Framework and those of Roy's Adaptation Model, which are listed in Table 1–1, illustrate the differences in the research rules of different conceptual models.

Conceptual Models and Theory Generation

Conceptual models act as guides for the generation of new middle-range theories by focusing attention on certain concepts. More specifically, each conceptual model guides theory generation through application of its research rules. The rules identify the phenomena to be studied and help the investigator to focus on particular problems, and they also facilitate selection of methods for the discovery of new theories. Thus, as can be seen in Figure 1–2, theory generation proceeds from the

Table 1–1 ■ THE RESEARCH RULES OF TWO CONCEPTUAL MODELS

Orem's Self-Care Framework	Roy's Adaptation Model
Rule 1. The phenomena to be studied encompass theoretical and practical components of self-care; dependent-care; self-care agency; dependent-care agency; the universal, developmental, and health deviation self-care requisites that make up the therapeutic self-care demand; self-care deficits; dependent-care deficits; nursing agency; nursing systems; and methods of helping.	**Rule 1.** The phenomena to be studied include basic life processes and how nursing enhances those processes. The particular focus of inquiry is (1) focal, contextual, and residual stimuli; (2) regulator and cognator coping processes; and (3) responses in the physiological, self-concept, role function, and interdependence modes.
Rule 2. The clinical problems to be studied are those that reflect actual or predictable self-care or dependent-care deficits. The ultimate purpose of research is to identify the effects of nursing systems of regulatory care on the exercise of self-care agency and dependent-care agency.	**Rule 2.** Researchers study problems in adaptation to constantly changing environmental stimuli. The purpose of research is to describe how people adapt to environmental stimuli, explain how adaptive processes affect health, and predict the effects of nursing interventions on adaptive life processes and functioning.
Rule 3. Research participants are people who may be considered legitimate patients of nursing, that is, people with deficit relationships between their current or projected capability for providing self-care or dependent-care and the therapeutic self-care demand of the person requiring care. Data may be collected in people's homes, hospitals, clinics, and resident-care institutions, and other settings in which nursing occurs.	**Rule 3.** The people who might serve as research participants may be well or have acute or chronic illnesses. Particular interest is in individuals in situations in which adaptive processes are threatened by health technologies and behaviorally induced health problems. Data can be gathered in any health care setting.
Rule 4. Inductive and deductive research using both qualitative and quantitative research designs and associated instrumentation is appropriate.	**Rule 4.** Research is directed toward the development of both basic and clinical science. Basic research designs involve investigation of human life processes with emphasis on adaptation that occurs as the human being interacts with the environment. Clinical research designs involve study of the effects of nursing care on adaptive life processes. Both qualitative and quantitative approaches can be used.
Rule 5. Data analysis techniques associated with both qualitative and quantitative research designs are appropriate.	**Rule 5.** Data analysis techniques encompass qualitative content analysis and nonparametric and parametric statistical procedures.
Rule 6. Research will advance knowledge by enhancing understanding of patient and nurse variables that affect the exercise of continuing therapeutic self-care and dependent-care.	**Rule 6.** Research enhances understanding of the person's use of adaptive mechanisms and the role of nursing intervention in the promotion of adaptation to constantly changing environmental stimuli.

Source: Adapted from Fawcett, J. (1995). Analysis and evaluation of conceptual models of nursing (3rd ed., pp. 310–311, 467–468). Philadelphia: F.A. Davis, with permission.

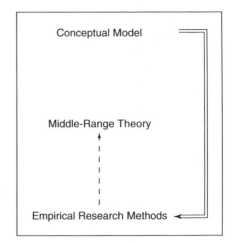

Figure 1–2 ■ Conceptual-theoretical-empirical structure for theory generation: from conceptual model to empirical research methods to middle-range theory.

conceptual model directly to the empirical research methods (═══). The obtained data then are analyzed and a new theory emerges (– – –). The conceptual model then can be judged as credible in the sense of its utility for theory generation.

The use of a conceptual model to guide middle-range theory generation is exemplified by Breckenridge's (1997a) study of dialysis modality decision making. As depicted in Figure 1–3, she used the research rules of Neuman's Systems Model to identify a relevant phenomenon, a method for data collection, and a structure for a secondary content analysis of interview data (═══) from her earlier study of why, how, and by whom the decision was made about the dialysis treatment modality (Breckenridge, 1997b). The theory of dialysis modality decision making emerged from the data analysis (– – –). Breckenridge concluded that Neuman's Systems Model provided a comprehensive framework for the secondary analysis.

Some proponents of what Lowenberg (1993) called interpretive research methods—such as phenomenology, ethnography, and grounded theory—may not agree that a conceptual model guides theory generation. They fail, however, to recognize that without some kind of underlying frame of reference, "a researcher would not know where to begin looking" (Judd, Smith, and Kidder, 1991, p. 25). They also fail to take into account that these methods actually are part of the research rules of interpretive or naturalistic paradigms (Dootson, 1995). In other words, the interpretive methods represent the methodological research rules of certain conceptual models. For example, the phenomenological research method represents the methodological rules of a conceptual model that focuses on the lived experiences of human beings from the perspective of those who have lived the experiences.

Furthermore, as Bunkers, Petardi, Pilkington, and Walls (1996) and Morse, Hupcey, Mitcham, and Lenz (1996) pointed out, some proponents of interpretive methods do not agree that such methods can be considered techniques to collect and analyze data within the context of another conceptual model. Schaefer's (1995, 1996) study serves as an example of the linkage of a conceptual model of nursing with an interpretive method. More specifically, she used the data-collection and data-analysis techniques of grounded the-

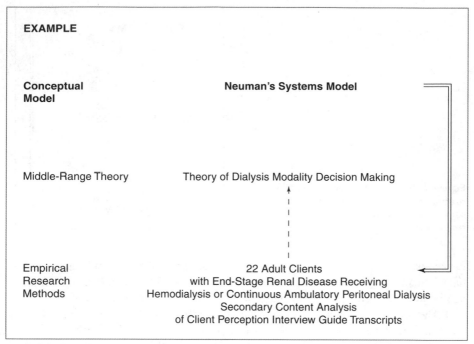

Figure I-3 ■ Example of a conceptual model used to guide middle-range theory generation. (Diagram for example constructed from Breckenridge, 1997a.)

ory in a Levine's Conservation Model-based study designed to generate a theory of how women live with fibromyalgia.

Conceptual Models and Theory Testing

Each conceptual model also guides middle-range theory testing through application of its research rules. In this case, a new theory is derived directly from, or an existing theory is linked with, one or more concepts and propositions of the conceptual model and then is empirically tested by using a research design, participants, setting, instruments, and procedures that are in keeping with the research rules. Thus, as can be seen in Figure 1–4, theory testing proceeds from the conceptual model to the theory (═══), and from the theory to the empirical research methods (– – –). The data then are analyzed and interpreted by following the research rules, the theory is found to be adequate or inadequate, and the conceptual model is judged as credible or not credible.

An example of middle-range theory testing from an explicit conceptual model is Mock and colleagues' (1997) experimental study, which tested the predictive theory of the effects of walking exercise for women undergoing radiation therapy for breast cancer. As can be seen in Figure 1–5, the theory was derived from Roy's Adaptation Model (═══). The theory concepts then were linked to appropriate empirical research methods (– – –) to permit theory testing. Mock and colleagues con-

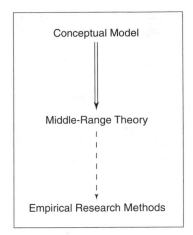

Figure 1–4 ■ Conceptual-theoretical-empirical structure for theory testing: from conceptual model to middle-range theory to empirical research methods.

cluded that the study findings supported the adequacy of the predictive theory of the effects of walking exercise for women undergoing radiation therapy for breast cancer and the credibility of Roy's Adaptation Model.

KINDS OF THEORY AND RESEARCH

The definitions of theory and research used in this book permit discussion of various kinds of theories and various kinds of research or, more generally, modes

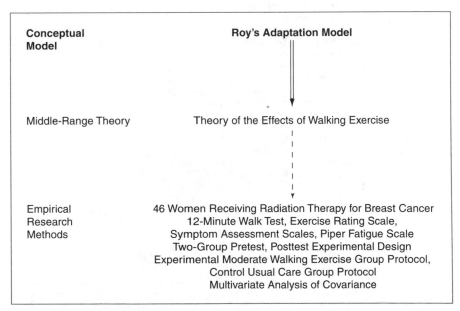

Figure 1–5 ■ Example of middle-range theory testing from an explicit conceptual model. (Diagram for example constructed from Mock et al., 1997.)

of inquiry. A comprehensive typology of theory and inquiry has been developed by Carper (1978) and refined by Chinn and Kramer (1995) and White (1995). Although this typology was derived from the nursing literature, it is likely that the same or a similar typology could be extracted from the literature of other disciplines with a practice component, such as education, engineering, social work, physical therapy, occupational therapy, or medicine.

Carper proposed that practice requires four patterns of knowing: empirics, ethics, personal knowledge, and esthetics. White added the sociopolitical pattern. Each pattern of knowing can be viewed as a different kind of theory that is generated and tested by a different mode of inquiry (Table 1–2).

Each kind of theory is an essential component of the integrated knowledge base for professional practice, and no one kind of theory should be used in isolation from

Table 1–2 ■ FIVE KINDS OF THEORY AND MODES OF INQUIRY

Kind of Theory	Characteristics	Mode of Inquiry
Empirics	Factual descriptions, explanations, or predictions based on subjective or objective group data. Publicly verifiable. Discursively written as empirical theories.	Empirical research
Ethics	Emphasizes the values of nurses and nursing. Focuses on the value of changes and outcomes in terms of desired ends. Addresses questions of moral obligation, moral value, and nonmoral value. Discursively written as standards, codes, and normative ethical theories.	Dialogue and justification
Personal knowledge	Concerned with the knowing, encountering, and actualizing of the self. Also concerned with wholeness and integrity in the personal encounter between nurse and patient. Addresses the quality and authenticity of the interpersonal process between each nurse and each patient. Expressed as realizing the authentic genuine self.	Reflection and response from others on the actualization of the authentic self
Esthetics	Focuses on particulars rather than universals. Emphasizes the nurse's perception of what is significant in the individual patient's behavior. Also addresses manual and technical skills. Expressed as envisioning the art-act of nursing.	Criticism and consensus about the act of nursing
Sociopolitical knowledge	Provides the context or cultural location for nurse-patient interactions and the broader context in which nursing and health care take place. Focuses on exposing and exploring alternate constructions of reality. Expressed as transformation and critique.	Critique and hearing all voices

Source: Constructed from Carper, B.A. (1978). Fundamental patterns of knowing in nursing. *Advances in Nursing Science, 1*(1), 13–23; Chinn, P.L., & Kramer, M.K. (1995). *Theory and nursing. A systematic approach* (4th ed.). St. Louis: Mosby Year Book; and White, J. (1995). Patterns of knowing: Review, critique, and update. *Advances in Nursing Science, 17*(4), 73–86.

the others. Furthermore, the five kinds of theory and inquiry should be used with the understanding that other ways of knowing and being are relevant to professional practice, including what Silva, Sorrell, and Sorrell (1995) called the inexplicable and the unknowable. The inexplicable pattern of knowing refers to experiences that are indescribable. The unknowable pattern refers to situations that are experienced outside of or between normal areas of awareness.

The emphasis in this book, however, is on empirics and empirical research. Readers are referred to Carper (1978), Chinn and Kramer (1995), and White (1995) for detailed discussions about ethics, personal knowledge, esthetics, and sociopolitical knowledge, and to Silva et al. (1995) for a provocative discussion of the inexplicable and the unknowable.

EMPIRICAL THEORIES AND RESEARCH

Middle-range empirical theories generally are classified as descriptive, explanatory, or predictive. The empirical research designs that generate and test these three types of middle-range theories are, respectively, descriptive, correlational, and experimental.

Descriptive Theory and Descriptive Research

Descriptive theories are the most basic type of middle-range theory. They describe or classify specific dimensions or characteristics of individuals, groups, situations, or events by summarizing the commonalities found in discrete observations. They state "what is." Descriptive theories are needed when nothing or very little is known about the phenomenon in question.

There are two categories of descriptive middle-range theory: naming and classification (Barnum, 1998). A *naming theory* is a description of the dimensions or characteristics of some phenomenon. A *classification theory* is more elaborate in that it states that the dimensions or characteristics of a given phenomenon are structurally interrelated. The dimensions may be mutually exclusive, overlapping, hierarchical, or sequential. Classification theories frequently are referred to as typologies or taxonomies. Examples of descriptive naming and classification theories follow.

Descriptive theories are generated and tested by *descriptive research.* This type of research is also called exploratory research. It is directed toward answering such questions as:

■ What are the characteristics of the phenomenon?

■ What is the prevalence of the phenomenon?

■ What is the process by which the phenomenon is experienced? (Polit and Hungler, 1995, p. 12)

In general, descriptive research involves observation of a phenomenon in its natural setting. Data are gathered by participant or nonparticipant observation, as well as by open-ended or structured interview schedules or questionnaires. The raw data gathered in a descriptive study may be qualitative and/or quantitative. Qualitative data typically are analyzed by means of some version of content analysis, which involves sorting data into a priori categories or into categories that emerge during the analysis. Content analysis can employ a strictly qualitative approach, such as the constant comparative strategy of grounded theory, or a combination of qualitative and quantitative approaches can be used to identify the categories and determine the frequency of each. Quantitative data are analyzed by calculation of simple frequencies, as well as by various measures of central tendency and variability, such as the mean, median, mode, standard deviation, and range.

Descriptive research employs many different methods, including concept analysis, psychometric analyses, case studies, surveys, phenomenology, ethnography, grounded theory, and historical inquiry. Concept analysis is the first step in the description of any phenomenon. The method of concept analysis encompasses several different approaches that are used to understand and clarify the properties of a phenomenon, including the evolutionary method (Rodgers, 1993), the Wilson method (Walker and Avant, 1995), the hybrid approach (Schwartz-Barcott and Kim, 1993) and the empirical/inductive approach (Morse, 1995). Rosenthal-Dichter (1996), for example, used the Wilson method to generate a descriptive classification theory of the concept of the pediatric physiologic stress response. Moreover, she identified various conceptual models that undergird the diverse descriptions of this concept (Institute of Medicine, 1981; Levine and Ursin, 1991; Selye, 1993).

Psychometric methodology is directed toward the development and testing of instruments used in empirical research. Each instrument reflects a descriptive theory about a concept, as well as the parent conceptual model. Newman (1997), for example, developed the Inventory of Functional Status—Caregiver of a Child in a Body Cast to measure the descriptive classification theory of categories of usual activities performed by the primary caregiver of a young child at home in a body cast. Newman used the role function response mode of Roy's Adaptation Model to guide the generation of the theory and the development of the instrument.

The case-study method involves an intensive and systematic investigation of many factors for one or a small number of individuals, a group, or a community. The case study is an excellent research method for the initial exploration of clinical problems. Janelli and colleagues (1995), for example, used the case-study method to describe the behaviors of a 76-year-old hospitalized man, who had been physically restrained, while he was out of restraints and was listening to tape-recorded music. The descriptive naming theory in this example addressed behaviors that the investigators linked to the physiological, self-concept, and interdependence response modes of Roy's Adaptation Model.

Surveys yield descriptions of an intact phenomenon, such as attributes, attitudes, knowledge, and opinions. Surveys use both open-ended and structured interview schedules or questionnaires for data collection. An example of survey research using an open-ended approach is Pollock and Sands's (1997) study, which yielded a descriptive classification theory of stressors and helpful strategies used by individuals with multiple sclerosis. The theory included hierarchical categorization of the individuals' experiences of suffering. This research was guided by a conceptual framework that linked the notion of focal, contextual, and residual stimuli in Roy's Adaptation Model, Frankl's (1963) conceptualization of meaning psychology, Lazarus and Folkman's (1984) conceptualization of coping, and Battenfield's (1984) levels of adaptation to suffering. An example of survey research using structured questionnaires is Artinian's (1991, 1992) research, which tested a descriptive classification theory of spouses' life stressors, supports, perceptions of illness severity, role strain, physical and mental symptoms of stress, and marital quality 48 hours, 6 weeks, and 1 year after the mate's coronary artery bypass graft surgery. Her research was guided by Roy's Adaptation Model.

The method of phenomenology yields a description of the lived experiences of human beings. Emphasis is placed on understanding individuals' cognitive and subjective perceptions of their experiences. Semple (1995), for example, used a phenomenological method to develop a descriptive naming theory of the lived experiences of family members of people with Huntington's disease. The research was based on the ideas of the client system central core and lines of defense and resistance found in Neuman's Systems Model.

The method of ethnography yields a theory of cultural behavior for a particular society or societal group. Emphasis is placed on describing ways of life from the perspectives of the members of the society or cultural group of interest. For example, Villarruel (1996) conducted an ethnographic study that generated a descriptive naming theory of Mexican-American people's meanings and expressions of pain and associated self-care and dependent-care actions. The research was guided by the central ideas of Orem's Self-Care Framework, including self-care agency and dependent-care agency, self-care and dependent-care, self-care requisites, and basic conditioning factors. The study findings lend credibility to Orem's Self-Care Framework and also provide data that can be used to refine the framework for use in diverse cultures (Villarruel and Denyes, 1997).

The method of grounded theory yields a description of processes occurring in social situations. Every piece of data is constantly compared with every other piece to discover the processes that characterize the phenomenon of interest. An example of this method is Rodriguez and Jones's (1996) study, which generated a descriptive naming theory of the adaptation of foster parents to a child with developmental disabilities. Rodriguez and Jones linked the foster parents' responses to the physiological, self-concept, role function, and interdependence response modes of Roy's Adaptation Model.

The method of historical inquiry focuses on the past and the way the present has evolved, as well as on influences on the flow of events over time. Historical inquiry is considered empirical research because the data typically are obtained from existing documents and transcripts of interviews with individuals who were involved with, or observers of, the phenomenon of interest. An example of historical inquiry is Baer and Frederickson's (1995) study of the alumni of the Columbia-Presbyterian School of Nursing. Their study, which was guided by the conceptual model of social history (Stearns, 1988), yielded a descriptive naming theory of ways in which the development of the discipline of nursing has reflected the social history of America.

Explanatory Theory and Correlational Research

Explanatory theories specify relations between dimensions or characteristics of individuals, groups, situations, or events. They explain why and the extent to which, one phenomenon is related to another phenomenon. Middle-range explanatory theories can be developed only after the parts of the phenomenon have been identified, that is, only after descriptive theories have been generated and tested.

Explanatory theories are generated and tested by *correlational research*. This type of research seeks to answer the following question:

■ Why does the phenomenon exist? (Polit and Hungler, 1995, p. 12)

Correlational research requires measurement of the dimensions or characteristics of phenomena in their natural states. Data usually are gathered by nonparticipant observation or self-report instruments. Instruments include fixed-choice observation checklists, rating scales, or standardized questionnaires, as well as open-ended questionnaires or interview schedules. The use of fixed-choice instruments is possible because the dimensions or characteristics of the phenomenon are thought to be known. Instruments used for correlational research yield qualitative or quantitative data. When quantitative explanations are desired and qualitative data have been collected, numbers must be attached to the raw data so that statistical procedures can be used. For example, the initial analysis of qualitative data may yield categories or themes. Then a number must be assigned to each category or theme if statistical procedures are to be performed. Statistical analyses employ various nonparametric or parametric measures of association, such as the contingency coefficient or the Pearson product moment coefficient of correlation. More sophisticated statistical analyses include multiple regression, canonical correlation, path analysis, and structural equation modeling.

Gaffney and Moore's (1996) study is an example of correlational research. They tested an explanatory theory derived directly from Orem's Self-Care Framework. The explanatory theory addressed Orem's proposition that asserts a relation between basic conditioning factors and dependent-care-agent performance. Basic conditioning factors were represented at the theory level by maternal and child age, child gender, number of children, marital status, child status (adopted, biological, stepchild), birth order, ethnic group, socioeconomic status, maternal employment status, and child health problems. Dependent-care-agent performance was represented by health promotion and self-care activities performed by adults for children.

Another example of correlational research is Yarcheski and Mahon's (1995) test of an explanatory theory that addressed the relation of human field motion, human field rhythms, creativity, and sentience to adolescents' perceived health status. The theory was derived from Rogers' Science of Unitary Human Beings; human field motion, human field rhythms, creativity, and sentience represented the Rogerian notion of human-environmental field patterning.

Predictive Theory and Experimental Research

Predictive theories move beyond explanation to the prediction of precise relations between the dimensions or characteristics of a phenomenon or differences between groups. This type of middle-range theory addresses how changes in a phenomenon occur. Predictive theories may be developed only after explanatory theories have been generated and tested.

Predictive theories are generated and tested by *experimental research.* The question answered by this type of research is:

■ Does an intervention result in the intended effect? (Polit and Hungler, 1995, p. 12)

Experimental research involves the manipulation of some phenomenon to determine how it affects or changes some dimension or characteristic of another phenomenon. Experimentation encompasses many different designs, including preexperiments such as the pretest-posttest-no control group design, quasi-experiments such as the nonequivalent pretest-posttest-control group design and time series analysis, and true experiments such as the Solomon Four Group and the posttest-only designs.

Like correlational research, experimental research requires quantifiable data. That is because numbers are needed to determine if an experimental treatment makes a difference and, if so, how much difference. Typically, these data are collected by standardized research instruments with calibrated scores. Statistical analyses involve various nonparametric and parametric measures of differences, such as the McNemar test, Mann-Whitney U-test, t-test, analysis of variance, and multivariate analysis of variance. Qualitative data also can be collected as a part of experimental research. These data can be used to amplify and clarify the reactions of experimental research participants to the experimental conditions (Sandelowski, 1996). Bobbitt (1990) pointed out that qualitative and quantitative data are mutually supportive. She explained, "Qualitative knowing can benefit from quantitative knowing, and together they can provide a depth of perception or a binocular vision that neither can provide alone" (p. 4).

Experimental research is exemplified by Roberts and colleagues' (1994) study. Their crossover experimental design tested a Levine's Conservation Model-based predictive theory of the effects of special "boomerang" pillows on respiratory vital capacity. Another example of experimental research is Hagopian's (1996) study. Her posttest-only control group experiment, which was guided by Orem's Self-Care Framework, was designed to test a predictive theory of the effects of informational audiotapes on knowledge and management of side effects experienced by cancer patients undergoing radiation therapy.

Lev's (1995) study, which was also guided by Orem's Self-Care Framework, exemplifies experimental research that includes the collection and analysis of both quantitative and qualitative data. She used the quantitative data to test a predictive theory of the effects of a self-efficacy-enhancing intervention on cancer patients' quality of life, self-care self-efficacy, mood distress, and symptom distress. The qualitative data were used to understand more fully the responses of the participants to the study.

ISSUES IN THE PROGRESSION OF THEORY AND RESEARCH

The choice of the kind of research to conduct depends on the question asked. The question asked, in turn, depends on the content of the conceptual model that is guiding the research. This means that the crucial issue in the design of a study is the selection of a question that is within the domain of a particular conceptual model. This also means that "methods that are best suited to meet the stated aims or purposes of the study" must be selected (Ford-Gilboe, Campbell, and Berman, 1995, p. 19). Accordingly, "the method chosen should not become an end in itself, but rather must be appropriate for answering the question" (Moody and Hutchinson, 1989, p. 292). In turn, the question asked depends on the current state of knowledge as expressed in the theory. Thus, if little is known about the phenomenon to be investigated, descriptive theory-generating research is needed. If the phenomenon has been adequately described but its relation to other phenomena is not known, correlational research designed to generate and test explanatory theories is required. If the phenomenon has been adequately described and its relation to other phenomena is well known, experimental research designed to generate and test predictive theories would be appropriate.

Thus, theory development is primarily a sequential process that begins with the generation of descriptive theories by means of descriptive research. The initial descriptive theories then could be tested by means of additional descriptive research. Theory development proceeds to the generation and testing of explanatory theories by means of correlational research. Finally, experimental research is employed to generate and test predictive theories (Fig. 1–6).

Dodd's (1997) program of research is an especially good example of the progression of theory and research. Her research program, which is guided by Orem's Self-Care Framework, focuses on cancer patients' self-care activities related to treatment side effects. The research program progressed from the generation of descriptive theories by means of descriptive research to the testing of explanatory theories by means of correlational research and, eventually, to the testing of predictive theories by means of experimental research.

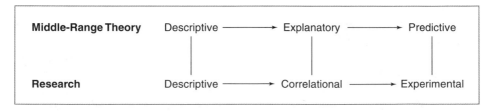

Figure 1–6 ■ Progression of theory and research.

The linear progression of theory development from descriptive through explanatory to predictive may seem self-evident. In the real world of empirical research, however, the progression is not always linear. Duffy's (1984, 1994) studies exemplify an initially linear and later nonlinear progression of theory and research. Her program of research began with generation of the descriptive classification theory of transcending options and progressed to a test of that theory by means of correlational research. Duffy (1994) concluded that the results of the theory-testing study indicate the need for refinement of the theory through additional descriptive research. Clearly, then, the theory of transcending options has not developed to the point where generation and testing of a predictive theory through experimental research would be appropriate. Furthermore, the rudimentary conceptual model that undergirds Duffy's research program—and links the concepts of family and levels of prevention—requires further development.

The nonlinear progression of research also is seen when a program of research begins with experimentation. Indeed, because the pressure to solve practical problems is so great and funding priorities are so compelling, it is tempting to begin with experiments designed to generate or test predictive theories about the efficacy of actions taken by practitioners, despite the absence of comprehensive descriptions of the actions and explanations for the effects of those actions. Although the heuristic value of such studies cannot be denied, the temptation to rush to experiments should be resisted if the goal of the discipline is development of logical and meaningful theories. As Cook and Shadish (1986) pointed out, although experiments can determine the connections between various treatments or interventions and outcomes, "they cannot by themselves explain why a treatment is or is not effective" (p. 218). Brooten's (1995) work is an example of a program of research that began with an experimental study. The program of research has been guided by an evolving conceptual model that focuses attention on the quality and cost of health care (Brooten et al., 1988). The first study was a test of the effects of interventions that were implemented by clinical nurse specialists (CNS) (Brooten et al., 1986). Later descriptive research was required to generate and test descriptive classification theories about specific CNS functions (Brooten et al., 1991; Cohen, Arnold, Brown, and Brooten, 1991). Additional research is needed to generate and test explanatory and predictive theories that will permit understanding of why and how the CNS interventions led to the specific outcomes observed in the initial experimental studies.

CONCLUSION

This chapter lays the groundwork for the remainder of the book. Here, the close connection between conceptual models, theories, and research was described as a hierarchy that begins with the abstract and general conceptual model. Each conceptual model provides a distinctive frame of reference that guides the generation and testing of middle-range theories by means of empirical research. The results of research, in turn, provide the evidence needed to determine the adequacy and utility of the theory and the credibility of the conceptual model. The close connection between conceptual models, theories, and research will continue to be emphasized in subsequent chapters by focusing on the analysis and evaluation of conceptual-theoretical-empirical structures for research.

References

Ajzen, I. (1991). The theory of planned behavior. *Organizational Behavior and Human Decision Processes, 50*, 179–211.

Alligood, M.R. (1991). Testing Rogers' theory of accelerating change: The relationships among creativity, actualization, and empathy in persons 18 to 92 years of age. *Western Journal of Nursing Research, 13*, 84–96.

Artinian, N.T. (1991). Stress experience of spouses of patients having coronary artery bypass during hospitalization and 6 weeks after discharge. *Heart and Lung, 20*, 52–59.

Artinian, N.T. (1992). Spouse adaptation to mate's CABG surgery: 1-year follow-up. *American Journal of Critical Care, 1*(2), 36–42.

Babbie, E. (1998). *The practice of social research* (8th ed.). Belmont, CA: Wadsworth.

Baer, E.D., & Frederickson, K.C. (1995). Columbia-Presbyterian nursing alumni: A case study in American social history. *Journal of the New York State Nurses Association, 26*(4), 8–13.

Barnum, B.J.S. (1998). *Nursing theory. Analysis, application, evaluation* (5th ed.). Philadelphia: Lippincott.

Barrett, E.A.M. (Ed.) (1990). *Visions of Rogers' science-based nursing.* New York: National League for Nursing.

Batey, M.V. (1997). Conceptualizing the research process. In L.H. Nicoll (Ed.), *Perspectives on nursing theory* (pp. 684–692). Philadelphia: Lippincott. (Original work published 1971).

Battenfield, B.L. (1984). Suffering: A conceptual description and content analysis of an operational schema. *Image: Journal of Nursing Scholarship, 16*, 36–41.

Bobbitt, N. (1990). A holistic profession requires holistic research. *Home Economics Forum, 4*(2), 3–5.

Breckenridge, D.M. (1997a). Decisions regarding dialysis treatment modality: A holistic perspective. *Holistic Nursing Practice, 12*(1), 54–61.

Breckenridge, D.M. (1997b). Patients' perceptions of why, how, and by whom dialysis treatment modality was chosen. *American Nephrology Nurses Association Journal, 24*, 313–319.

Brooten, D. (1995). Perinatal care across the continuum: Early discharge and nursing home follow-up. *Journal of Perinatal and Neonatal Nursing, 9*, 38–44.

Brooten, D., Brown, L., Munro, B.H., York, R., Cohen, S.M., Roncoli, M., & Hollingsworth, A. (1988). Early discharge and specialist transitional care. *Image: Journal of Nursing Scholarship, 20*, 64–68.

Brooten, D., Gennaro, S., Knapp, H., Jovene, N., Brown, L., & York, R. (1991). Functions of the CNS in early discharge and home follow-up of very low birth weight infants. *Clinical Nurse Specialist, 5*, 196–201.

Brooten, D., Kumar, S., Brown, L.P., Butts, P., Finkler, S.A., Bakewell-Sachs, S., Gibbons, A., & Delivoria-Papadopoulos, M. (1986). A randomized clinical trial of early hospital discharge and home follow-up of very-low-birth-weight infants. *New England Journal of Medicine, 315*, 934–939.

Bunkers, S.S., Petardi, L.A., Pilkington, F.B., & Walls, P.A. (1996). Challenging the myths surrounding qualitative research in nursing. *Nursing Science Quarterly, 9*, 33–37.

Burton, A. (Ed.). (1974). *Operational theories of personality.* New York: Brunner/Mazel.

Carper, B.A. (1978). Fundamental patterns of knowing in nursing. *Advances in Nursing Science, 1*(1), 13–23.

Chinn, P.L., & Kramer, M.K. (1995). *Theory and nursing. A systematic approach* (4th ed.). St. Louis: Mosby Year Book.

Cohen, S.M., Arnold, L., Brown, L., & Brooten, D. (1991). Taxonomic classification of transitional follow-up care nursing interventions with low birth weight infants. *Clinical Nurse Specialist, 5*, 31–36.

Collin, F. (1992). Nursing science as an interpretive discipline: Problems and challenges. *Vård i Norden, 12*, 14–23.

Cook, T.D., & Shadish, W.R., Jr. (1986). Program evaluation: The worldly science. *Annual Review of Psychology, 37*, 193–232.

Dodd, M.J. (1997). Self-care: Ready or not! *Oncology Nursing Forum, 24*, 981–990.

Dootson, S. (1995). An in-depth study of triangulation. *Journal of Advanced Nursing, 22*, 183–187.

Downs, F.S. (1994). Hitching the research wagon to theory [Editorial]. *Nursing Research, 43*, 195.

Duffy, M.E. (1984). Transcending options: Creating a milieu for practicing high level wellness. *Health Care for Women International, 5,* 145–161.

Duffy, M.E. (1994). Testing the theory of transcending options: Health behaviors of single parents. *Scholarly Inquiry for Nursing Practice, 8,* 191–202.

Fawcett, J. (1993). From a plethora of paradigms to parsimony in worldviews. *Nursing Science Quarterly, 6,* 56–58.

Fawcett, J. (1997). The structural hierarchy of nursing knowledge: Components and their definitions. In I.M. King & J. Fawcett (Eds.), *The language of nursing theory and metatheory* (pp. 11–17). Indianapolis: Sigma Theta Tau International Center Nursing Press.

Feigl, H. (1970). The "orthodox" view of theories: Remarks in defense as well as critique. In M. Radner & S. Winokuk (Eds.), *Minnesota studies in the philosophy of science. Volume IV: Analyses of theories and methods of physics and psychology* (pp. 3–16). Minneapolis: University of Minnesota Press.

Ford-Gilboe, M., Campbell, J., & Berman, H. (1995). Stories and numbers: Coexistence without compromise. *Advances in Nursing Science, 18*(1), 14–26.

Frank, L.K. (1968). Science as a communication process. *Main Currents in Modern Thought, 25,* 45–50.

Frankl, V.E. (1963). *Man's search for meaning: An introduction to logotherapy.* New York: Holt, Rinehart and Winston.

Frey, M.A., & Sieloff, C.L. (Eds.). (1995). *Advancing King's systems framework and theory of nursing.* Thousand Oaks, CA: Sage.

Gaffney, K.F., & Moore, J.M. (1996). Testing Orem's theory of self-care deficit: Dependent care agent performance for children. *Nursing Science Quarterly, 9,* 160–164.

Gibbs, J. (1972). *Sociological theory construction.* Hinsdale, IL: Dryden Press.

Hagopian, G.A. (1996). The effects of informational audiotapes on knowledge and self-care behaviors of patients undergoing radiation therapy. *Oncology Nursing Forum, 23,* 697–700.

Hanson, M.J.S. (1995). *Beliefs, attitudes, subjective norms, perceived behavioral control, and cigarette smoking in white, African-American, and Puerto Rican-American teenage women.* Unpublished doctoral dissertation, University of Pennsylvania. 1995.

Hanson, N.R. (1958). *Patterns of discovery.* New York: Cambridge University Press.

Hempel, C.G. (1970). On the "standard conception" of scientific theories. In M. Radner & S. Winokuk (Eds.), *Minnesota studies in the philosophy of science. Volume IV: Analyses of theories and methods of physics and psychol-*

ogy (pp. 142–163). Minneapolis: University of Minnesota Press.

Homans, G.C. (1964). Bringing men back in. *American Sociological Review, 29,* 809–818.

Institute of Medicine. (1981). *Report of a study: Research on stress and human health.* Washington, DC: National Academy Press.

Janelli, L.M., Kanski, G.W., Jones, H.M., & Kennedy, M.C. (1955). Exploring music intervention with restrained patients. *Nursing Forum, 30*(4), 12–18.

Jennings, K.M. (1997). *Predicting intentions to obtain a Pap smear among African American and Latina women.* Unpublished doctoral dissertation, University of Pennsylvania.

Johnson, D.E. (1990). The behavioral system model for nursing. In M. E. Parker (Ed.), *Nursing theories in practice* (pp. 23–32). New York: National League for Nursing.

Judd, C.M., Smith, E.R., & Kidder, L.H., (1991). *Research methods in social relations* (6th ed.). New York: Holt, Rinehart and Winston.

Kerlinger, F.N. (1986). *Foundations of behavioral research* (3rd ed.). New York: Holt, Rinehart and Winston.

Kim, H.S. (1997). Terminology in structuring and developing nursing knowledge. In I.M. King & J. Fawcett (Eds.), *The language of nursing theory and metatheory* (pp. 27–36). Indianapolis: Sigma Theta Tau International Center Nursing Press.

King, I.M. (1997). Knowledge development for nursing: A process. In I.M. King & J. Fawcett (Eds.), *The language of nursing theory and metatheory* (pp. 19–25). Indianapolis: Sigma Theta Tau International Center Nursing Press.

Kramer, M.K. (1997). Terminology in nursing: Definitions and comments. In I.M. King & J. Fawcett (Eds.), *The language of nursing theory and metatheory* (pp. 61–71). Indianapolis: Sigma Theta Tau International Center Nursing Press.

Laudan, L. (1981). A problem-solving approach to scientific progress. In I. Hacking (Ed.), *Scientific revolutions* (pp. 144–155). New York: Oxford University Press.

Lavee, Y., & Dollahite, D.C. (1991). The linkage between theory and research in family science. *Journal of Marriage and the Family, 53,* 361–373.

Lazarus, R.S., & Folkman, S. (1984). *Stress, appraisal, and coping.* New York: Springer.

Lev, E.L. (1995). Triangulation reveals theoretical linkages and outcomes in a nursing intervention study. *Clinical Nurse Specialist, 9,* 300–305.

Levine, S., & Ursin, H. (1991). What is stress? In M.R. Brown, G.F. Koob, & C. Rivier (Eds.), *Stress: Neurobiology and neuroendocrinology* (pp. 3–21). New York: Marcel Dekker.

Lowenberg, J.S. (1993). Interpretive research methodology: Broadening the dialogue. *Advances in Nursing Science, 16*(2), 57–69.

Margenau, H. (1972). The method of science and the meaning of reality. In H. Margenau (Ed.), *Integrative principles of modern thought* (pp. 3–43). New York: Gordon and Breach.

Mock, V., Dow, K.H., Meares, C.J., Grimm, P.M., Dienemann, J.A., Haisfield-Wolfe, M.E., Quitasol, W., Mitchell, S., Chakravarthy, A., & Gage, I. (1997). Effects of exercise on fatigue, physical functioning, and emotional distress during radiation therapy for breast cancer. *Oncology Nursing Forum, 24*, 991–1000.

Moody, L.E., & Hutchinson, S.A. (1989). Relating your study to a theoretical context. In H.S. Wilson, *Research in nursing* (2nd ed., pp. 275–332). Redwood City, CA: Addison-Wesley Health Sciences.

Morse, J.M. (1995). Exploring the theoretical basis of nursing using advanced techniques of concept analysis. *Advances in Nursing Science, 17*(3), 31–46.

Morse, J.M., Hupcey, J.E., Mitcham, C., & Lenz, E.R. (1996). Concept analysis in nursing research: A critical appraisal. *Scholarly Inquiry for Nursing Practice, 10*, 253–277.

Nagel, E. (1961). *The structure of science.* New York: Harcourt, Brace and World.

Neuman, B. (1995). *The Neuman systems model* (3rd ed.). Norwalk, CT: Appleton and Lange.

Newman, D.M.L. (1997). The Inventory of Functional Status-Caregiver of a Child in a Body Cast. *Journal of Pediatric Nursing, 12*, 142–147.

Newman, M.A. (1994). *Health as expanding consciousness* (2nd ed.). New York: National League for Nursing Press.

Orem, D.E. (1995). *Nursing: Concepts of practice* (5th ed.). St. Louis: Mosby YearBook.

Parse, R.R. (1997). The language of nursing knowledge: Saying what we mean. In I.M. King & J. Fawcett (Eds.), *The language of nursing theory and metatheory* (pp. 73–77). Indianapolis: Sigma Theta Tau International Center Nursing Press.

Payton, O.D. (1994). *Research: The validation of clinical practice* (3rd ed.). Philadelphia: F.A. Davis.

Polit, D.F., & Hungler, B.P. (1995). *Nursing research: Principles and methods* (5th ed.). Philadelphia: Lippincott.

Pollock, S.E., & Sands, D. (1997). Adaptation to suffering: Meaning and implications for nursing. *Clinical Nursing Research, 6*, 171–185.

Popper, K.R. (1965). *Conjectures and refutations: The growth of scientific knowledge.* New York: Harper and Row.

Roberts, K.L., Brittin, M., Cook, M-A., &

deClifford, J. (1994). Boomerang pillows and respiratory capacity. *Clinical Nursing Research, 3*, 157–165.

Rodgers, B.L. (1993). Concept analysis: An evolutionary view. In B.L. Rodgers & K.A. Knafl (Eds.), *Concept development in nursing: Foundation, techniques, and applications* (pp. 73–92). Philadelphia: Saunders.

Rodriguez, J.A., & Jones, E.G. (1996). Foster parents' early adaptation to the placement of a child with developmental disabilities in their home. *Journal of Pediatric Nursing, 11*, 111–118.

Rogers, M.E. (1986). Science of unitary human beings. In V.M. Malinski (Ed.), *Explorations on Martha Rogers' science of unitary human beings* (pp. 3–8). Norwalk, CT: Appleton-Century-Crofts.

Rosenthal-Dichter, C.H. (1996). The pediatric physiologic stress response: A concept analysis. *Scholarly Inquiry for Nursing Practice, 10*, 211–234.

Roy, C., & Andrews, H.A. (1991). *The Roy adaptation model. The definitive statement.* Norwalk, CT: Appleton and Lange.

Sandelowski, M. (1996). Using qualitative methods in intervention studies. *Research in Nursing and Health, 19*, 359–364.

Schaefer, K.M. (1995). Struggling to maintain balance: A study of women living with fibromyalgia. *Journal of Advanced Nursing, 21*, 95–102.

Schaefer, K.M. (1996). Levine's conservation model: Caring for women with chronic illness. In P. Hinton-Walker & B. Neuman (Eds.), *Blueprint for use of nursing models: Education, research, practice, and administration* (pp. 187–227). New York: NLN Press.

Schaefer, K.M., & Pond, J.B. (Eds.). (1991). *Levine's conservation model: A framework for nursing practice.* Philadelphia: F. A. Davis.

Schlotfeldt, R.M. (1975). The need for a conceptual framework. In P.J. Verhonick (Ed.), *Nursing research I* (pp. 1–24). Boston: Little, Brown.

Schumacher, K.L., & Gortner, S.R. (1992). (Mis)conceptions and reconceptions about traditional science. *Advances in Nursing Science, 14*(4), 1–11.

Schwartz-Barcott, D., & Kim, H.S. (1993). An expansion and elaboration of the hybrid model of concept development. In B.L. Rodgers & K.A. Knafl (Eds.), *Concept development in nursing: Foundation, techniques, and applications* (pp. 107–133). Philadelphia: Saunders.

Selye, H. (1993). History of the stress concept. In L. Goldberger & S. Breznitz (Eds.), *Handbook of stress: Theoretical and clinical aspects* (2nd ed., pp. 7–18). New York: The Free Press.

Semple, O.D. (1995). The experiences of family members of persons with Huntington's Disease. *Perspectives, 19*(4), 4–10.

Silva, M.C., Sorrell, J.M., & Sorrell, C.D. (1995). From Carper's patterns of knowing to ways of being: An ontological philosophical shift in nursing. *Advances in Nursing Science, 18*(1), 1–13.

Slife, B.D., & Williams, R.N. (1995). *What's behind the research? Discovering hidden assumptions in the behavioral sciences.* Thousand Oaks, CA: Sage.

Stearns, P. (1988). Introduction: Social history and its evolution. In P. Stearns (Ed.), *Expanding the past: A reader in social history* (pp. 3–15). New York: New York University Press.

Villarruel, A.M. (1995). Mexican-American cultural meanings, expressions, self-care and dependent-care actions associated with experiences of pain. *Research in Nursing and Health, 18,* 427–436.

Villarruel, A.M., & Denyes, M.J. (1997). Testing Orem's theory with Mexican Americans. *Image: Journal of Nursing Scholarship, 29,* 283–288.

Walker, L.O., & Avant, K.C. (1995). *Strategies for theory construction in nursing* (3rd ed.). Norwalk, CT: Appleton and Lange.

Whall, A.L. (1986). *Family therapy theory for nursing: Four approaches.* Norwalk, CT: Appleton-Century-Crofts.

White, J. (1995). Patterns of knowing: Review, critique, and update. *Advances in Nursing Science, 17*(4), 73–86.

Yarcheski, A., & Mahon, N.E. (1995). Rogers's pattern manifestations and health in adolescents. *Western Journal of Nursing Research, 17,* 383–397.

Additional Readings

Achinstein, P. (1974). Theories. In A.C. Michalos, *Philosophical problems of science and technology* (pp. 280–297). Boston: Allyn and Bacon.

Acton, G.J., Irvin, B.L., & Hopkins, B.A. (1991). Theory-testing research: Building the science. *Advances in Nursing Science, 14*(1), 52–61.

Avant, K.C. (1991). The theory-research dialectic: A different approach. *Nursing Science Quarterly, 4,* 2.

Babbie, E.R. (1990). *Survey research methods* (2nd ed.). Belmont, CA: Wadsworth.

Beck, C.T. (1997). Developing a research program using qualitative and quantitative approaches. *Nursing Outlook, 45,* 265–269.

Blegen, M.A., & Tripp-Reimer, T. (1997). Implications of nursing taxonomies for middle-range theory development. *Advances in Nursing Science, 19*(3), 37–49.

Brown, H.I. (1977). *Perception, theory and commitment. The new philosophy of science.* Chicago: Precedent Publishing.

Campbell, D.T., & Stanley, J.C. (1963). *Experimental and quasi-experimental designs for research.* Chicago: Rand McNally.

Connelly, L.M., Bott, M., Hoffart, N., & Taunton, R.L. (1997). Methodological triangulation in a study of nurse retention. *Nursing Research, 46,* 299–302.

Diesing, P. (1971). *Patterns of discovery in the social sciences.* New York: Aldine, Atherton.

Donnelly, E., & Deets, C.A. (1990). Theory-laden observation: Two examples. In N.L. Chaska (Ed.), *The nursing profession: Turning points* (pp. 156–164). St. Louis: Mosby.

Fitzpatrick, J.J. (Ed.). (1998). *Encyclopedia of nursing research.* New York: Springer Publishing Company, Inc.

Frank-Stromborg, M., & Olsen, S.J. (Eds.). (1997). *Instruments for clinical health-care research* (2nd ed.). Boston: Jones and Bartlett.

Gift, A.G. (Ed.). (1997). *Clarifying concepts in nursing research.* New York: Springer Publishing Company, Inc.

Grant, J.S., Kinney, M.R., & Davis, L.L. (1993). Using conceptual frameworks or models to guide nursing research. *Journal of Neuroscience Nursing, 25,* 52–56.

Krippendorff, K. (1980). *Content analysis. An introduction to its methodology.* Newbury Park, CA: Sage.

Kuhn, T.S. (1977). Second thoughts on paradigms. In F. Suppe (Ed.), *The structure of scientific theories* (2nd ed., pp. 459–482). Chicago: University of Illinois Press.

Lusk, B. (1997). Historical methodology for nursing research. *Image: Journal of Nursing Scholarship, 29,* 355–359.

Munhall, P.L., & Boyd, C.O. (1993). *Nursing research: A qualitative perspective.* New York: National League for Nursing Press.

Newman, M.A. (1979). *Theory development in nursing.* Philadelphia: F.A. Davis.

Paley, J. (1996). How not to clarify concepts in nursing. *Journal of Advanced Nursing, 24,* 572–578.

Pearson, P. (1991). Clients' perceptions: The use of case studies in developing theory. *Journal of Advanced Nursing, 16,* 521–528.

Sandelowski, M. (1996). One is the liveliest number: The case orientation of qualitative research. *Research in Nursing and Health, 19,* 525–529.

2 Analyzing Conceptual-Theoretical-Empirical Structures for Research

■ The close connection between conceptual models, theories, and research mandates analysis of the conceptual, theoretical, and empirical elements of a research document. This chapter presents a description of the content of each section of a research document and a comprehensive format for analysis of the conceptual-theoretical-empirical structure for the research. The chapter draws on the discussion of the components of conceptual-theoretical-empirical structures presented in Chapter 1. Emphasis is placed on analysis of the content of existing research documents that address the generation or testing of middle-range theories.

CONTENT OF RESEARCH DOCUMENTS

Research designed to generate or test a middle-range theory typically is presented in a written document, such as a proposal for a thesis or dissertation, an application for funding, or a report of the completed research. Regardless of their form, all research documents contain similar content. More specifically, all middle-range theory-generating and theory-testing research documents typically include introductory and method sections. Reports of completed research also include the results and discussion sections.

THEORY-GENERATING RESEARCH DOCUMENTS

The introductory section of a middle-range theory-generating research document may be labeled the conceptual framework or conceptual model, the theoretical framework, the rationale, the review of the literature, the background, or the significance of the research. In this section, the research purpose is presented, the conceptual model that guides the research is described, and the reasons why the research should be or was undertaken and how it fills gaps in current theories or extends a previously developed theory are explained. In particular, this section contains the purpose of the study in the form of a narrative statement, research questions, or specific aims. Furthermore, it includes discussion of the social and theoretical significance of the research, a description of the conceptual model that guides the research, and an explanation of the links between the conceptual model, the theory, and the empirical research methods.

The method section of theory-generating research documents presents a detailed discussion of how the study will be or was conducted. The subsections under method include descriptions of the sample of study participants or literary documents, the research instruments and equipment, the procedures for data collection, and the methods of data interpretation.

The results section of a report of completed theory-generating research presents the theory that was induced from the data. The theory frequently is presented in the form of one or more newly discovered concepts, the dimensions of the concept(s), and relevant propositions. For example, data from Schaefer's (1995, 1996) descriptive study of how women live with fibromyalgia led to articulation of the descriptive naming theory of struggling to maintain balance. The theory is made up of five concepts and their dimensions, along with the propositions that define and describe the concepts and their dimensions. The study was guided by Levine's Conservation Model (Schaefer and Pond, 1991), and employed the interpretive research method of grounded theory for data collection and analysis. In-person and follow-up telephone interviews were conducted with 36 women. The concepts and dimensions of the theory are listed in Table 2–1.

The discussion section of theory-generating research documents presents an interpretation of the results and their implications. More specifically, the theory that was generated is compared with other theories, and the credibility of the conceptual model is discussed.

THEORY-TESTING RESEARCH DOCUMENTS

The introductory section of a middle-range theory-testing research document also may be labeled the conceptual framework or conceptual model, the theoretical framework, the rationale, the review of the literature, the background, or the significance of the research. As in theory-generating research documents, this section includes the purpose of the research and a description of the conceptual model that guides the research, as well as an explanation of the reasons why the research should be or was undertaken and how it fills gaps in current theories or extends a previ-

---

Table 2–1 ■ **THE THEORY OF STRUGGLING TO MAINTAIN BALANCE: Concepts and Their Dimensions**

Concepts
   Dimensions of the Concepts
Recalling perceived normality
Searching for a diagnosis
      Noticing something is wrong
      Fearing the worst
      Convincing others
      Losing my marbles
      Depleting resources
      Taking forever to find out
Finding out
      Making attributions
      Denying
      Trying everything
Moving on
      Finding meaning
      Living day by day
      Creating a safe environment
      Transcending the illness
Relinquishing the struggle

Source: Adapted from Schaefer, 1995, p. 97, with permission.

ously developed theory. More specifically, this section of theory-testing research documents contains the presentation of the purpose of the study in the form of a narrative statement, research questions, specific aims, or hypotheses. In addition, this section contains discussion of the social and theoretical significance of the research, a description of the conceptual and theoretical components of the research, an explanation of the links between the conceptual model and the middle-range theory, and critical discussion of previous research that both supports and refutes the theoretical assertions under investigation.

Various forms of middle-range theories are evident in theory-testing research documents. One form is the established theory, such as role theory, body-image theory, the theory of planned behavior, or self-efficacy theory, that is tested in a new setting or with a new population. Research designed to test an established theory is evident in Hanson's (1995, 1997) correlation study, which was guided by Neuman's (1995) Systems Model. Hanson used the statistical technique of path analysis to test the generalizability of the explanatory theory of planned behavior (Ajzen, 1991) to the cigarette smoking intentions of 141 African-American, 146 Puerto Rican, and 143 non–Hispanic white teenage females (Fig. 2–1). A structured questionnaire directly derived from the theory of planned behavior was used to collect data.

Another form of theory, usually referred to as a theoretical rationale or theoretical framework, uses the findings from previous empirical research to develop testable propositions. For example, although Mock et al.'s (1997) study was guided

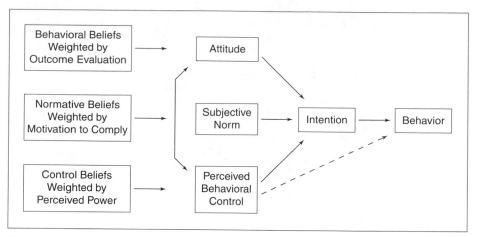

Figure 2–1 ■ The theory of planned behavior. (From Hanson, 1997, p. 156, with permission.)

by Roy's Adaptation Model (Roy and Andrews, 1991), they used the findings from the available research literature to formulate a predictive theory of the effects of walking exercise on physical functioning, exercise level, emotional distress, and symptom experience of women with breast cancer who were receiving radiation therapy. The experimental study employed the statistical technique of multivariate analysis of covariance to analyze data from structured questionnaires and tests of physical function. The sample included 46 women with newly diagnosed Stage I or II breast cancer.

In some instances, the theoretical framework combines some elements of an established theory with findings from previous research. An example is Lev's (1995) predictive theory of the effects of an efficacy-enhancing intervention on the quality of life, self-care efficacy, mood distress, and symptom distress of cancer patients who were receiving chemotherapy. The theory, which was guided by Orem's (1991) Self-Care Framework, is made up of concepts and propositions from self-efficacy theory (Bandura, 1986) and other concepts and propositions identified through a review of previous research dealing with responses to chemotherapy. A sample of 49 men and women with cancer completed structured questionnaires and responded to an open-ended interview schedule. The experimental research employed the statistical technique of multivariate analysis of variance to analyze the quantitative data and content analysis to analyze the qualitative data.

The method section of theory-testing research documents also presents a detailed discussion of how the study will be or was conducted. The subsections under method include descriptions of the sample of study participants or literary documents, the research instruments and equipment, the procedures for data collection, and the techniques used to analyze the data.

The results section of a report of completed theory-testing research includes a summary of the data that were collected and a presentation of the outcomes of statistical calculations. The results section also includes conclusions regarding hypotheses. The discussion section presents an interpretation of the results and their implications. Here, conclusions are drawn about the adequacy and utility of the theory and the credibility of the conceptual model.

FORMALIZATION OF CONCEPTUAL-THEORETICAL-EMPIRICAL STRUCTURES

Analysis of the conceptual, theoretical, and empirical components of a research document is accomplished by the technique of *conceptual-theoretical-empirical (C-T-E) formalization*, which sometimes is called theory formalization or theoretical substruction. C-T-E formalization is used to determine exactly what a conceptual model and a theory say, and to identify the methods used to conduct the research. It is a way of extracting an explicit statement and diagram of the conceptual-theoretical-empirical structure from the narrative research document, which may be somewhat "untidy and inelegant" prior to formalization (Marx, 1976, p. 235).

C-T-E formalization is similar to grammatical parsing of a sentence. Just as parsing identifies the nouns, verbs, adjectives, adverbs, and other parts of a sentence, so C-T-E formalization permits identification of the concepts and propositions that make up a conceptual model and those that make up a middle-range theory, and identification of the empirical research methods. The result of C-T-E formalization is a concise and polished version of the conceptual-theoretical-empirical structure that sets forth its components clearly, concisely, and pictorially.

STEP ONE: IDENTIFICATION OF CONCEPTS

The first step in formalization of a conceptual-theoretical-empirical structure is the identification of concepts. Inasmuch as conceptual models and theories both contain concepts, this step encompasses naming the conceptual model and identifying the conceptual model concepts that guided the theory development effort, as well as identifying and classifying the concepts of the middle-range theory that was generated or tested.

Concepts summarize actual observations and experiences that seem to be related. Babbie (1998) explained:

> ■ Although the observations and experiences are real, . . . concepts are only mental creations. The terms associated with concepts are merely devices created for the purposes of filing and communication. (p. 122)

A concept, then, is a tool and not a real entity. It facilitates observation and understanding of the properties that comprise a phenomenon (Bates, 1987). Furthermore, a concept gives meaning to phenomena that can be directly or indirectly seen, heard, tasted, smelled, and touched. Thus, a concept provides a mental image that enables us to categorize, interpret, and impose a structure on a phenomenon. The concepts of a conceptual model and a theory represent their special vocabularies. Conceptual model concepts are, of course, more abstract and general than those of a theory. Examples of conceptual model concepts and theory concepts are given in Table 2–2.

Concepts have one or multiple dimensions. The dimensions of a concept represent its component parts. For example, as can be seen in Table 2–1, the middle-range theory of struggling to maintain balance is made up of two unidimensional concepts—recalling perceived normality and relinquishing the struggle, and three multidimensional concepts—searching for a diagnosis, finding out, and moving on (Schaefer, 1995, 1996).

Pragmatics of Concept Identification

Concept identification begins with identification of the name of the conceptual model that guided the research and continues with identification of the particular conceptual model concepts used in that research. Many research documents do not contain even the name of the conceptual model that guided the study. By failing to identify the conceptual model, the investigator does not fully inform readers of the distinctive intellectual and sociohistorical context of the study. The omission may lead to a critique of the research that is inappropriate because it reflects an entirely different perspective. Moreover, the omission creates difficulties in identifying groups of related studies and programs of research and, therefore, in integrating the results (Polit and Hungler, 1995). Consequently, the narrative of a research document must be analyzed systematically to identify the name of the conceptual model and the particular concepts of that conceptual model that were used to guide the

---

Table 2–2 ■ **EXAMPLES OF CONCEPUAL MODEL CONCEPTS AND THEORY CONCEPTS**

Conceptual Model Concepts	Theory Concepts
King's General Systems Framework	General health behavior
Personal system	Illness management behavior
Interpersonal system	Perception of illness severity
Social system	
Levine's Conservation Model	Respiratory capacity
Energy	Pressure ulcers
Structural integrity	Confusion
Personal integrity	
Social integrity	
Neuman's Systems Model	Risk factors
Client system	Patients' needs
Stressors	Emotional distress
Lines of defense	
Orem's Self-Care Framework	Activities of daily living
Self-care agency	Treatment side effects self-management
Dependent-care agency	Child care
Self-care deficit	
Roy's Adaptation Model	Self-esteem
Stimuli	Functional status
Coping mechanisms	Interpersonal relationships
Response modes	

study. If the conceptual model that guided the study is not explicitly identified in the research document and cannot be extracted from the narrative, identification of the conceptual model concepts that guided the study may not be possible. Sometimes a review of the investigator's other publications or direct communication with the investigator may reveal the parent conceptual model. For example, Schaeffer (1995) did not mention Levine's Conservation Model in the initial report of her theory-generating study of women with fibromyalgia. In a later publication, however, she clearly explained the linkage between Levine's model and the theory of struggling to maintain balance (Schaefer, 1996).

Concept identification continues with identification of the concepts of the middle-range theory that was generated or tested. The research document must be read carefully to identify the concepts and to categorize them as concepts of the conceptual model or concepts of the theory.

At times, it may be difficult to distinguish between the ideas that are integral to the conceptual model and the theory and those that are part of the supporting narrative. Furthermore, it may be difficult to distinguish between concepts and their dimensions. Consider the example of the multidimensional concept "quality of life." The dimensions of this concept may include "physical health," "psychological state," "functional ability," and "social relationships." These dimensions should not be classified as separate concepts when they are considered components of the concept "quality of life." Consider also the example of "types of information" in a predictive theory. Here, the dimensions of the concept that are the experimental and control treatments, such as "audiotaped information" and "printed information," must not be classified as separate concepts when the actual concept is "types of information."

Accurate identification of concepts and their dimensions may require repeated readings of the research document. The final selection of relevant concepts and the dimensions of those concepts is aided by identifying the concepts contained in the title of the document, the stated purpose of the research, the research questions, the hypotheses (if any), and the conceptual or theoretical framework. In theory-generating research documents, the theory concepts and their dimensions frequently are not evident until the results of the data analysis are presented. In theory-testing research documents, the concepts typically are found in the introduction, although some concepts also may be extracted from other sections of the document.

STEP TWO: CLASSIFICATION OF MIDDLE-RANGE THEORY CONCEPTS

The second step in formalization of a conceptual-theoretical-empirical structure is the classification of the middle-range theory concepts. Concept classification is applicable only to the middle-range theory concepts because the schemata for classification of concepts are not appropriate or particularly meaningful for the abstract and general concepts that make up conceptual models. The concepts of the middle-range theory that was generated or tested are classified on the basis of the extent of their observability and their measurement characteristics.

Classification by Observability

Classification of middle-range theory concepts on the basis of their observability refers to the degree to which a phenomenon can be directly experienced or observed. Kaplan's (1964) concept classification schema is a continuum of observability, whereas Willer and Webster's (1970) schema is a dichotomy of observability.

KAPLAN'S CONTINUUM. At one end of Kaplan's (1964) continuum is the *observational term*, which refers to a phenomenon that is a directly observable empirical referent. The phenomenon is observed by means of the senses, especially the visual and auditory senses. A woman's statement that she feels depressed because she has breast cancer is an observational term because the statement can be directly observed through the sense of hearing. Clinicians cannot see the woman's depression, but they have no difficulty in recognizing it when she reports it: the woman says she is depressed. The precise concept in this example, then, is "report of depression."

Next in line on Kaplan's continuum is the *indirect observable term*, which refers to a phenomenon that must be inferred. In contrast to the concept "report of depression," the concept "depression" cannot be directly observed, but it can be inferred by a combination of signs and symptoms exhibited by a person, such as insomnia and weight gain. The indirect observable term is more subject to misinterpretation than is the observational term. For example, insomnia and weight gain may be experienced by nondepressed students who study intensely during midterm and final examination periods, as well as by individuals who are depressed about an illness.

Misinterpretation of the indirect observable term can be reduced or eliminated by designating a proxy observational term. For example, the observational term "report of depression" can be designated as the proxy for the indirect observable term "depression." Alternatively, the responses to a questionnaire that measures depression can be used as the proxy. Thus, when a concept is classified as an indirect observable term, the observable proxy also must be identified.

The third point on Kaplan's continuum is the *construct*, which refers to a phenomenon that is neither directly nor indirectly observed. Constructs are invented for special scientific purposes. Although they have intrinsic theoretical meaning, they have empirical meaning only when proxy observational terms are designated. An example of a construct is "psychosocial adjustment," which was invented to describe the quality of a person's psychological and social adaptation to a situation or event. The construct "psychosocial adjustment" cannot be observed, but it can be inferred through designation of a proxy observational term, such as "report of the quality of psychological and social adaptation to a situation." Or, the proxy can be the responses to a questionnaire that measures psychosocial adjustment. As with the indirect observable term, then, when a concept is classified as a construct, the observable proxy also must be identified.

At the opposite end of Kaplan's continuum is the *theoretical term*, which refers to a complex, global phenomenon that is even more abstract than a construct. A theoretical term is impossible to observe, but it can be interpreted through its relation to a construct. Thus, a theoretical term ultimately is observed through its connection to the proxy observational term designated for the construct. "Quality of life," for example, cannot be observed, but it can be interpreted in a theory through its relation to constructs such as the "satisfaction with physical health," "satisfaction with psychological state," "satisfaction with functional ability," and "satisfaction with social relationships," all of which are regarded as dimensions of quality of life. These constructs, in turn, can be observed through such proxy observational terms as "report of satisfaction with physical health state," "report of satisfaction with current mood state," "report of satisfaction with ability to perform usual activities," and "report of satisfaction with the quality of communication with family members and friends." Alternatively, the proxy can be the responses to one or more questionnaires that measure satisfaction with physical health state, mood state, functional ability, and interpersonal relationships. Thus, as with the indirect observable term and the construct, when a concept is classified as a theoretical term, the observable proxy also must be identified.

Kaplan's classification schema, although widely cited, is not particularly easy to use. Distinctions among the four types of concepts are somewhat unclear and can be confusing. Acknowledging this lack of clarity, Kaplan (1964) stated:

> ■ These four types of terms are usually treated as two, the first two being combined as "observational" and the last two as "symbolic;" or else, the first three are lumped together as "empirical" or "descriptive" and contrasted with the "theoretical." However the lines are drawn, it is important to recognize that drawing them is to a significant degree arbitrary. The distinctions are vague, and in any case a matter of degree. (p. 57)

WILLER AND WEBSTER'S DICHOTOMY. Willer and Webster (1970) argued that there is no justification for the assumption that concepts exist in any sort of continnum. They classified concepts as either observables or constructs. *Observables*, which also are called descriptive terms, are the result of sensation. They are, then, phenomena that are immediately accessible to or very close to being immediately accessible to direct sensory observations; "gender" and "race" are examples.

Constructs, which refer to abstract phenomena, are the result of thought. They are not immediately accessible to direct sensory observation and, therefore, must be connected to observable phenomena to test a theory empirically. Constructs, according to Willer and Webster, can be generalized to diverse situations, whereas observables tend to be tied to a specific situation. They pointed out that most mature sciences use constructs to build theory, and they offered the examples of "mass" and "specific gravity" from physics, "bonds" and "valences" from chemistry, and "heredity," "natural selection," and "genes" from biology. Another example is "psychosocial adjustment."

Classification by Measurement Characteristics

Classification of middle-range theory concepts on the basis of their measurement characteristics refers to the way in which phenomena are manifested. One way of classifying concepts according to their measurement characteristics is on the basis of variability. Another way is on the basis of Dubin's (1978) schema.

CLASSIFICATION BY VARIABILITY. Concepts represent nonvariable or variable phenomena. When a phenomenon has just one form, when the mental image evoked is of one and only one form of the phenomenon, the concept is referred to as a *non-variable*. An example of a nonvariable concept is "women with breast cancer." The nonvariable "women with breast cancer" is simply present; nothing is implied about the severity of breast cancer or about men who might have breast cancer.

When a phenomenon has more than one form, when the mental image evoked is of diverse forms or fluctuations in the phenomenon, the concept is referred to as a *variable*. A variable can be thought of as a rule or way of classifying a phenomenon into different categories (Judd, Smith, and Kidder, 1991). Numerical scores usually are assigned to the fluctuations in or categories of a concept that is a variable. That is, of course, mandatory when statistical analyses are required to generate or test a theory. For example, the concept "cancer status" is a variable because it can fluctuate or be classified into different categories. One type of fluctuation of "cancer status" might be the categorical scores 0, 1, 2, and 3, representing the categories of "no cancer," "cancer in remission," "localized cancer," and "metastatic cancer," respectively. Another type of fluctuation might be continuous scores ranging from 1 to 10, wherein a score of 1 represents "the least severe cancer" and a score of 10, "the most severe cancer."

Many of the concepts that make up middle-range theories are variables. For example, the concept "report of depression" can take the categorical scores of "0 = No" and "1 = Yes." Furthermore, the experimental and control conditions of predictive theories and experimental research represent categories of a concept. For example, the categories of the concept "cancer support groups" could be an experimental condition that consists of psychological support from health professionals and group participants, as well as information about cancer provided by health professionals; one control condition that consists only of psychological support; and another control condition that consists only of information.

Nonvariable concepts that are part of middle-range theories typically are confined to the characteristics of the individuals to whom the theory is addressed. For example, the theory could be limited to "married women" or "African-American men." Sometimes, a term may be a nonvariable concept in one theory and a dimension of a variable concept in another theory. For example, in a descriptive theory of changes in women's usual activities during pregnancy, a concept is the nonvariable "pregnant women." In a theory addressing the usual activities of pregnant and nonpregnant women, however, a concept is the variable "reproductive status"; "pregnant" is one of the two dimensions of the concept, and "nonpregnant" is the other.

Furthermore, occasionally a concept that is a variable in a theory takes only one score when subjected to empirical research and, therefore, must be classified as a nonvariable. Suppose, for example, that an investigator who is testing a theory of breast cancer–related depression expects that from a randomly selected sample of 100 women with breast cancer, some women will report that they feel depressed and others will report that they do not. Suppose, however, that none of the 100 women report that they do, in fact, feel depressed. In that case, the concept "report of depression" would be classified as a nonvariable on the basis of the research results. Consequently, the classification of a concept as a nonvariable or a variable depends on how the concept is used in the theory and on the empirical research results.

DUBIN'S SCHEMA. Dubin (1978) offered another way to classify phenomena according to their measurement characteristics. He identified five types of units, the term he used for concept. The *enumerative unit* refers to a phenomenon that is always present, regardless of its condition; it can never take a zero or absent value. If the enumerative unit is nonvariable, it is always present. "Female" is an example of a nonvariable enumerative unit. In contrast, if the enumerative unit is a variable, it is always present in some form. "Ethnicity" is an example of a variable enumerative unit.

The *associative unit* refers to a phenomenon that can have a real zero or absent value, as well as positive and negative numerical values. An associative unit that is nonvariable, such as "women with breast cancer," is either present or absent. More specifically, a woman can have breast cancer or not have breast cancer, and a person can be a woman or a man. An associative unit that is a variable is either present to some degree or not present at all. "Severity of breast cancer" is an example; the person can have no breast cancer or can have a particular level of severity of breast cancer.

The *relational unit* refers to a phenomenon that can be determined only by the relations between its components parts. One type of relational unit reflects an interaction between the component parts of a phenomenon; for example, when a mother and her infant communicate, they reflect one phenomenon called "maternal-infant communication."

Another type of relational unit reflects a combination of component parts. For example, "critically ill child" is a combination of the components "health state" and "developmental stage."

Relational units also may encompass plural components and entities. "Sibling rivalry" is an example; the plural components are the "child-child relationship" and the "parent-child relationship," and the plural entities are "children" and "parents."

The *statistical unit* refers to a phenomenon that summarizes its distribution. The label for this unit comes from the statistical terms for measures of central tendency and dispersion. There are three classes of statistical units.

One class of statistical units summarizes the central tendency in the distribution of a phenomenon. An example is "mean extent of problem solution," which is calculated from the score the individual receives for each item on a questionnaire, divided by the number of items answered by that individual; that is, a mean score is determined for each individual (see Spitzer, Bar-Tal, and Ziv, 1996a).

The second class of statistical units summarizes the dispersion of a phenomenon in a group as a whole. For example, the "ethnicity of people in a town" may be designated as homogeneous or diverse.

The third class of statistical units designates the relative position in the distribution of a phenomenon. An example is the "percentage of time an individual received hospice care from onset of terminal illness until death."

It is important to understand that the statistical unit is the unit of analysis for certain quantitative data that are collected as part of a study. For example, the individual's mean score could be the unit of analysis. A mean of all individuals' mean scores then would be calculated for descriptive and inferential purposes.

The *summative unit* is a global unit that refers to an entire complex phenomenon. Like Kaplan's theoretical term, this unit draws together several properties of the phenomenon and gives them a label that summarizes those properties. An example is "quality of life," which encompasses the individual's satisfaction with his or her life in the realms of physical health, psychological state, functional ability, and social relationships.

Comparison of Classification Schemas

Kaplan's (1964) and Willer and Webster's (1970) schemata emphasize the empirical observability of the properties of phenomena, whereas the measurement schemata are based on established canons of measurement theory. As can be seen in Table 2–3, there are some overlaps among the various schemata. Together, the two types of schemata—observability and measurement characteristics—provide a comprehensive method of concept classification.

Pragmatics of Concept Classification

Classification of the concepts of middle-range theories involves determination of the observability and the measurement characteristics of the properties of a phenomenon that are summarized by the concept name. The observability of the concept is determined by applying Kaplan's or Willer and Webster's schema, or both schemata. If a concept is not an observational term, then the way it is made observable has to be determined. For example, if the concept "depression" is determined to be Kaplan's indirect observable term and Willer and Webster's construct, the research document must be reviewed to determine how "depression" actually was observed.

Table 2–3 ■ **COMPARISON OF SCHEMATA FOR CONCEPT CLASSIFFICATION**

Kaplan	Willer and Webster	Dubin	Variability
Observational term	Observable		Nonvariable or variable
Indirect observable term	Construct		Nonvariable or variable
Construct	Construct		Nonvariable or variable
Theoretical term	Construct	Summative unit	Nonvariable or variable

The measurement characteristics of middle-range theory concepts are determined by identifying the variability of the concept and by applying Dubin's schema. The classification of the concept as a nonvariable or a variable is determined by identifying the number of forms the concept takes in the particular conceptual-theoretical-empirical structure being analyzed. Dubin's schema then is applied to further determine the measurement characteristics of each concept. Once again, classification is determined by how the concept was used in the conceptual-theoretical-empirical structure. For example, the concept "depression" is classified as an enumerative unit in a theory limited to individuals who exhibit signs of depression. In contrast, "depression" is classified as an associative unit in a theory that encompasses both depressed and nondepressed individuals.

Care must be taken in the classification of relational units because these concepts often appear to be associative or enumerative. Care also must be taken to classify statistical units correctly. In that case, the measure of central tendency or dispersion must be the raw score for each individual in the study sample; group means, for example, are not the basis for classification.

Successful classification of concepts according to their measurement characteristics is dependent on the information given in the research document. If the ranges for possible and obtained scores on a measurement device are not described, and if the interpretation of scores is not explained, it may not be possible to determine whether a concept is a nonvariable or variable or to apply Dubin's schema. Furthermore, if investigators who present the results of theory-generating research that employed such interpretative methods as phenomenology or grounded theory do not provide the number of study participants whose responses reflected a particular concept, it probably is not possible to determine whether every participant expressed this concept or only some of the participants did. Consequently, it probably is not possible to determine whether the concept is nonvariable or variable, and it may not be possible to apply Dubin's schema.

STEP THREE: IDENTIFICATION AND CLASSIFICATION OF PROPOSITIONS

The third step in formalization of a conceptual-theoretical-empirical structure is identification and classification of the propositions as they are given in the research document. A proposition is a declarative statement about one or more concepts, a statement that purports or asserts what is thought to be the case (Achinstein, 1974).

Types of Propositions

The statements that describe or link concepts encompass nonrelational and relational propositions. Although definitions are sometimes treated as separate components of a conceptual model or a middle-range theory, here they are more accurately identified as one category of nonrelational propositions.

Both conceptual models and theories contain nonrelational and relational propositions. The propositions of a conceptual model are written at a greater level of abstraction and generality than those of a middle-range theory. Furthermore, conceptual model propositions that are definitions typically are very broad, and those that assert relations rarely go beyond the statement that a relation exists.

NONRELATIONAL PROPOSITIONS. Propositions that say something about one concept are called nonrelational propositions. There are two categories of nonrelational propositions—those that state the existence of a concept and those that define a concept.

Existence propositions. Existence propositions assert the existence or level of existence of a phenomenon. A proposition that asserts the *existence* of a phenomenon simply states that a name or label has been attached to a phenomenon. This type of proposition is found in both conceptual models and middle-range theories. The general form of a nonrelational existence proposition found in a conceptual model or a theory is:

There is a phenomenon known as X.

An example of a conceptual model proposition that asserts the existence of a phenomenon is:

There is a phenomenon known as response mode.

This proposition was extracted from Roy's Adaptation Model.

An example of a middle-range theory proposition that asserts the existence of a phenomenon is:

There is a phenomenon known as physical health status.

This proposition was extracted from Brydolf and Segesten's (1994) descriptive naming theory of long-term adaptation to colectomy in young persons, which was derived from Roy's Adaptation Model.

A nonrelational proposition that asserts the *level of existence* of a phenomenon addresses the amount of that phenomenon. Due to its specificity, this type of proposition usually is not found in conceptual models but may be found in middle-range theories. The general form of a nonrelational level of existence proposition is:

The amount of the phenomenon known as X is small (moderate, large).

An example of a nonrelational proposition that asserts the level of existence of a phenomenon is:

The prevalence rate for a phenomenon known as pressure ulcers was 25%.

This proposition was extracted from Hunter and colleagues' (1992) descriptive naming theory of the prevalence and incidence of pressure ulcers experienced by patients in a rehabilitation hospital. Their theory is based on Levine's Conservation Model concept "structural integrity."

Another example of a nonrelational proposition that asserts the level of existence of a phenomenon is:

Four of the 22 clients expressed the phenomenon known as "To Live."

This example was extracted from Breckenridge's (1997) descriptive classification theory of dialysis modality decision making, which was guided by Neuman's Systems Model.

Definitional propositions. Definitional propositions go beyond statements of existence and level of existence by describing the characteristics of a phenomenon. A definition is a statement of the meaning of a concept and the intention to use that concept in a particular way. Furthermore, definitions are arbitrary labels that are not verifiable, and they usually are determined by convention. The definitions of conceptual model concepts are very broad, whereas the concepts of middle-range theories are more precisely defined.

Three types of definitional propositions are evident in fully specified conceptual-theoretical-empirical structures. Constitutive definitions are evident in both conceptual models and middle-range theories. Representational definitions link the concepts of a conceptual model to those of a middle-range theory. Operational definitions link middle-range theory concepts to empirical research methods.

The *constitutive definition* provides concepts with meaning. This type of definition also is called a theoretical definition, a nominal definition, or a rational definition. A constitutive definition states what a concept means by defining it with one or more other concepts. In addition, a constitutive definition indicates whether a concept is unidimensional or multidimensional. The general form of a nonrelational proposition that is a constitutive definition is:

X is defined as . . . .

The phrase "is defined as," should be included in the proposition so that the statement is immediately recognized as the constitutive definition.

An example of a constitutive definition for a conceptual model concept that is unidimensional is:

Health is defined as the dynamic life experiences of a human being.

This constitutive definition is from King's General Systems Framework (Frey and Sieloff, 1995). Here, the concept "health" is defined by the concept "dynamic life experiences."

An example of a constitutive definition for a conceptual model concept that is multidimensional is:

Response mode is defined as a multidimensional concept that encompasses physiological mode responses, self-concept mode responses, role function mode responses, and interdependence mode responses.

In this example, extracted from the content of Roy's Adaptation Model, the concept "response mode" is defined by the concepts "physiological mode responses," "self-concept mode responses," "role function mode responses," and "interdependence mode responses," which then become the dimensions of the concept "response mode."

An example of a constitutive definition for a theory concept that is unidimensional is:

General health behavior is defined as actions directed toward health promotion.

This example was extracted from Frey's (1996) explanatory theory of the relation of general-health behavior and illness-management behavior to health status and illness outcomes, which was derived from King's General Systems Framework. In this example, the concept "general-health behavior" is defined by the concepts "action" and "health promotion."

An example of a constitutive definition for a theory concept that is multidimensional is:

Physical-health status is defined as a multidimensional concept that encompasses four dimensions—nutrition, elimination, activity and rest, and protection.

In this example, the concept "physical-health status" is defined by the concepts "nutrition," "elimination," "activity and rest," and "protection," which then become the dimensions of the concept "physical-health status." The example was extracted from Brydolf and Segesten's (1994) descriptive naming theory of physical-health status.

The *representational definition* states the linkage between a particular conceptual model concept or one of its dimensions and a theory concept. This type of definition, then, forges a link between the more abstract and general conceptual model and the more concrete and specific middle-range theory or the even more concrete and specific empirical research methods. The general forms of a nonrelational proposition that is a representational definition are:

Conceptual model concept X is represented by theory concept X.

Conceptual model concept X is represented by empirical research method X'.

The phrase "is represented by" should be included in the proposition so that the statement is immediately recognized as the representational proposition.

An example of the first general form of a representational definition is a proposition that was extracted from Brydolf and Segesten's (1994) descriptive classification theory of physical health status, which was derived from Roy's Adaptation Model. The representational definition is:

The physiological response mode is represented by physical health status.

In this example, the dimension of Roy's Adaptation Model concept "response mode" called "physiological response mode" is linked to the theory concept "physical-health status."

The second general form of a representational definition is more likely to be found in documents dealing with theory-generating research than in documents about theory-testing research. An example of this form of a representational definition is:

Client perceptions are represented by data from the Client Perception Interview Guide provided by 22 clients with end-stage renal disease who were receiving hemodialysis or continuous ambulatory peritoneal dialysis.

This representational definition was extracted from Breckenridge's (1997) report of her theory-generating research. The empirical research methods and the descriptive classification theory that was generated were based on Neuman's Systems Model. The Neuman's model concept "client perceptions" is represented by the empirical research methods, including the Client Perception Interview Guide and the dialysis clients who served as study participants. The theory emerged from a secondary content analysis of the interview guide transcripts.

The *operational definition* provides a middle-range theory concept with empirical meaning and asserts the intention to use the concept in a particular way by defining it in terms of observable data, such as the activities necessary to measure the concept or to manipulate it. This type of definition also is called an epistemic definition, a real definition, or rules of correspondence or interpretation. Operational definitions identify the proxies for nonobservable concepts. They are measurement-oriented interpretations of the constitutive definitions of middle-range theory concepts. In particular, operational definitions are the means by which numbers or categories are assigned to theory concepts, "the sequence of steps or procedures a researcher follows to obtain a measurement" (Judd et al., 1991, p. 43).

Kerlinger (1986) identified two classes of operational definitions, which he called measured and experimental. The *measured operational definition* states how a concept will be measured. The general form of a nonrelational proposition that is a measured operational definition is:

Theory concept X is measured by X'.

The phrase "is measured by" should be included in the proposition so that the statement is immediately recognized as a measured operational definition.

An example of a measured operational definition is:

Self-care behaviors used to manage radiation therapy side effects were measured by the Radiation Side Effects Profile.

This definition was extracted from Hagopian's (1996) predictive theory of the effects of informational audiotapes on knowledge and management of side effects experienced by cancer patients undergoing radiation therapy. The theory is based on Orem's (1995) Self-Care Framework.

The *experimental operational definition* spells out the details or operations required to manipulate or vary the dimensions of a concept that typically is the independent variable in an experimental study. The general form of a nonrelational proposition that is an experimental operational definition is:

The experimental treatment(s) consisted of . . . .

The control treatment(s) consisted of . . . .

An example of an experimental operational definition, which was extracted from Hagopian's (1996) predictive theory, is:

The experimental treatment subjects received standard care and listened to audiotapes. Standard care was defined as the typical care received by patients undergoing radiation therapy where the study was conducted. The typical care consisted of providing literature from the National Cancer Institute and information about the department and the nature of radiation therapy, as well as weekly visits with the physician to discuss progress and side effects. Six audiotapes addressed the topics of radiation therapy, skin care, nutrition, fatigue, mouth care, diarrhea, and urinary frequency. The tapes covered several side effects that patients might experience and suggested self-care activities to relieve them. Other content included pertinent information about the nature of radiation therapy, special procedures in the radiation therapy department, nutrition information, and care after completion of treatment. The scripts for the tapes were written by the principal investigator. All audiotapes were narrated by the same nurse. The reading level of the tapes ranged from grade five to grade seven. The audiotapes ranged in length from 7 to 10 minutes. Subjects received the audiotapes of their choice, which they were allowed to keep as long as they wanted, and a tape player.

The control treatment subjects received standard care, which was defined as the typical care received by patients undergoing radiation therapy where the study was conducted. The typical care consisted of providing literature from the National Cancer Institute and information about the department and the nature of radiation therapy, as well as weekly visits with the physician to discuss progress and side effects.

The concept in this example is "type of information," and the two dimensions are "standard care plus informational audiotapes" and "standard care." The descriptions of the dimensions of the concept, that is, the experimental and control treatments, sometimes are referred to as protocols.

Operational definitions are necessary regardless of the type of research. This is true whether the operational definition identifies the paper-and-pencil questionnaire used in a survey, the experimental and control treatment protocols of an experiment, or the domain of the researcher-informant experience of an ethnography. Although operational definitions are needed for all kinds of research, they are a legacy of experimental research. More specifically, because development of theory by experimentation depends on actual operations with the concepts involved, Bridgman (1927), the originator of operationism, viewed a concept as nothing more than a set of unique operations or procedures necessary to produce an observation. His view of the one-to-one correspondence of concepts and operational definitions has been superseded by the view that no one operational definition can capture the richness and complexity of a concept (Judd et al., 1991). Indeed, many concepts have multiple operational definitions. Functional status, for example, is measured by a plethora of instruments (Richmond, McCorkle, Tulman, and Fawcett, 1997).

Operational definitions state how concepts are to be observed or measured and how the middle-range theory is to be generated or tested. Their crucial function is to link middle-range theory concepts to the real world; that is, to forge a link between the relatively concrete and specific theory and the very concrete and specific tools and techniques employed to generate or test the theory.

Empirical research methods are the actual tools and techniques of research, that is, the actual research design, subjects, instruments, data-collection procedures, and data-analysis techniques that are used in a study. The term *empirical indicator* typically is used to refer specifically to the research instruments used in any kind of research, as well as to the experimental treatment and control treatment protocols of experimental research. Operational definitions and empirical research methods, including the empirical indicators, complete the conceptual-theoretical-empirical structure for theory-generating or theory-testing research.

RELATIONAL PROPOSITIONS. Propositions that link two or more concepts are referred to as relational propositions. They are declarative statements that express an association or connection between concepts. More specifically, relational propositions state patterns of covariation between concepts that are variables; that is, they state that fluctuations in one concept are systematically accompanied by fluctuations in another. In explanatory theories, the relation between concepts is expressed as a correlation. In predictive theories, the relation frequently is expressed as the effects of the experimental and control treatments. Thus, the phrases used to indicate a relation include "relation between," "relationship between," "related to," "associated with," "correlated with," and "effect of."

The use of the phrase "effect of" may connote a causal or deterministic relation, that is, a proposition that asserts what always happens in a given situation. Contemporary philosophy of science, however, suggests that deterministic relations do not exist, even in the physical sciences. Furthermore, those individuals who qualify a proposition asserting a deterministic relation by adding, "all things being equal," fail to recognize that all things are rarely, if ever, equal (Schumacher and Gortner, 1992). Accordingly, propositions that purport to assert deterministic relations are not considered in this book. Instead, all relational propositions are regarded as probabilistic. Thus, all relational propositions are founded on the chances or probability of something happening in a given situation. In empirical research, probability typically is addressed by tests of statistical significance.

A relational proposition can make several types of assertions. In fact, the more assertions a proposition can make, the more that is known about the nature of the relation between the concepts.

Existence of a relation. The most basic assertion that can be made about a relation is that it exists. A relational proposition asserting the existence of a relation indicates that the association between two or more concepts is a recurring phenomenon rather than a unique event. Relational existence propositions are found in both conceptual models and middle-range theories. The general form of this assertion is:

There is a relation between X and Y.

An example of a conceptual model proposition asserting the existence of a relation, which was extracted from Roy's Adaptation Model, is:

There is a relation between stimuli and response mode.

An example of a theory proposition asserting the existence of a relation is:

There is a relation between loneliness and cognitive functioning.

This proposition was extracted from Ryan's (1996) explanatory theory of the relations of loneliness, social support, and depression to cognitive functioning, which was derived from Roy's Adaptation Model. The proposition simply asserts that a relation between "loneliness" and "cognitive functioning" exists.

Direction of a relation. A proposition that asserts the direction of a relation states that the association between two concepts is positive (direct) or negative (indirect, inverse). Directional relational propositions usually are not found in conceptual models but are a part of many middle-range theories. The two general forms of a directional relational proposition are:

There is a positive (negative) relation between X and Y.

X is positively (negatively) related to Y.

An example of a directional relational proposition is:

There is a negative relation between loneliness and cognitive functioning.

This proposition was extracted from Ryan's (1996) explanatory theory. Earlier, the relation between loneliness and cognitive functioning was given as an example of the existence of a relation. Now it can be asserted that the relation exists and is negative, such that the greater the loneliness, the lower the cognitive functioning, or, conversely, the less the loneliness, the greater the cognitive functioning.

Another example of a directional relational proposition is:

There is a positive relation between type of information and the number of self-care behaviors used to manage radiation therapy side effects, such that standard care plus informational audiotapes is associated with use of a greater number of self-care behaviors than standard care only.

This proposition was extracted from Hagopian's (1996) predictive theory of the effects of informational audiotapes on knowledge and management of side effects experienced by cancer patients undergoing radiation therapy, which is based on Orem's Self-Care Framework. The example illustrates how details beyond the specification of "negative" or "positive" can clarify the meaning of a directional relational proposition that is part of a predictive theory.

Shape of a relation. A proposition that asserts the shape of a relation states that the association between concepts is linear or curvilinear; and, if curvilinear, is quadratic, cubic, quartic, or another shape. A quadratic relational proposition is one that includes a second-power term (X^2) in the equation for the proposition. A cubic relational proposition is one that includes a third-power term (X^3) in the equation. A quartic relational proposition is one that includes a fourth-power term (X^4) in the equation. Relational propositions that assert shape usually are not found in conceptual models but may be found in middle-range theories.

The general form of a proposition that asserts a linear relation is:

There is a linear relation between X and Y such that as the numerical values of X increase, the numerical values of Y also increase (decrease).

An example of a proposition that asserts a linear relation is:

> There is a linear relation between loneliness and cognitive functioning, such that an increase in loneliness is associated with a decrease in cognitive functioning, and decrease in loneliness is associated with an increase in cognitive functioning.

This proposition was extracted from information given in Ryan's (1996) report of the test of her explanatory theory of the relations of loneliness, social support, and depression to cognitive functioning. Earlier in this chapter, the relation between loneliness and cognitive functioning was given as an example of the existence of a relation and as an example of the direction of a relation. Now it can be asserted that a linear negative relation exists.

The general form of a proposition that asserts a quadratic relation is:

> There is a quadratic relation between X and Y such that, when the values of X are low and high, the values of Y are low (high), and when the values of X are moderate, the values of Y are high (low).

An example of a proposition that asserts a quadratic relation is:

> There is a quadratic relation between prenatal anxiety and length of labor, such that low and high levels of anxiety are associated with longer labor than a moderate level of anxiety.

This proposition was extracted from McCool's (1997) provisional explanatory theory of biopsychosocial correlates of the outcomes of pregnancy, which is based on a conceptual model of human development.

Propositions about relations taking other shapes are stated in the same general form as linear and quadratic relational propositions, and the particular shape is specified.

Strength of a relation. A proposition that asserts the strength of a relation identifies the magnitude of the relation between two concepts. Magnitude is quantified by the effect size of a relation, which is a standardized measure of the association between concepts or the difference between conditions. Formulas for the effect sizes for several statistics and the designation of these effect sizes as small, medium, or large, are given by Cohen (1988), among others. Relational propositions that assert strength usually are not found in conceptual models but may be found in middle-range theories. If the strength of the relation is not stated explicitly in a theory, the effect size sometimes can be calculated from the data given in the report of the research that generated or tested that theory. The general form of a proposition that asserts the strength of a relation is:

> There is a weak (moderate, strong) relation between X and Y.

An example of this type of proposition is:

> There is a moderate relation between type of information and number of self-care behaviors used to manage radiation therapy side effects, such that standard care plus informational audiotapes is associated with use of a greater number of self-care behaviors to manage radiation therapy side effects than standard care only.

This proposition was extracted from information about sample size calculations given in Hagopian's (1996) report of a test of her predictive theory.

Another example of a relational proposition asserting strength is:

> There is a strong relation between walking and physical functioning, such that moderate walking exercise is associated with much better physical functioning than usual care.

This proposition was extracted from information about sample size calculations given in Mock et al.'s (1997) report of a test of their predictive theory of the effects of walking exercise on physical functioning, exercise level, emotional distress, and symptom experience of women with breast cancer who were receiving radiation therapy. The theory was based on Roy's Adaptation Model and findings from previous research.

Still other examples, which illustrate the explicit use of effect size metrics to assert the strength of a relation, are:

> The effect size (ES) for the relation between interpersonal relations and functional status was large at both Time 1 ($ES_r = .67$) and Time 2 ($ES_r = .53$).

> The ES for the relation between depression and functional status at Time 1 was small ($ES_r = .11$). In contrast, the ES for the relation between those two concepts at Time 2 was large ($ES_r = .83$).

> The ES for the relation between stage of breast cancer and functional status was extremely small ($ES_r = .03$).

> A relatively large ES was found for the relation between employment status and functional status ($ES_{t\text{-test}} = .63$).

These propositions were found in Tulman and Fawcett's (1996) report of the results of a longitudinal pilot test of an explanatory theory of the correlates of functional status in women with breast cancer, which was derived from Roy's Adaptation Model.

Symmetry of a relation. A proposition asserting the symmetry of a relation states that the association between two concepts is either asymmetrical or symmetrical. Assertions about the symmetry of a relational proposition are found in both conceptual models and middle-range theories.

An *asymmetrical relation* is irreversible; only one idea is conveyed (X is related to Y). The general form of a proposition that asserts an asymmetrical relation is:

> If X, then Y; but if no X, no conclusion can be drawn about Y.

An example of a conceptual model proposition asserting an asymmetrical relation is:

> Coping mechanism is related to response mode.

This proposition is part of Roy's Adaptation Model.

An example of a theory proposition asserting an asymmetrical relation is:

> Type of coping is related to functional ability.

This asymmetrical relational proposition was extracted from an explanatory theory of adaptation to spinal cord injury (Barone, 1993; Barone and Roy, 1996), which was derived from Roy's Adaptation Model. The theory concept "type of coping" represents Roy's conceptual model concept "cognator coping mechanism," and the theory concept "functional ability" represents the physiological mode dimension of Roy's model concept "response mode."

A *symmetrical relation* is also called a reversible or reciprocal relation; it contains two separate ideas (X is related to Y and Y is related to X) that require two separate empirical tests. The general form of a proposition that asserts a symmetrical relation is:

If X, then Y; and if Y, then X.

An example of a conceptual model proposition asserting a symmetrical relation is:

There is a reciprocal relation between the personal system and the interpersonal system.

This relational proposition was extracted from King's General Systems Theory.

An example of a proposition asserting a symmetrical relation in a theory is:

There is a reciprocal relation between child health and family health.

This relational proposition was extracted from Frey's (1993) explanatory theory of family and child health, which was derived from King's General Systems Framework. King's conceptual model concept "personal system" is represented by the theory concept "child health," and King's model concept "interpersonal system" is represented by "family health."

Concurrrent and sequential relations. A proposition that asserts the concurrent or sequential nature of a relation refers to the period of time that elapses between the appearance of one concept and the appearance of another. Concurrent and sequential relational propositions typically are not part of a conceptual model but may be found in a middle-range theory.

If both concepts appear at the same time, the relation is said to be *concurrent* or *coextensive*. The general form of a proposition that asserts a concurrent relation is:

If X, then also Y.

An example of a proposition asserting a concurrent relation is:

There is a concurrent relation between depression and cognitive functioning.

This proposition was extracted from Ryan's (1996) explanatory theory.

If one concept appears prior to the other, the relation is said to be *sequential.* The general form of a sequential relational proposition is:

If X, then Y follows later.

An example of a proposition asserting a sequential relation, which was extracted from Hagopian's (1996) predictive theory, is:

> There is a sequential relation between type of information and number of self-care behaviors used to manage radiation therapy side effects.

This proposition is another example of the fact that several assertions can be made about the relations between concepts. The information given by Hagopian (1996) indicates that the relation between "type of information" and "self-care behaviors used to manage radiation therapy side effects" exists and is positive, moderate in strength, asymmetrical, and sequential.

Necessary and substitutable relations. A proposition asserting a necessary or substitutable relation refers to the need for a particular concept in the relation. Propositions asserting the necessary or substitutable nature of relations usually are not found in a conceptual model but may be part of a middle-range theory.

Propositions that assert a *necessary* relation state that if one concept occurs, and only if that concept occurs, will the other concept occur. The first concept must be present to bring about the relation. The general form of a proposition that asserts a necessary relation is:

> If X, and only if X, then Y.

An example of such a relational proposition is:

> Type of preparatory information is related to mood state, such that concrete, objective information consisting of physical sensations, temporal features, environmental features, and causes of the sensations is necessary to increase positive mood.

This relational proposition was extracted from Johnson, Fieler, Wlasowicz, Mitchell, and Jones's (1997) predictive theory of the effects of information given by nurses on coping with radiation therapy. The proposition is part of the self-regulation theory, which was derived from a conceptual model of stress and coping (Johnson, Fieler, Jones, Wlasowicz, and Mitchell, 1997).

Propositions that assert a *substitutable* relation state that if one concept occurs the other concept will occur. In this kind of relation, however, if some other similar concept occurs the second concept also will occur. The general form of a proposition that asserts a substitutable relation is:

> If X_1, but also if X_2, then Y.

An example of such a relational proposition is:

> Loneliness or depression is negatively related to cognitive functioning.

This relational proposition was extracted from Ryan's (1996) explanatory theory. The proposition indicates that either a high (low) level of loneliness or a high (low) level of depression is associated with a low (high) level of cognitive functioning.

Sufficient and contingent relations. A proposition that asserts a sufficient or contingent relation refers to the conditional nature of a concept in the relation. Such propositions rarely are found in any conceptual model and only occasionally in a middle-range theory.

Propositions that assert a sufficient relation state that when one (or more) particular concept occurs, a certain other concept will occur, regardless of anything else. The general form of this type of relational proposition is:

If X, then Y, regardless of anything else.

An example of a proposition asserting a sufficient relation, which was extracted from Johnson, Fieler, Wlasowicz, Mitchell, and Jones's (1997) predictive theory, is:

Type of preparatory information and outcome expectancies are related to mood state, such that concrete, objective information consisting of physical sensations, temporal features, environmental features, and causes of the sensations as well as pessimistic expectations about outcomes are sufficient to increase positive mood.

Previously, the need for concrete, objective information was given as an example of a proposition asserting a necessary relation. Now it can be asserted that concrete, objective information is necessary for an increase in positive mood, but it is not sufficient. Rather, both concrete, objective information and pessimistic outcome expectancies are required to increase positive mood.

Propositions that assert a *contingent* relation state that the relation between the two concepts X and Y is influenced by the presence of some third concept. The third concept is referred to as an intervening concept C. The general form of a proposition that asserts a contingent relation is:

If X, then Y, in the presence of C.

One form of a contingent relation occurs when the intervening concept C is directly in the path between two other concepts X and Y; thus, the three concepts form a chain. An example of a conceptual model proposition asserting this form of a contingent relation is:

Stimuli are related to type of coping mechanism, which in turn is related to response mode.

This contingent relational proposition was extracted from Roy's Adaptation Model. It is one of the very few such propositions found in conceptual models of nursing.

An example of a theory proposition asserting this form of a contingent relation is:

Sociodemographic characteristics and hardiness are related to type of coping, which in turn is related to functional ability.

This contingent relational proposition was extracted from Barone's (1993; Barone and Roy, 1996) explanatory theory of adaptation to spinal cord injury. The theory concepts "sociodemographic characteristics" and "hardiness" represent Roy's Adaptation Model concept "stimuli," and, as noted earlier, the theory concept "type of coping" represents Roy's model concept "cognator coping mechanism," and the theory concept "functional ability" represents the physiological mode dimension of Roy's model concept "response mode."

Other forms of contingent relations occur when the numerical values taken by the intervening concept C affect the existence, direction, or strength of the relation between X and Y. An example of a theory proposition asserting the form of a contingent relation that involves the existence of the relation between X and Y is:

> The relation between self-care and perception of extent of problem solution is contingent on age, such that the relation does not exist for younger individuals and is relatively strong for older individuals.

This proposition states how the existence of a relation between the two concepts "self-care" and "perception of extent of problem solution" is influenced by the numerical values of a third concept "age." The study participants ranged in age from 20 to 95 years (median = 65 years). The proposition was tested by dividing the participants according to the median for age. It was extracted from Spitzer, Bar-Tal, and Ziv's (1996a) explanatory theory of the association of chronically ill patients' age on the relation of symptom severity, self-care, and others' care to perception of the extent of problem solution, satisfaction with problem solution, and perception of control over health, which was based on Orem's (1991) Self-Care Framework.

An example of a theory proposition asserting the form of a contingent relation that involves the direction of the relation between X and Y is:

> The relation between psychosocial resources and perceived stress is contingent on gender, such that the relation is positive for males and negative for females.

This proposition states how the direction of a relation between the two concepts "psychosocial resources" and "perceived stress" is influenced by a third concept, in this case the fluctuation in the concept "gender," which was measured by the categorical scores given to the dimensions "male" and "female." The proposition was extracted from Leidy's (1990) explanatory theory of the relations among psychosocial resources, perceived stress, disease severity, and symptomatic experience in men and women with chronic obstructive pulmonary disease, which was derived from Erickson, Tomlin, and Swain's (1983) Modeling and Role-Modeling conceptual framework.

An example of a theory proposition asserting the form of a contingent relation that involves the strength of the relation between X and Y is:

> The positive relation between perceived social support and general well-being is contingent on hopefulness, such that the lower the hopefulness, the stronger the positive relation between perceived social support and general well-being. Conversely, the strength of the positive relation between perceived social support and general well-being decreases when hopefulness increases.

The proposition states how the strength of a relation between the two concepts "perceived social support" and "general well-being" is influenced by the numerical values of a third concept "hopefulness." The proposition was extracted from Yarcheski, Scoloveno, and Mahon's (1994) explanatory theory of social support, well-being, and hopefulness in adolescents, which was derived from Baron and Kenny's (1986) conceptual model of mediation.

Another example of a theory proposition asserting the form of a contingent relation that involves the strength of the relation between X and Y is:

> The relation between self-care and well-being in daily living is contingent on gender, such that the relation is stronger for women than for men.

This proposition states how the strength of a relation between the two concepts "self-care" and "well-being in daily living" is influenced by the fluctuation in a third concept, in this case the categorical scores given to the "male" and "female" dimensions of the concept "gender." The proposition was extracted from Spitzer, Bar-Tal, and Ziv's (1996b) explanatory theory of the association of the gender of chronically ill patients on the relation of symptom severity, self-care, and others' care to psychosocial well-being, daily living well-being, and physical well-being, which was based on Orem's (1991) Self-Care Framework.

THE HYPOTHESIS. Hypotheses are special types of propositions that represent conjectures about the concepts of middle-range theories stated in empirically testable forms. They are expectations about the way things are in the world if the assertions of middle-range theory propositions are empirically adequate. A hypothesis is derived from a proposition by linking one or more constitutively defined concepts with the empirical indicators identified in the operational definitions. Technically, a hypothesis is a conjecture about one or more empirical indicators; more specifically, it is a conjecture about the scores obtained from the empirical indicator(s) (Dubin, 1978; Gibbs, 1972). The numerical scores from the empirical indicators are what are compared when statistical tests are conducted. Although most research documents state the hypotheses by using only the names of the concepts, examination of the document should reveal what empirical indicators are included in the actual hypotheses.

A hypothesis can state a conjecture about a nonrelational or relational proposition. The general form of a nonrelational proposition and its derived hypothesis is:

Proposition: There is a phenomenon known as X.

Hypothesis: The phenomenon known as X is empirically demonstrated by X'.

An example of a nonrelational proposition and its derived hypothesis is:

Proposition: The phenomenon known as functional status-caregiver of a child in a body cast encompasses the dimensions of personal-care activities, household activities, child-care activities, occupational activities, and social and community activities; the dimension of child-care activities encompasses the two subdimensions of child in body cast and other child(ren).

Hypothesis: The 49 items of the Inventory of Functional Status—Caregiver of a Child in a Body Cast are categorized into six subscales: personal-care activities, 10 items; household activities, 9 items; care of child in body cast activities, 8 items; care of other child(ren) activities, 9 items; occupational activities, 7 items; and social and community activities, 6 items.

The proposition and hypothesis in this example were extracted from Newman's (1997) descriptive classification theory of the functional status of the caregivers of children in body casts. Newman used the role function dimension of Roy's Adaptation Model concept "response mode" to guide the generation of the theory and the development of the empirical indicator. Here, each dimension of the theory concept "functional status—caregiver of a child in a body cast" was measured by a subscale of the empirical indicator, the Inventory of Functional Status—Caregiver of a Child in a Body Cast. The hypothesis stipulates both the subscales and the number of items on each subscale that are expected to make up the empirical indicator for the theory concept. Although this type of hypothesis rarely is explicated, it represents exactly what is tested when the psychometric properties of an instrument are being established.

The general form of a relational proposition and its derived hypothesis is:

Proposition: There is a relation between X and Y.

Hypothesis: X′ and Y′ are related.

An example of a relational proposition from an explanatory theory and its derived hypothesis is:

Proposition: There is a negative relation between loneliness and cognitive functioning.

Hypothesis: The higher the score on the Revised UCLA Loneliness Scale, the lower the score on the Mini Mental Status Examination.

This proposition and hypothesis were extracted from Ryan's (1996) explanatory theory, which was derived from Roy's Adaptation Model. Here, the theory concept "loneliness" was measured by the empirical indicator Revised UCLA Loneliness Scale, and the theory concept "cognitive functioning" was measured by the empirical indicator Mini Mental Status Examination. The hypothesis stipulates the statistical relation between the scores on the two empirical indicators.

An example of a relational proposition from a predictive theory and its derived hypothesis is:

Proposition: Type of preparation for chemotherapy is related to mood distress, such that efficacy-enhancing preparation has a statistically significantly greater effect ($p < .05$) on reduction of mood distress than usual preparation.

Hypothesis: Compared with the control usual preparation group, the experimental efficacy-enhancing preparation group has statistically significantly lower ($p < .05$) scores on the Profile of Mood States.

This proposition and hypothesis were extracted from Lev's (1995) predictive theory, which was based on Orem's (1991) Self-Care Framework. Here, the theory concept "type of preparation for chemotherapy" was measured by the empirical indicators experimental efficacy-enhancing preparation group protocol and control usual preparation group protocol, and the theory concept "mood distress" was measured by the empirical indicator Profile of Mood States. The hypothesis stipulates the level of probability required for the statistical test used to determine the difference between the experimental group and the control group on the empirical indicator used to measure mood distress.

Another example of a relational proposition from a predictive theory and its derived hypothesis is:

Proposition: There is a strong positive relation between walking exercise and physical functioning, such that moderate walking exercise is associated with much better physical functioning than usual care.

Hypothesis: The difference in scores on the 12-Minute Walk Test between the experimental moderate walking exercise program group and the control usual care group signify a large effect size, with higher scores for the experimental group.

This proposition and hypothesis were extracted from Mock et al.'s (1997) predictive theory of the effects of walking exercise on physical functioning, exercise level, emotional distress, and symptom experience of women with breast cancer who were receiving radiation therapy, which was based on Roy's Adaptation Model and findings from previous research. Here, the theory concept "walking exercise" was measured by the empirical indicators experimental moderate walking exercise program group protocol and control usual care group protocol, and the theory concept "physical functioning" was measured by the empirical indicator 12-Minute Walk Test. The hypothesis stipulates the direction and magnitude of the difference between the experimental and control groups on the empirical indicator measuring physical functioning. This example illustrates the fact that a hypothesis may be used to empirically test more than one assertion about concepts. In this case, three explicit assertions are made—the existence of a relation between walking exercise and physical functioning, the direction of that relation, and its strength. Although the effect size rarely is included in the hypothesis, it can be incorporated into hypotheses easily when a power analysis is done to determine sample size (Cohen, 1988).

Pragmatics of Proposition Identification and Classification

Propositions are not always presented explicitly or clearly in documents dealing with theory-generating or theory-testing research. Therefore, the research document may have to be reviewed several times before all propositions are identified. More specifically, identification of propositions requires careful and repeated reading to screen out extraneous narrative. Only the narrative that deals directly with the particular conceptual model propositions that guided the study and with the particular propositions of the middle-range theory that was generated or tested is of interest.

Propositions are identified by listing all statements—sentences or phrases—that include the concepts already identified as central to the conceptual model that guided the research and to the middle-range theory that was generated or tested. The propositions should be listed exactly as they are stated in the research document. After all propositions are listed, they can be restated in a more formal manner (e.g., X is defined as . . . ; X is related to Y) if that facilitates the analysis. However, only the propositions presented in the research document should be listed, even if some concepts included in the theory are not accounted for in the list. Although it may be tempting to add the needed propositions, that should not be done as part of the analysis of a conceptual-theoretical-empirical structure.

In theory-testing research documents, all propositions that are part of the theory must be identified so that the version of the theory that was tested can be compared with the version of the theory that was retained after the test. The propositions that are part of the version of the theory that was tested are more likely to be found in the introductory and method sections of the research document. Those that are part of the theory that was retained after the test are found in the results and discussion sections of the report of the completed research.

Identification of the propositions is followed by their classification. Classification involves separating the propositions that are part of the conceptual model from those that are part of the theory. Classification also involves determining whether each proposition is nonrelational or relational.

Nonrelational propositions frequently are the major statements in theory-generating research documents and are found in the results or discussion section of the report of the completed research. In theory-testing research documents, nonrelational propositions typically are found in the introductory and method sections.

Nonrelational propositions are classified as either existence or definitional propositions. Nonrelational existence propositions frequently are implicit and rarely stated in the formal manner of "There is a phenomenon known as . . . ."; instead, they are reflected in the substance of the research document. For example, formalization of Brydolf and Segesten's (1994) conceptual-theoretical-empirical structure revealed an existence proposition dealing with the phenomenon of physical health status.

Definitions of concepts, like concepts themselves, may not be readily identifiable. That is because definitional propositions are not always labeled as such in a research document. The research document, therefore, needs to be carefully reviewed to determine which concepts are defined and how they are defined. The type of definition—constitutive, representational, or operational—also must be determined.

Constitutive definitions, if given, typically can be extracted from the narrative discussion of the concepts in the introductory section of the research document, or from the description of the empirical indicators in the method section. Representational definitions typically can be extracted from the introductory section discussion of the conceptual model that guided the research or, on occasion, from the discussion of the empirical research methods. In theory-generating research documents, an effort should be made to identify how the representational definitions link the conceptual model concepts to the empirical research methods. In theory-testing research documents, the effort is directed toward identifying how the representational definitions link the conceptual model concepts directly to the theory concepts.

Operational definitions usually can be determined from the description of the empirical indicators or the research procedure in the method section of the research report. In theory-generating research documents, an effort should be made to identify how the operational definitions link the empirical research methods to the theory. In theory-testing research documents, the effort is directed toward identifying how the operational definitions link the theory concepts to the empirical indicators and other components of the empirical research methods.

Relational propositions may be found in the introductory, results, and discussion sections of the research document. In theory-generating research documents, relational propositions usually are found in the results or discussion section. In theory-testing research documents, relational propositions usually are found in the introductory section, although some may not appear until the results or discussion section.

Relational propositions are classified according to the assertions that can be made about them (existence, direction, strength, and so on). The direction of a relation, if not stated explicitly, usually can be extracted from the results section. More specifically, the direction of a relation can be determined from the sign of a correlation coefficient or the difference in the mean scores of the experimental and control groups. The strength of a relation sometimes can be extracted from the research document by reviewing the description of the sample size calculations, which include the effect size, or by calculating the effect size from data given in the results section.

Classification of propositions concludes with identification of those that are hypotheses. If desired, the hypotheses can be restated by substituting the empirical indicators for the concept names. The results section of a research document may reveal relational propositions that were not initially presented as part of the theory. In particular, the results section may yield propositions that are implicit hypotheses. Such propositions can be extracted from the report of any inferential statistical tests. Suppose, for example, that an investigator reported that a *t*-test was performed to determine the difference in scores on a perceived health status questionnaire of the men and women who participated in a study designed to test a predictive theory of the effects of types of information on perceived health status. Suppose also that the initial statement of the theory did not include the concept "gender." The implicit hypothesis, stated in concept names in this example, would be: There is a relation between gender and perceived health status.

STEP FOUR: HIERARCHICAL ORDERING OF PROPOSITIONS

The fourth step in formalization of a conceptual-theoretical-empirical structure is the hierarchical ordering of the propositions into sets. A proposition set provides a concise justification for the existence of a phenomenon or an explanation of why a particular relation exists. Proposition sets can be arranged hierarchically according to level of abstraction, inductive reasoning, or deductive reasoning. Hierarchies based on level of abstraction typically include conceptual model propositions and middle-range theory propositions. Those based on inductive or deductive reasoning are limited to the propositions of the middle-range theory that was generated or tested.

Hierarchies by Level of Abstraction

Propositions can be arranged on a continuum from abstract to concrete. The abstract propositions are concerned with more general phenomena or a wider class of objects than are the concrete propositions, which are concerned with more specific phenomena or a narrower class of objects. Gibson (1960) referred to abstract statements as unrestricted propositions and to concrete statements as restricted propositions. He noted that the distinction arises from the limits of space and time within which the proposition applies. Abstract propositions are found in conceptual models, whereas somewhat concrete propositions are found in middle-range theories, and the most concrete propositions are those that identify or link empirical research methods. The proposition set, therefore, consists of statements arranged from most abstract to most concrete.

Hierarchies of propositions that can be arranged according to level of abstraction are most often found in documents that identify the conceptual model that guided the research, as well as the middle-range theory that will be or was generated or tested. Such hierarchies are, in essence, the narrative for a conceptual-theoretical-empirical structure. An example of a hierarchy of propositions based on level of abstraction is:

Abstract proposition: Stimuli are related to coping mechanisms, which in turn are related to response mode.

Somewhat concrete proposition: Sociodemographic characteristics and hardiness are related to type of coping, which in turn is related to functional ability in spinal-cord-injured individuals.

Most concrete proposition: Scores from a Sociodemographic Data Sheet and the Health-Related Hardiness Scale are related to scores on the Ways of Coping Checklist, which in turn are related to scores on the FONE Functional Independence Measure in a sample of 243 adults with quadriplegia or paraplegia of at least 4 weeks' duration.

This example was extracted from the reports of a test of an explanatory theory of adaptation to spinal cord injury (Barone, 1993; Barone and Roy, 1996), which was derived from Roy's Adaptation Model. This example illustrates how propositions become more narrow and specific in scope as they become more concrete. The most abstract proposition is part of Roy's conceptual model. The somewhat concrete proposition narrows the relation to the particular situation of spinal cord injury and to particular middle-range theory concepts. The most concrete proposition specifies the particular empirical indicators used to measure the theory concepts and the particular sample of study subjects.

Hierarchies by Inductive Reasoning

Inductive reasoning is evident when a conclusion summarizes a series of discrete observations about a phenomenon. Each observation represents evidence for the conclusion (Crossley and Wilson, 1979). Inductive reasoning is most often found in reports of theory-generating research that employed interpretative methods yielding qualitative data. The inductive proposition set consists of a series of observations followed by a conclusion. Its general form is:

Observation$_1$: . . .

Observation$_2$: . . .

Observation$_n$: . . .

Conclusion: *Observations*$_{1-n}$ make up the phenomenon known as X.

An example of a hierarchy of propositions based on inductive reasoning is:

Observation$_1$: That's part of life.

Observation$_2$: I have to suffer.

Observation$_3$: You're supposed to live with it.

Observation$_4$: It's something from God.

Conclusion: Acceptance of pain was a prevailing attitude of Mexican-Americans. (Villarruel, 1995, p. 431)

This example was taken from Villarruel's (1995) descriptive naming theory of Mexican-American people's meanings and expressions of pain and associated self-care and dependent-care actions. The theory-generating ethnographic research was guided by Orem's (1991) Self-Care Framework. The theory, which encompasses four themes (concepts) and two or more patterns within each theme (dimensions of the concepts), was induced from the data provided by 20 key informants and 14 general informants. The example includes four observations from which a pattern called "acceptance of pain" was induced. This pattern is part of the theme called "Pain is an accepted obligation of life and of one's role within the family: A burden one must bear so as not to inflict pain on others."

Hierarchies by Deductive Reasoning

Deductive reasoning is evident when a conclusion necessarily follows from one or more statements that are taken as empirically adequate (Crossley and Wilson, 1979). This type of reasoning is found most frequently in theory-testing research documents. Hierarchical ordering of the propositions of a deductively developed theory requires that some statements be identified as initial starting points and others as deductions from the starting points.

The propositions that represent the starting points for deduction are called axioms, premises, or postulates. They are taken as givens in a theory and, therefore, do not have to be tested. A proposition that is deduced from two or more axioms is called a theorem or a supposition. Its logical and empirical adequacy must be determined. Thus, the deductive proposition set is made up of a series of axioms followed by a theorem. The transitive rule of relations is used to deduce a theorem from axioms. The general form of a deductive proposition set, using the transitive rule, is:

Axiom$_1$: If X is related to Y, and

Axiom$_2$: if Y is related to Z, then

Theorem: X is related to Z.

An example of a hierarchy of propositions based on deductive reasoning and using the transitive rule is:

Axiom$_1$: If there is a relation between hardiness and job stress, and

Axiom$_2$: if there is a relation between job stress and burnout, then

Theorem: there is a relation between hardiness and burnout.

This example was constructed on the basis of information given in Collins's (1996) report of her correlational research, which was designed to test an explanatory theory of the relations between hardiness, burnout, and job stress. The theory was derived from Neuman's Systems Model. In this example, X is represented by "hardiness"; Y, by "job stress"; and Z, by "burnout."

Although axioms usually are statements of relations, sometimes one or more axioms may be nonrelational definitional propositions. Hypotheses stated in the vocabulary of empirical indicators are developed through this form of deduction. In this case, the nonrelational definitional propositions are axioms that identify the empirical indicators X′ and Y′ for concepts X and Y. The proposition set in this case consists of axioms and the hypothesis. The general form of this type of deductive proposition set is:

Axiom$_1$: If X is related to Y, and

Axiom$_2$: if X is measured by X′, and

Axiom$_3$: if Y is measured by Y′, then

Hypothesis: the scores for X′ are related to the scores for Y′.

An example of a deductive hierarchy for a hypothesis is:

Axiom$_1$: If depression is negatively related to cognitive functioning, and

Axiom$_2$: if depression is measured by the Hayes and Lohse Depression Scale, and

Axiom$_3$: if cognitive functioning is measured by the Mini Mental Status Examination, then

Hypothesis: the higher the scores on the Hayes and Lohse Depression Scale, the lower the scores on the Mini Mental Status Examination and, conversely, the lower the scores on the Hayes and Lohse Depression Scale, the higher the scores on the Mini Mental Status Examination.

This example was extracted from Ryan's (1996) explanatory theory. The example illustrates the derivation of the hypothesis testing the relation between the concepts "depression" and "cognitive functioning." Here, X is represented by "depression"; X′, by the Hayes and Lohse Depression Scale; Y, by "cognitive functioning"; and Y′, by the Mini Mental Status Examination.

SIGN OF A RELATIONAL PROPOSITION. The direction, or sign, of an axiom, if known, was established in previous research. The sign of a deduced theorem, however, must be calculated by means of the so-called sign rule, which is based on mathematical logic. This rule states that the sign of the deduced theorem is the algebraic product of the signs of the axioms. That is, the sign of the deduced relation between X and Z is found by multiplying the sign of the relation between X and Y by the sign of the relation between Y and Z. Four possible combinations of signs are given in Table 2–4.

Use of the sign rule is exemplified by adding the directions and signs for the deductive proposition set drawn from Collins's (1996) explanatory theory:

Axiom₁: If there is a negative relation ($-$) between hardiness and job stress, and

Axiom₂: if there is a positive relation ($+$) between job stress and burnout, then

Theorem: there is a negative relation ($-$) between hardiness and burnout.

Pragmatics of Hierarchical Ordering of Propositions

Selection of the method of hierarchy development depends on the information given in the research document and the purpose of the research. Arrangement of propositions according to level of abstraction is possible when the conceptual model propositions are given. In addition, if the purpose of the research was to generate a

---

Table 2–4 ■ **FOUR COMBINATIONS OF SIGNS FOR RELATIONAL PROPOSITIONS**

Combination 1
Axiom₁: If X is positively ($+$) related to Y, and
Axiom₂: if Y is positively ($+$) related to Z, then
Theorem: X is positively ($+$) related to Z.
Combination 2
Axiom₁: If X is negatively ($-$) related to Y, and
Axiom₂: if Y is negatively ($-$) related to Z, then
Theorem: X is positively ($+$) related to Z.
Combination 3
Axiom₁: If X is negatively ($-$) related to Y, and
Axiom₂: if Y is positively ($+$) related to Z, then
Theorem: X is negatively ($-$) related to Z.
Combination 4
Axiom₁: If X is positively ($+$) related to Y, and
Axiom₂: if Y is related to Z in an unknown (?) direction, then
Theorem: X is related to Z in an unknown (?) direction.

---

theory by using inductive reasoning, then an attempt should be made to arrange the propositions as inductive sets of observations and conclusions. On the other hand, if the research purpose was to test a theory, then an attempt should be made to arrange the propositions as deductive sets of axioms, theorems, and hypotheses. Arrangement of propositions as deductive sets of axioms and theorems requires that some statements are regarded as givens and others are deduced from those statements. Arrangement of propositions are deduced from those statements. Arrangement of propositions as deductive sets of axioms and hypotheses requires that at least one relational proposition can be extracted from the document and that operational definitions are given for the concepts that make up that proposition.

The task of hierarchical ordering is accomplished by first arranging the propositions found in the research document in groups according to the concept or concepts included in each proposition. For example, all propositions about concept X could be placed in one group, all propositions about concept Y could be placed in another group, and all propositions about concepts X and Y could be placed in still another group.

Once the propositions are grouped, they can be arranged according to the type of hierarchy that is evident. If level of abstraction is evident, then the more abstract propositions are separated from the more concrete ones. If induction has been used, then the propositions that are observations are separated from those that are conclusions. If deduction has been used, then the propositions that are used as axioms are separated from those that are theorems and those that are hypotheses. Finally, the proposition sets are created by listing the propositions in the appropriate hierarchical order.

The arrangement of deductive proposition sets in appropriate hierarchical order is facilitated by listing each hypothesis in its narrative form (i.e., the theorem) or in its operational form (i.e., using empirical indicators for concept names). Inasmuch as the hypothesis is the last part of the deductive process, the other propositions are arranged in the order that leads to that end point.

The arrangement of propositions in hierarchical order is frequently the most difficult step in the formalization of a conceptual-theoretical-empirical structure. That is because research documents usually do not present the conceptual model and the theory in the formal manner of proposition sets. Furthermore, a hierarchical arrangement of proposition sets according to inductive or deductive reasoning may not be possible because space limitations in journals often preclude the development of full inductive or deductive arguments.

STEP FIVE: CONSTRUCTION OF DIAGRAMS

The fifth and final step in the formalization of a conceptual-theoretical-empirical structure is the construction of a diagram of the entire structure, as well as one or more diagrams of the propositions of the conceptual model and the middle-range theory. A diagram helps to determine how all the concepts and propositions of the conceptual model and the theory were brought together. It is the final aid to understanding exactly what the conceptual-theoretical-empirical structure says and does not say. A diagram also facilitates the identification of gaps and overlapping ideas or redundancies in the structure.

Diagramming Conventions

Conventions for diagramming the relations between concepts have been given by several authors (Blalock, 1969; Burr, Hill, Nye, and Reiss, 1979; Hardy, 1974; Lin, 1976). The general forms of conceptual-theoretical-empirical structures for theory-generating and theory-testing research were developed for this book and were first given in Chapter 1 (Fig. 1–2; Fig. 1–4). More elaborate versions of those diagrams are given here.

Figure 2–2 displays the general form of a conceptual-theoretical-empirical structure for theory generation. The representational definition linking the concepts of the conceptual model that guided the theory-generating research to the empirical research methods is depicted by a double line ($=\!=$), with an arrowhead pointing to the left ($\blacktriangleleft$) to indicate that theory generation proceeds from the conceptual model concepts to the empirical research methods. The operational definition that links the empirical research methods and empirical indicators to the concepts and propositions that make up the newly discovered theory is depicted by a broken line ($-\,-\,-$), with an arrowhead pointing up ($\blacktriangle$) to indicate that the research proceeds from the data obtained from the empirical research methods to the new theory. The diagram may depict any number of conceptual model concepts (CMC_{1-n}), middle-range theory concepts (TC_{1-n}), operational definitions ($-\,-\,-$), and empirical research methods (ERM_{1-n}).

The example of the diagram of a conceptual-theoretical-empirical-structure for theory generation in Figure 2–3 was taken from Breckenridge's (1997) report of her descriptive study of dialysis modality decision making. Breckenridge explained that

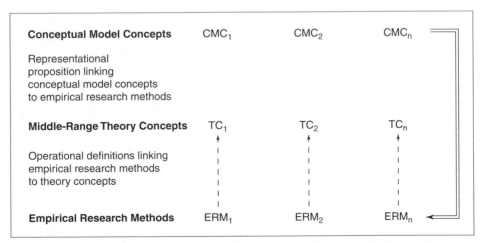

Figure 2–2 ■ General form of a conceptual-theoretical-empirical structure for theory-generating research.

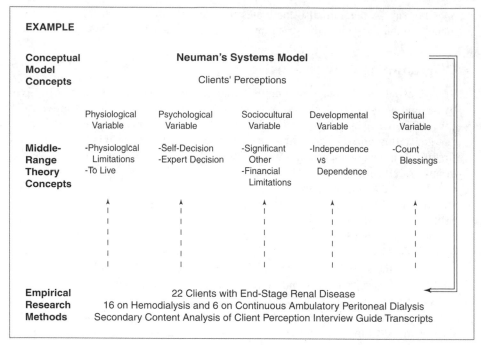

EXAMPLE

| Conceptual Model Concepts | Neuman's Systems Model |
| Clients' Perceptions |

| | Physiological Variable | Psychological Variable | Sociocultural Variable | Developmental Variable | Spiritual Variable |

Middle-Range Theory Concepts
- -Physiological Limitations
- -To Live
- -Self-Decision
- -Expert Decision
- -Significant Other
- -Financial Limitations
- -Independence vs Dependence
- -Count Blessings

Empirical Research Methods

22 Clients with End-Stage Renal Disease
16 on Hemodialysis and 6 on Continuous Ambulatory Peritoneal Dialysis
Secondary Content Analysis of Client Perception Interview Guide Transcripts

Figure 2–3 ■ Example of a conceptual-theoretical-empirical structure for theory generation. (Reprinted/adapted with permission from Decisions regarding dialysis treatment modality: A holistic perspective. *Holistic Nursing Practice, 12*(1), 54–61. © 1997 Aspen Publishers, Inc.)

Neuman's Systems Model directed her to consider the client's perceptions about dialysis treatment modality, which she elicited by means of an open-ended Client Perception Interview Guide. In her secondary content analysis, Breckenridge specifically looked for data that reflected five of Neuman's conceptual model concepts, including "physiological variables," "psychological variables," "sociocultural variables," "developmental variables," and "spiritual variables." A descriptive classification theory of clients' perceptions of dialysis modality decision making emerged from the secondary content analysis. Neuman's concept "physiological variables" was evident in the theory concepts "physiological limitations" and "to live." Neuman's model concept "psychological variables" was evident in the theory concepts "self-decision" and "expert decision." Neuman's model concept "sociocultural variables" was evident in the theory concepts "significant others" and "financial limitations." Neuman's model concept "developmental variables" was evident in the theory concept "independence versus dependence." Neuman's model concept "spiritual variables" was evident in the theory concept "count blessings."

Figure 2–4 displays the general form of a conceptual-theoretical-empirical structure for theory testing. The representational definitions linking the concepts of the conceptual model that guided the research to the concepts of the theory that was tested are depicted by double lines (⚌), with arrowheads pointing down (▼) to indicate that the theory testing proceeds from the conceptual model concepts to the

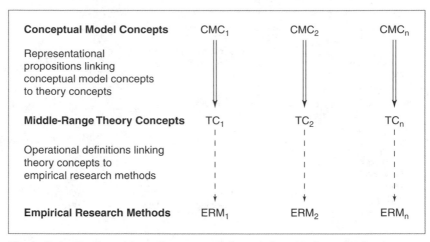

Figure 2–4 ■ General form of a conceptual-theoretical-empirical structure for theory-testing research.

theory concepts. The operational definitions that link the theory concepts to the empirical research methods are depicted by broken lines (– – –), with arrowheads pointing down (▼) to indicate that the research proceeds from the theory concepts to the empirical research methods. Once again, the diagram may depict any number of conceptual model concepts (CMC_{1-n}), theory concepts (TC_{1-n}), operational definitions (– – –), and empirical research methods (ERM_{1-n}).

The example of the diagram of a conceptual-theoretical-empirical structure for theory testing given in Figure 2–5 was extracted from Mock et al.'s (1997) report of their experimental study, which was based on Roy's Adaptation Model and findings from previous research. The study was designed to test a predictive theory of the differential effects of an experimental moderate walking exercise program and a control usual care program, which did not include walking exercise. The physiological mode dimension of Roy's model concept "response mode" was represented by the theory concepts "physical functioning" and "level of exercise," which were measured by the 12-Minute Walk Test and the Exercise Rating Scale, respectively. The personal self subdimension of the self-concept mode dimension of Roy's model concept "response mode" was represented by the theory concept "emotional distress," which was measured by the Symptom Assessment Scales. The physical self subdimension of the self-concept mode dimension of Roy's model concept "response mode" was represented by the theory concept "symptom experience," which was measured by the Symptom Assessment Scales and the Piper Fatigue Scale.

Diagrams for Nonrelational and Relational Propositions

The diagram of a conceptual-theoretical-empirical structure may be expanded by other diagrams that illustrate the nonrelational constitutive definitional proposi-

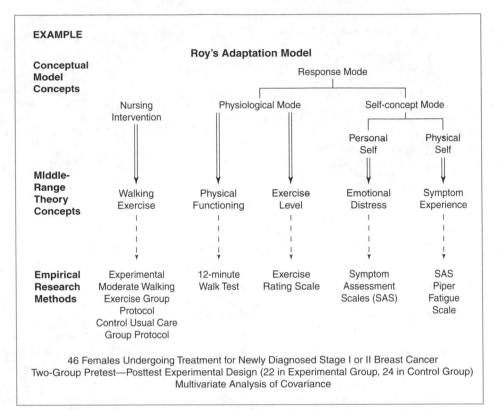

EXAMPLE

Roy's Adaptation Model

Conceptual Model Concepts

Response Mode

Nursing Intervention | Physiological Mode | Self-concept Mode

Personal Self | Physical Self

Middle-Range Theory Concepts

Walking Exercise | Physical Functioning | Exercise Level | Emotional Distress | Symptom Experience

Empirical Research Methods

Experimental Moderate Walking Exercise Group Protocol Control Usual Care Group Protocol | 12-minute Walk Test | Exercise Rating Scale | Symptom Assessment Scales (SAS) | SAS Piper Fatigue Scale

46 Females Undergoing Treatment for Newly Diagnosed Stage I or II Breast Cancer
Two-Group Pretest—Posttest Experimental Design (22 in Experimental Group, 24 in Control Group)
Multivariate Analysis of Covariance

Figure 2–5 ■ Example of a conceptual-theoretical-empirical structure for theory testing. (Diagram for example adapted from Mock et al., 1997, p. 993, with permission.)

tions for multidimensional concepts and the relational propositions at each level of abstraction. A diagram of a constitutive definition illustrates each dimension of a concept with a vertical unbroken line (|). The general form of a nonrelational constitutive definitional proposition and an example constructed from Newman's (1997) descriptive classification theory of functional status—caregiver of a child in a body cast, which was discussed on p. 54, are given in Figure 2–6 and 2–7.

Diagrams of relational propositions use horizontal unbroken lines (——) to depict the linkage of conceptual model concepts with each other, theory concepts with each other, and the scores on the empirical indicators with each other. If desired, the sign (+ − ?) for the direction of each relation could be added to the diagram. Arrowheads pointing to the right (▶) and the left (◀) also could be added to depict the symmetry of the relation.

The conventions for illustrating the existence and direction of a relation and for asymmetrical and symmetrical relations are shown in Figures 2–8, 2–9, 2–10, 2–11, 2–12, and 2–13, along with examples from Ryan (1996), Barone (1993; Barone

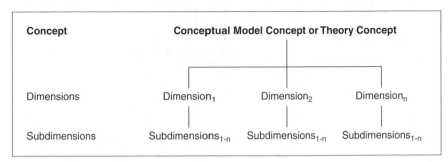

Figure 2–6 ■ Diagram of a nonrelational proposition: constitutive definition of a multidimensional concept.

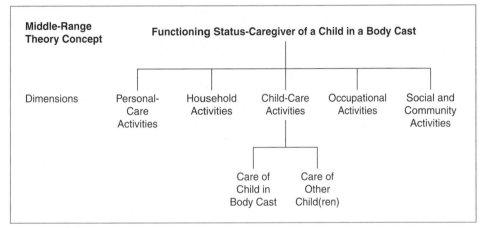

Figure 2–7 ■ Example of a nonrelational proposition: constitutive definition of a multidimensional concept. (Diagram for example adapted from Newman, 1997, p. 143, with permission.)

and Roy, 1996), and Frey (1993), which were discussed earlier in this chapter. The existence of a relation is illustrated by an unbroken line (———) connecting the two concepts X and Y (Fig. 2–8). An arrowhead at one end of the line indicates an asymmetrical relation (———→) (Fig. 2–10). Arrowheads at both ends of the line indicate a symmetrical relation (←——→) (Fig. 2–12). The direction of the relation is indicated by a plus sign (+) for a positive relation or a minus sign (−) for a negative, or inverse, relation. If the direction of the relation is not known, a question mark (?) may be used.

Conventions for diagramming contingent relations and examples of these types of relations are illustrated in Figures 2–14, 2–15, 2–16, 2–17, 2–18, and 2–19. Figure 2–14 shows the three concepts in a chain. The intervening concept C comes between concepts X and Y. The direction of each relation is indicated by a plus (+) or minus (−) sign. The first example (Fig. 2–15) was extracted from Barone's (1993; Barone and Roy, 1996) explanatory theory, discussed on p. 51.

Chains can include more than three concepts. Diagrams that depict explanatory theories tested by means of path analysis and structural equation modeling, for

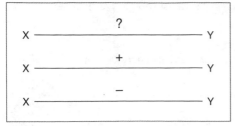

Figure 2–8 ■ Diagram of a relational proposition: existence and direction of a relation. (Diagramming convention adapted from Burr, Hill, Nye, & Reiss, 1979, p. 23, with permission.)

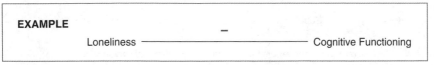

Figure 2–9 ■ Example of a relational proposition: existence and direction of a relation. (Diagram for example constructed from Ryan, 1996.)

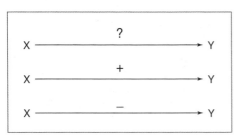

Figure 2–10 ■ Diagram of a relational proposition: asymmetrical relation. (Diagramming convention adapted from Burr, Hill, Nye, & Reiss, 1979, p. 23, with permission.)

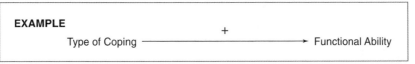

Figure 2–11 ■ Example of a relational proposition: asymmetrical relation. (Diagram for example constructed from Barone & Roy, 1996.)

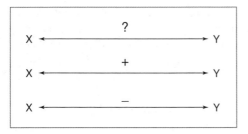

Figure 2–12 ■ Diagram of a relational proposition: symmetrical relation. (Diagramming convention adapted from Burr, Hill, Nye, & Reiss, 1979, p. 23, with permission.)

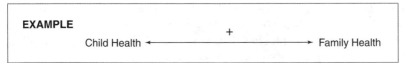

Figure 2–13 ■ Example of a relational proposition: symmetrical relation. (Diagram for example adapted from Frey, 1993, p. 32, with permission.)

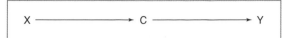

Figure 2–14 ■ Diagram of a contingent relation chain. (Diagramming conventions adapted from Burr, Hill, Nye, & Reiss, 1979, p. 23, with permission.)

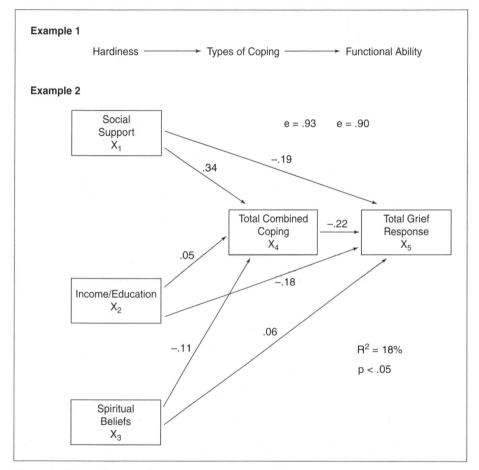

Figure 2–15 ■ Example of a contingent relation: chain. (Diagram for example 1 constructed from Barone & Roy, 1996; diagram for example 2 from Robinson, 1995, p. 162, with permission.)

example, are chains that contain many intervening concepts (Pedhazur, 1982). The second example in Figure 2–15 illustrates the concepts and propositions of Robinson's (1995) explanatory theory of the correlates of grief responses. The theory was derived from Roy's Adaptation Model, and the statistical technique of path analysis was used to test the theory. Roy's conceptual model concept "stimuli" was represented by the theory concepts "bereavement event," "social support," "social network," "spiritual beliefs," "education," and "income." Roy's model concept "cognator coping

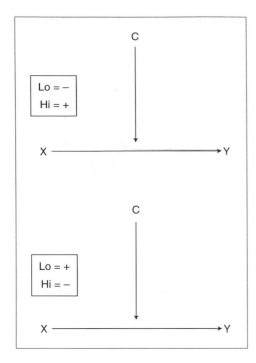

Figure 2–16 ■ Diagram of a contingent relation: existence or direction of the relation. (Diagramming conventions adapted from Burr, Hill, Nye, & Reiss, 1979, pp. 23–24, with permission.)

mechanism" was represented by the theory concept "coping process." Roy's model concept "response mode" was represented by the theory concept "grief response." The diagram depicts only those theory concepts that were used in the path analysis.

Figure 2–16 shows the diagramming conventions for a contingent relational proposition where the intervening concept C influences the existence or direction of the relation between X and Y. The symbols Lo = − and Hi = + indicate that if the magnitude of C is low, the relation between X and Y is negative and if the magnitude of C is high, the relation between X and Y is positive. In contrast, the symbols Lo = + and Hi = − indicate that if the magnitude of C is low, the relation between X and Y is positive and if the magnitude of C is high, the relation between X and Y is negative. If the intervening concept is a characteristic of the study subjects, the characteristic is substituted for Hi and Lo. The symbol 0 is used when a certain value taken by the intervening concept eliminates the existence of the relation between X and Y.

The first example in Figure 2–17 was constructed from Spitzer and colleagues' (1996a) explanatory theory, discussed on p. 52. The second example was constructed from Leidy's (1990) explanatory theory, discussed on p. 52.

Figure 2–18 shows the diagramming conventions for a contingent relational proposition in which the intervening concept C influences the strength of the relation between X and Y. The symbol ↑S indicates that as the intervening concept C increases in magnitude, the strength of the relation between X and Y increases. The symbol ↓S indicates that as C decreases in magnitude, the strength of the relation

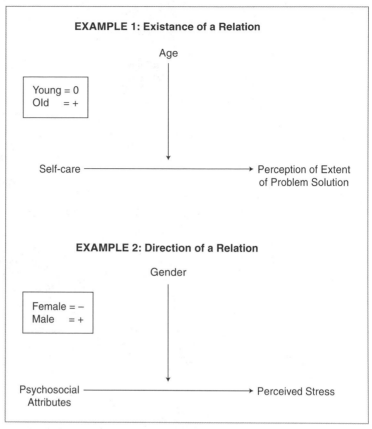

Figure 2–17 ■ Example (*I*) of the existence of a relation and example (2) of the direction of a relation. (Diagram for example I constructed from Spitzer, Bar-Tal, & Ziv, 1996a; diagram for example 2 constructed from Leidy, 1990.)

between X and Y increases. A plus (+) or minus (−) sign is used to indicate the direction of the relation. The example in Figure 2–19 was constructed from Yarcheski, Scoloveno, and Mahon's (1994) explanatory theory, discussed on p. 52.

Inventories of Concepts and Propositions

The diagramming conventions also can be used in inventories that depict all of the concepts and propositions that make up a theory. Inventories take four different forms.

MATRIX OF CONCEPTS. One form of an inventory is a matrix of concepts. The matrix, which is adapted from the matrix format used to display correlation coefficients, is used to illustrate the stated relation between concepts in a theory and to uncover the unstated relations. The number of cells in the matrix is determined by the number of concepts in the theory. The matrix may include check marks (√) to

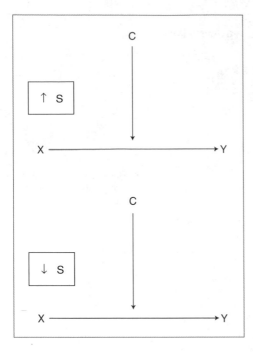

Figure 2–18 ■ Diagram of a contingent relation: strength of the relation. (Diagramming conventions adapted from Burr, Hill, Nye, & Reiss, 1979, p. 23, with permission..)

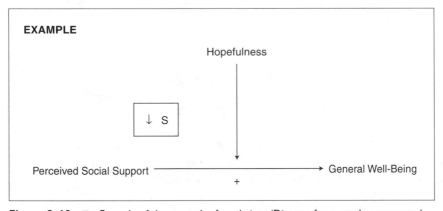

Figure 2–19 ■ Example of the strength of a relation. (Diagram for example constructed from Yarcheski, Scoloveno, & Mahon, 1994.)

indicate which concepts have been linked. It may also include the signs for the direction of the relations (+ −) if they are known or a question mark (?) if the direction of a relation is not known. Use of "x" indicates that the concepts are not linked in the theory. The matrix format is shown in Figure 2–20, along with an example (Fig. 2–21) extracted from Gaffney and Moore's (1996) explanatory theory. Their theory was derived from Orem's (1995) Self-Care Framework. The theory concepts "maternal age," "socioeconomic status," "marital status," "maternal em-

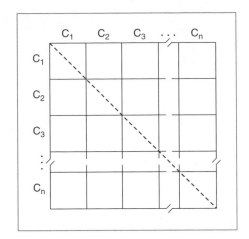

Figure 2–20 ■ The matrix form of inventory. (Diagram adapted from Hardy, 1974, p. 103, with permission.)

ployment hours," "ethnic group," "only child," "child age," "child gender," "birth order," "number of children," "child health problems," and "child status (biologic, adopted, stepchild)" represent Orem's conceptual model concept "basic conditioning factors." The theory concept "mothers' performance," which was defined as health promotion and child self-care activities performed by mothers, represent Orem's model concept "dependent-care agency."

INVENTORY OF ANTECEDENTS. The second form of an inventory, displayed in Figure 2–22, is a diagram of the relations between a concept of interest (Y) and its antecedents (X_{1-n}). The antecedent form of an inventory links the concept of interest to other concepts that precede it either theoretically or in time. The unbroken lines with arrowheads (⟶) indicate asymmetrical relations. The sign for the direction of the relation (+ −) may be included if known, or a question mark (?) may be used if the direction is unknown. The concept of interest is the dependent variable, and the antecedent concepts are the independent variables. The example given in Figure 2–23 was developed from Gaffney and Moore's (1996) explanatory theory, which also was the example for a matrix of concepts (Fig. 2–21).

INVENTORY OF CONSEQUENCES. The third form of an inventory, shown in Figure 2–24, is a diagram of the relations between a concept of interest (Y) and its consequent concepts (Z_{1-n}). This inventory links the concept of interest with other concepts that follow it either theoretically or in time. The unbroken lines with arrowheads (⟶) indicate asymmetrical relations. The sign for the direction of the relation (+ −) may be included if it is known, or a question mark (?) may be used if the direction is unknown. Here, the concept of interest is the independent variable and the consequent concepts are the dependent variables. The example given in Figure 2–25 was developed from Mock et al's (1996) predictive theory, which was discussed on pp. 29–30, and was the example used for a theory-testing conceptual-theoretical-empirical structure (Fig. 2–5, p. 66).

	Maternal Age	Socioeconomic Status	Marital Status	Maternal Employment Hours	Ethnic Group	Only Child	Child Age	Child Gender	Birth Order	Number of Children	Child Health Problems	Child Status	Mother Performance
Maternal Age		+	?	+	?	?	+	?	+	+	?	?	–
Socioeconomic Status			?	–	?	?	–	?	–	+	?	?	+
Marital Status				?	?	?	?	?	?	?	?	?	?
Maternal Employment Hours					?	?	+	?	–	–	?	?	–
Ethnic Group						?	?	?	?	?	?	?	?
Only Child							?	?	?	?	?	?	–
Child Age								?	–	+	?	?	–
Child Gender									?	?	?	?	+
Birth Order										+	?	?	+
Number of Children											?	?	–
Child Health Problems												?	–
Child Status													?

Figure 2–21 ■ Example of the matrix form of inventory. (Diagram for example constructed from Gaffney & Moore, 1996.)

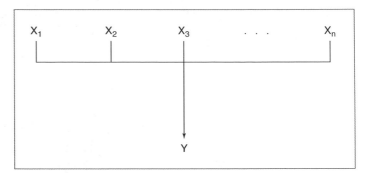

Figure 2–22 ■ Inventory of antecedents. (Diagram adapted from Blalock, 1969, p. 35, with permission.)

INVENTORY OF ANTECEDENTS AND CONSEQUENCES. The fourth form of an inventory, depicted in Figure 2–26, is a diagram of the relations between a concept of interest (Y) and both antecedent (X_{1-n}) and consequent (Z_{1-n}) concepts. The antecedent-consequent form of an inventory links the concept of interest with other concepts that precede it and still others that follow it theoretically or in time. As in the other inventories, the unbroken lines with arrowheads ($\longrightarrow$) indicate asymmetrical relations. Again, the sign for the direction of the relation ($+ \ -$) may be included if it is known, or a question mark (?) may be used if the direction is unknown. The example shown in Figure 2–27 illustrates antecedents and consequences for Barone's (1993; Barone and Roy, 1996) explanatory theory, discussed initially on p. 51. As noted earlier, the theory concepts "sociodemographic characteristics" and "hardiness" represent Roy's Adaptation Model concept "stimuli"; the theory concept "type of coping" represents Roy's conceptual model concept "cognator coping mechanism," and the theory concept "functional ability" represents the physiological mode dimension of Roy's model concept "response mode." The theory concept "medical complications" also represents the physiological mode dimension of Roy's model concept "response mode," and the theory concept "psychosocial adjustment" represents the self-concept mode, role function mode, and interdependence mode dimensions of Roy's model concept "response mode."

Pragmatics of Diagramming

Diagramming is done after the concepts and propositions of the conceptual model and the theory have been identified and the propositions have been hierarchically ordered. A diagram of the conceptual-theoretical-empirical structure should be done for all research documents. If the conceptual model that guided the research cannot be identified, the diagram should indicate that by use of a question mark (?) or the bracketed notation "[conceptual model implicit]."

In addition, the conceptual model concepts and propositions and the theory concepts and propositions can be diagrammed in greater detail than illustrated in

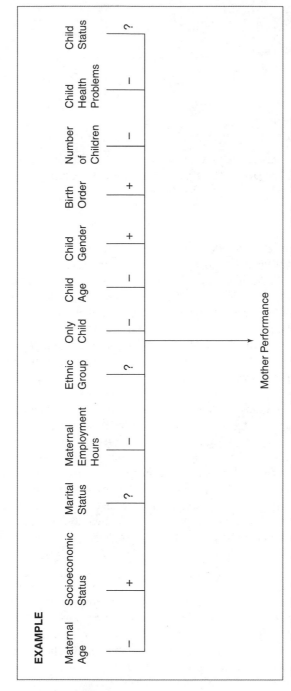

Figure 2–23 ■ Example of an inventory of antecedents. (Diagram for example constructed from Gaffney & Moore, 1996.)

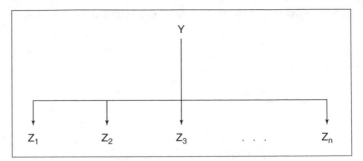

Figure 2–24 ■ Inventory of consequences. (Diagram adapted from Blalock, 1969, p. 41, with permission.)

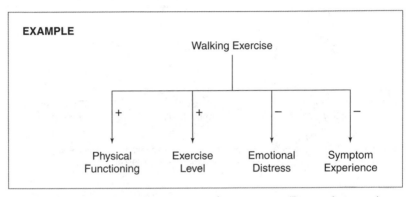

Figure 2–25 ■ Example of an inventory of consequences. (Diagram for example constructed from Mock et al., 1997.)

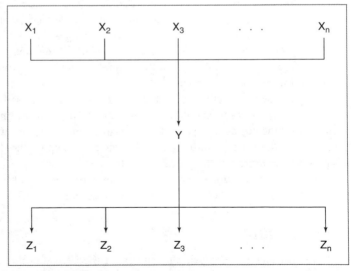

Figure 2–26 ■ Inventory of antecedents and consequences. (Diagram adapted from Blalock, 1969, p. 42, with permission.)

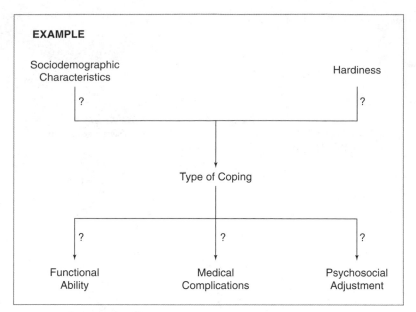

Figure 2–27 ■ Example of an inventory of antecedents and consequences. (Diagram for example constructed from Barone & Roy, 1996.)

the diagram of the conceptual-theoretical-empirical structure. The various approaches to diagramming beyond the basic conceptual-theoretical-empirical structure can be used separately or in combination. The choice of approach is an individual one. No one approach is better than another. Whatever approach makes clear what concepts are included in the conceptual model and the theory and which of these concepts are linked in propositions should be selected. Caution must be exercised, however, not to include in the diagram concepts or propositions that are not given in the research document.

Some research documents include one or more diagrams of concepts and propositions. Those diagrams should be examined carefully to determine if they are congruent with the narrative report. If a diagram is not congruent with the narrative description of the conceptual-theoretical-empirical structure, the decision to adjust the diagram to conform to the narrative or use the diagram as a source of additional concepts and propositions should be based on whichever approach will yield a more complete conceptual-theoretical-empirical structure.

CONCLUSION

In this chapter, analysis of conceptual-theoretical-empirical structures is described as a technique consisting of five steps that make up C-T-E formalization. Step One involves the identification of conceptual model and middle-range theory concepts. Step Two involves the classification of middle-range theory concepts. Step

Three involves the identification and classification of conceptual model and middle-range theory propositions. Step Four is the hierarchical ordering of propositions. Step Five is the construction of a diagram of the full conceptual-theoretical-empirical structure, as well as one or more diagrams of the concepts and propositions of the conceptual model and the theory. The five steps are outlined in Table 2–5, and work sheets that can be used to record the concepts and propositions as they are extracted from the research document are displayed in Figures 2–28 and 2–29.

The use of the technique of C-T-E formalization facilitates understanding of the exact content of a conceptual model and a middle-range theory and the way the theory was operationalized in research. Examples of formalization of the concep-

---

Table 2–5 ■ **STEPS OF FORMALIZAION OF A CONCEPTUAL-THEOREICAL-EMPIRICAL STRUCTURE**

Step One: Identification of Conceptual Model and Middle-Range Theory Concepts
- Name of the conceptual model
- Name and dimensions of each conceptual model concept
- Name and dimensions of each theory concept

Step Two: Classification of Middle-Range Theory Concepts
- Kaplan's schema
- Willer and Webster's schema
- Variability
- Dubin's schema

Step Three: Identification and Classification of Conceptual Model and Middle-Range Theory Propositions
- Nonrelational propositions
  - ☐ Existence
  - ☐ Level of existence*
  - ☐ Constitutive definition
  - ☐ Representational definition
  - ☐ Measured operational definition†
  - ☐ Experimental operational definition (experiments)†
- Relational propositions
  - ☐ Existence
  - ☐ Direction*
  - ☐ Shape*
  - ☐ Strength*
  - ☐ Symmetrical or asymmetrical
  - ☐ Concurrent or sequential*
  - ☐ Necessary or substitutable*
  - ☐ Sufficient or contingent*
- Hypotheses†

Step Four: Hierarchical Ordering of Propositions
- Hierarchy by level of abstraction
- Hierarchy by inductive reasoning (theory generation)†
- Hierarchy by deductive reasoning (theory testing)†

Step Five: Construction of Diagrams
- Diagram of full conceptual-theoretical-empirical structure
- Diagram(s) of conceptual model propositions
- Diagram(s) of theory propositions

---

*Applicable primarily to middle-range theory propositions
†Applicable only to middle-range theory propositions

Name of Concept and Page of Document	Conceptual-Model (CM) or Theory (T) Concept	Empirical Indicator and Scoring Method*	Kaplan*	Willer & Webster*	Nonvariable or Variable*	Dubin*

*Identification of empirical indicators and classification only for middle-range theory concepts.

Figure 2–28 ■ Work sheet for concept identification and classification.

tual-theoretical-empirical structures for theory-generating and theory-testing research are given in the Appendices.

The results of the formalization of conceptual-theoretical-empirical structures are drawn upon when the structure is evaluated. Evaluation of conceptual-theoretical-empirical structures is the focus of Chapter 3.

Proposition [Underline Concept (s)] and Page of Document	Conceptual Model (CM) or Theory (T) Proposition	Classification

Figure 2–29 ■ Work sheet for proposition identification and classification.

References

Achinstein, P. (1974). Theories. In A.C. Michalos, *Philosophical problems of science and technology* (pp. 280–297). Boston: Allyn and Bacon.

Ajzen, I. (1991). The theory of planned behavior. *Organizational Behavior and Human Decision Processes, 50,* 179–211.

Babbie, E. (1998). *The practice of social research* (8th ed.). Belmont, CA: Wadsworth.

Bandura, A. (1986). *Social foundations of thought and action.* Englewood Cliffs, NJ: Prentice-Hall.

Baron, R.M., & Kenny, D.A. (1986). The moderator-mediator variable distinction in social-psychological research: Conceptual, strategic, and statistical considerations. *Journal of Personality and Social Psychology, 51,* 1173–1182.

Barone, S.H. (1993). *Adaptation to spinal cord injury.* Unpublished doctoral dissertation, Boston College.

Barone, S.H., & Roy, C. (1996). The Roy adaptation model in research: Rehabilitation nursing. In P. Hinton-Walker & B. Neuman (Eds.), *Blueprint for use of nursing models: Education, research, practice, and administration* (pp. 64–87). New York: NLN Press.

Bates, J.E. (1987). Temperament in infancy. In J.D. Osofsky (Ed.), *Handbook of infant development* (2nd ed., pp. 1101–1149). New York: Wiley.

Blalock, H.M., Jr. (1969). *Theory construction: From verbal to mathematical formulations.* Englewood Cliffs, NJ: Prentice-Hall.

Breckenridge, D.M. (1997). Decisions regarding dialysis treatment modality: A holistic perspective. *Holistic Nursing Practice, 12*(1), 54–61.

Bridgman, P.W. (1927). *The logic of modern physics.* New York: Macmillan.

Brydolf, M., & Segesten, K. (1994). Physical health status in young subjects after colectomy: An application of the Roy model. *Journal of Advanced Nursing, 20,* 500–508.

Burr, W.R., Hill, R., Nye, F.I., & Reiss, I.L. (1979). Metatheory and diagramming conventions. In W.R. Burr, R. Hill, F.I. Nye, & I.L. Reiss (Eds.), *Contemporary theories about the family. Vol. I. Research-based theories* (pp. 17–24). New York: The Free Press.

Cohen, J. (1988). *Statistical power analysis for the behavioral sciences* (2nd ed.). Hillsdale, NJ: Lawrence Erlbaum.

Collins, M.A. (1996). The relation of work stress, hardiness, and burnout among full-time hospital staff nurses. *Journal of Nursing Staff Development, 12,* 81–85.

Crossley, D.J., & Wilson, P.A. (1979). *How to argue: An introduction to logical thinking.* New York: Random House.

Dubin, R. (1978). *Theory building* (rev. ed.). New York: The Free Press.

Erickson, H., Tomlin, E., & Swain, M.A. (1983). *Modeling and role-modeling: A theory and paradigm for nursing.* Englewood Cliffs, NJ: Prentice-Hall.

Frey, M.A. (1993). A theoretical perspective of family and child health derived from King's conceptual framework for nursing: A deductive approach to theory building. In S.L. Feetham, S.B. Meister, J.M. Bell, & C.L. Gilliss (Eds.), *The nursing of families: Theory/research, education/practice* (pp. 30–37). Newbury Park, CA: Sage.

Frey, M.A. (1996). Behavioral correlates of health and illness in youths with chronic illness. *Applied Nursing Research, 9,* 167–176.

Frey, M.A., & Sieloff, C.L. (Eds.). (1995). *Advancing King's systems framework and theory of nursing.* Thousand Oaks, CA: Sage.

Gaffney, K.F., & Moore, J.B. (1996). Testing Orem's theory of self-care deficit: Dependent care agent performance for children. *Nursing Science Quarterly, 9,* 160–164.

Gibbs, J. (1972). *Sociological theory construction.* Hinsdale, IL: Dryden Press.

Gibson, Q. (1960). *The logic of social enquiry.* New York: Humanities Press.

Hagopian, G.A. (1996). The effects of informational audiotapes on knowledge and self-care behaviors of patients undergoing radiation therapy. *Oncology Nursing Forum, 23,* 697–700.

Hanson, M.J.S. (1995). *Beliefs, attitudes, subjective norms, perceived behavioral control, and cigarette smoking in white, African-American, and Puerto Rican-American teenage women.* Unpublished doctoral dissertation, University of Pennsylvania.

Hanson, M.J.S. (1997). The theory of planned behavior applied to cigarette smoking in African-American, Puerto Rican, and non-Hispanic white teenage females. *Nursing Research, 46,* 155–162.

Hardy, M.E. (1974). Theories: Components, development, evaluation. *Nursing Research, 23,* 100–107.

Hunter, S.M., Cathcart-Silberberg, T., Langemo, D.K., Olson, B., Hanson, D., Burd, C., & Sauvage, T.R. (1992). Pressure ulcer prevalence and incidence in a rehabilitation hospital. *Rehabilitation Nursing, 17,* 239–242.

Johnson, J.E., Fieler, V.K., Jones, L.S., Wlasowicz, G.S., & Mitchell, M.L. (1997). *Self-regulation theory: Applying theory to your practice.* Pittsburgh: Oncology Nursing Press.

Johnson, J.E., Fieler, V.K., Wlasowicz, G.S., Mitchell, M.L., & Jones, L.S. (1997). The effects of nursing care guided by self-regulation theory on coping with radiation therapy. *Oncology Nursing Forum, 24,* 1041–1050.

Judd, C.M., Smith, E.R., & Kidder, L.H., (1991). *Research methods in social relations* (6th ed.). New York: Holt, Rinehart and Winston.

Kaplan, A. (1964). *The conduct of inquiry.* San Francisco: Chandler.

Kerlinger, F.N. (1986). *Foundations of behavioral research* (3rd ed.). New York: Holt, Rinehart and Winston.

Leidy, N.K. (1990). A structural model of stress, psychosocial resources, and symptomatic experience in chronic physical illness. *Nursing Research, 39,* 230–236.

Lev, E.L. (1995). Triangulation reveals theoretical linkages and outcomes in a nursing intervention study. *Clinical Nurse Specialist, 9,* 300–305.

Lin, N. (1976). *Foundations of social research.* New York: McGraw-Hill.

Marx, M.H. (1976). Formal theory. In M.H. Marx & F. E. Goodson (Eds.), *Theories in contemporary psychology* (2nd ed., pp. 234–260). New York: Macmillan.

McCool, W. (1997). [Biopsychosocial correlates of pregnancy outcome.] Unpublished raw data.

Mock, V., Dow, K.H., Meares, C.J., Grimm, P.M., Dienemann, J.A., Haisfield-Wolfe, M.E., Quitasol, W., Mitchell, S., Chakravarthy, A., & Gage, I. (1997). Effects of exercise on fatigue, physical functioning, and emotional distress during radiation therapy for breast cancer. *Oncology Nursing Forum, 24,* 991–1000.

Neuman, B. (1995). *The Neuman systems model* (3rd ed.). Norwalk, CT: Appleton and Lange.

Newman, D.M.L. (1997). The Inventory of Functional Status-Caregiver of a Child in a Body Cast. *Journal of Pediatric Nursing, 12,* 142–147.

Orem, D.E. (1991). *Nursing: Concepts of practice* (4th ed.). St. Louis: Mosby Year Book.

Orem, D.E. (1995). *Nursing: Concepts of practice* (5th ed.). St. Louis: Mosby Year Book.

Pedhazur, E.J. (1982). *Multiple regression in behavioral research* (2nd ed.). New York: Holt, Rinehart and Winston.

Polit, D.F., & Hungler, B.P. (1995). *Nursing research: Principles and methods* (5th ed.). Philadelphia: Lippincott.

Richmond, T., McCorkle, R., Tulman, L., & Fawcett, J. (1997). Measuring function. In M. Frank-Stromborg & S.J. Olsen (Eds.), *Instruments for clinical nursing research* (2nd ed., pp. 75–85). Boston: Jones and Bartlett.

Robinson, J.H. (1995). Grief responses, coping processes, and social support of widows: Research with Roy's model. *Nursing Science Quarterly, 8,* 158–164.

Roy, C., & Andrews, H.A. (1991). *The Roy adaptation model: The definitive statement.* Norwalk, CT: Appleton and Lange.

Ryan, M.C. (1996). Loneliness, social support and depression as interactive variables with cognitive status: Testing Roy's model. *Nursing Science Quarterly, 9,* 107–114.

Schaefer, K.M. (1995). Struggling to maintain balance: A study of women living with fibromyalgia. *Journal of Advanced Nursing, 21,* 95–102.

Schaefer, K.M. (1996). Levine's conservation model: Caring for women with chronic illness. In P. Hinton-Walker & B. Neuman (Eds.), *Blueprint for use of nursing models: Education, research, practice, and administration* (pp. 187–227). New York: NLN Press.

Schaefer, K.M., & Pond, J.B. (Eds.). (1991). *Levine's conservation model: A framework for nursing practice.* Philadelphia: F. A. Davis.

Schumacher, K.L., & Gortner, S.R. (1992). (Mis)conceptions and reconceptions about traditional science. *Advances in Nursing Science, 14*(4), 1–11.

Spitzer, A., Bar-Tal, Y., & Ziv, L. (1996a). The moderating effect of age on self-care. *Western Journal of Nursing Research, 18,* 136–148.

Spitzer, A., Bar-Tal, Y., & Ziv, L. (1996b). The moderating effect of gender on benefits from self- and others' health care. *Social Sciences in Health, 2,* 162–173.

Tulman, L., & Fawcett, J. (1996). Lessons learned from a pilot study of biobehavioral correlates of functional status in women with breast cancer. *Nursing Research, 45,* 356–358.

Villarruel, A.M. (1995). Mexican-American cultural meanings, expressions, self-care and dependent-care actions associated with experiences of pain. *Research in Nursing and Health, 18,* 427–436.

Willer, D., & Webster, M., Jr. (1970). Theoretical concepts and observables. *American Sociological Review, 35,* 748–757.

Yarcheski, A., Scoloveno, M.A., & Mahon, N.E. (1994). Social support and well-being in adolescents: The mediating role of hopefulness. *Nursing Research, 43,* 288–292.

Additional Readings

Beard, M.T. (Ed.). (1995). *Theory construction and testing.* Lisle: IL: Tucker Publications.

Cartwright, N. (1983). *How the laws of physics lie.* New York: Oxford University Press.

Dean, H. (1997). Multiple instruments for measuring quality of life. In M. Frank-Stromborg & S.J. Olsen (Eds.), *Instruments for clinical health-care research* (2nd ed., pp. 135–148). Boston: Jones and Bartlett.

Dulock, H.L., & Holzemer, W.L. (1991). Substruction: Improving the linkage from theory to method. *Nursing Science Quarterly, 4*, 83–87.

Hinshaw, A.S. (1979). Theoretical substruction: An assessment process. *Western Journal of Nursing Research, 1*, 319–324.

Jacox, A. (1974). Theory construction in nursing: An overview. *Nursing Research, 23*, 4–13.

McLaughlin, F.E., & Marascuilo, L.A. (1990). *Advanced nursing and health care research: Quantification approaches*. Philadelphia: Saunders.

McQuiston, C.M., & Campbell, J.C. (1997). Theoretical substruction: A guide for theory testing. *Nursing Science Quarterly, 10*, 117–123.

Padilla, G.V., & Frank-Stromborg, M. (1997). Single instruments for measuring quality of life. In M. Frank-Stromborg & S.J. Olsen (Eds.), *Instruments for clinical health-care research* (2nd ed., pp. 114–134). Boston: Jones and Bartlett.

Pasacreta, J. (1997). Measuring depression. In M. Frank-Stromborg & S.J. Olsen (Eds.), *Instruments for clinical health-care research* (2nd ed., pp. 342–360). Boston: Jones and Bartlett.

Reynolds, P.D. (1971). *A primer in theory construction*. Indianapolis: Bobbs-Merrill.

Rodgers, B.L., & Knafl, K.A. (1993). *Concept development in nursing: Foundations, techniques, and applications*. Philadelphia: Saunders.

Walker, L.O., & Avant, K.C. (1995). *Strategies for theory construction in nursing* (3rd ed.). Norwalk, CT: Appleton and Lange.

Zetterberg, H. (1965). *On theory and verification in sociology* (3rd ed.). Totowa, NJ: Bedminster Press.

3 Evaluating Conceptual-Theoretical-Empirical Structures for Research

■ The close connection between conceptual models, theories, and research mandates evaluation of the conceptual, theoretical, and empirical components of a research document. This chapter presents criteria for the evaluation of the conceptual, theoretical, and empirical components of research documents that draw on the results of the analysis of conceptual-theoretical-empirical structures, which was the subject of Chapter 2. Once again, the emphasis is on research that addresses the generation or testing of middle-range theories.

CRITERIA FOR EVALUATION OF CONCEPTUAL-THEORETICAL-EMPIRICAL STRUCTURES

Criteria for the evaluation of middle-range theories and empirical research methods are available in the literature of almost every discipline. Review of those criteria indicates considerable agreement about what should be expected of a theory and of empirical research methods. Few criteria, however, emphasize the relation between a middle-range theory and the research that generated or tested that theory. Moreover, very little attention has been paid to the evaluation of conceptual models and the relation of conceptual models to middle-range theories and empirical research methods. The evaluation criteria presented in this chapter highlight the commonalities found in the literature and emphasize the essential connection between the conceptual, theoretical, and methodological aspects of research. An attempt has been made to develop the criteria so that they are appropriate for evaluation of documents addressing descriptive, correlational, and experimental research designed to generate or test middle-range descriptive, explanatory, or predictive theories, respectively.

Judgments regarding the extent to which the content of a research document satisfies certain criteria are most readily and accurately made after an analysis of the conceptual-theoretical-empirical structure has been completed. A detailed discussion of the analytic technique of conceptual-theoretical-empirical (C-T-E) formalization was presented in Chapter 2. As explained there, C-T-E formalization yields a clear and concise listing of the concepts and propositions that make up a conceptual model and those that make up a middle-range theory. In theory-generating research, C-T-E formalization involves identification of the conceptual model concepts and propositions that guided the research, identification of the empirical research methods used to conduct the research, and identification and classification of the concepts and propositions of the middle-range theory that emerged from the research.

In theory-testing research, C-T-E formalization involves identification of the conceptual model concepts and propositions that guided the research, identification and classification of the concepts and propositions of the version of the middle-range theory that entered into the empirical test, and identification of the empirical research methods used to test the theory. Formalization of the conceptual-theoretical-empirical structure for theory testing research also involves identification and classification of the middle-range theory concepts and propositions that were retained after testing.

STEP ONE: EVALUATION OF THE CONCEPTUAL-THEORETICAL-EMPIRICAL LINKAGES

The first step in the evaluation of a conceptual-theoretical-empirical structure focuses on the linkage of the conceptual model to the middle-range theory and the empirical research methods. The criteria are specification adequacy and linkage adequacy.

Specification Adequacy

The criterion of specification adequacy requires the conceptual model to be identified explicitly and to be described clearly and concisely. The authors of some research textbooks have begun to highlight the importance of explicit identification of the conceptual model that guided the study (e.g., Polit and Hungler, 1995). In addition, the editors of at least two nursing journals have underscored the importance of identifying the conceptual basis for the work described in an article. Johnson

(1982) commented on the importance of using nursing actions and terms to organize the content of an article. Feeg (1989) called for the explicit identification of the conceptual basis of nursing practice, commenting that, "In this time of professional territoriality, it has become even more important to understand our identity in nursing and operationalize our practice from a theoretical knowledge base" (p. 450). Furthermore, the president of one nursing specialty organization called for the explicit identification of the conceptual models that guide nursing research and practice to "help nurses better communicate what they do" (Neff, 1991, p. 534).

It is not sufficient, however, to simply mention the name of the conceptual model that guided the work. Instead, a clear and concise overview of the conceptual model should be included. More specifically, the conceptual model should be described in sufficient detail to permit understanding of its distinctive focus and its major concepts and propositions.

APPLICATION OF THE CRITERION OF SPECIFICATION ADEQUACY. The application of the specification criterion is especially important because some researchers do little more than cite the name of a particular conceptual model in the research report (Silva, 1987). The same level of detail about the conceptual model should be included for both theory-generating and theory-testing research documents.

Linkage Adequacy

The criterion of linkage adequacy requires the particular conceptual model concepts and propositions that guide the theory-generating or theory-testing research to be identified and clearly linked with the theoretical and empirical components of the research. More specifically, the criterion of linkage adequacy requires that representational definitions are evident and complete.

In theory-generating research, the conceptual model concepts and propositions should be linked directly and logically to the empirical research methods. In this case, logical linkage means that the phenomenon selected for study is within the domain of the conceptual model, and that the methodological research rules of the conceptual model are reflected in the empirical research methods employed.

In theory-testing research, the conceptual model concepts and propositions should be linked directly and logically to the concepts and propositions of the middle-range theory. In this case, logical linkage means that the phenomenon selected for study is within the domain of the conceptual model, the constitutive definitions of the theory concepts are in keeping with the focus of the conceptual model, the theory propositions are in keeping with the focus of the conceptual model, and the methodological research rules of the conceptual model are reflected in the empirical research methods employed.

APPLICATION OF THE CRITERION OF LINKAGE ADEQUACY. As with the specification criterion, the same level of detail about the linkage of the conceptual model content with the theoretical and empirical components of the research should be included for both theory-generating and theory-testing research documents.

Conceptual Model Usage Rating Scale

Evaluation of specification adequacy and linkage adequacy can be summarized by application of the Conceptual Model Usage Rating Scale (Fig. 3–1). This scale permits the use of a number or verbal descriptor to signify the extent to which the conceptual model is identified and described in the research document, as well as the extent to which the conceptual model concepts and propositions are linked explicitly with the middle-range theory concepts and propositions and with the empirical research methods. The rating scale points are 0 = Missing, 1 = Insufficient Use, 2 = Minimal Use, and 3 = Adequate Use.

STEP TWO: EVALUATION OF THE THEORY

The second step in the evaluation of a conceptual-theoretical-empirical structure focuses on the middle-range theory. Criteria include the significance, internal consistency, parsimony, and testability of the middle-range theory.

Significance of the Theory

The significance criterion requires middle-range theories to reflect social significance and theoretical significance.

Title of Research Report: _____

CONCEPTUAL MODEL USAGE RATING SCALE

Directions: Review the content of the research document and circle the number that best describes the extent to which the investigator specified the conceptual model on which the study is based.

Rating Scale

0 = Missing
The conceptual model is not evident in the research document.

1 = Insufficient Use
The conceptual model is named and briefly summarized.

2 = Minimal Use
The conceptual model is named and briefly summarized. The linkage of the conceptual model concepts and propositions with the middle-range theory concepts and propositions and the empirical research methods is evident.

3 = Adequate Use
The conceptual model is named and summarized clearly and concisely. The linkage of the conceptual-model concepts and propositions with the middle-range theory concepts and propositions and the empirical research methods is clearly stated.

Figure 3–1 ■ Conceptual Model Usage Rating Scale.

SOCIAL SIGNIFICANCE. The criterion of significance requires a middle-range theory to be socially significant. Social significance is evident when a theory addresses a problem of particular interest to society. Such a problem frequently can be identified by reference to priorities for research that are set by expert panels sponsored by government agencies, professional organizations, or clinical specialty organizations.

Although it is generally agreed that a socially significant middle-range theory provides a new insight into a phenomenon or a new way to view a phenomenon, the judgment of significance can be relative: What seems significant to one person may not be significant to another. The ultimate jury usually is the relevant scientific community, and increasingly the public sector as well, neither of which is always unbiased. Indeed, some theories may generate considerable attention from the scientific community and the general public for reasons that have little or nothing to do with their intrinsic merit. For example, the predictive theory of the efficacy of support groups for a wide variety of life transitions and serious illnesses has been adopted enthusiastically by clinicians and clients despite little empirical evidence of beneficial outcomes of support group participation (Bottomley, 1997). Perhaps clinicians are so desperate to find ways to relieve clients' distress, and clients are so eager to find relief, that they are blinded to the lack of evidence of beneficial effects.

A similar situation is evident in predictive theories of the efficacy of a vast array of commonly used interventions for pregnancy and childbirth. Chalmers, Enkin, and Keirse (1989) found that only 35% of 285 interventions could be judged as effective on the basis of available evidence. Another 13% were judged to be possibly effective but required additional study. The available evidence indicated that still another 21% of the interventions had little beneficial effect and could even be dangerous. The outcomes of the remaining 31% were unknown.

Conversely, a theory may be scorned by scientists and/or the public sector because it goes against current thinking or because it represents such a major leap in knowledge that it cannot be comprehended. An example of the former is Darwin's theory of evolution; an example of the latter is McClintock's theory of gene transposition. Everyone knows about Darwin's theory; McClintock's may not be so familiar. McClintock, the winner of a 1983 Nobel Prize, found that genes are not fixed on the chromosome but rather can move around in an unpredictable manner and cause unexpected changes in heredity. Although her gene transposition ("jumping genes") theory was first published more than 35 years ago, its significance has been acknowledged only in recent years; indeed, the full significance of her work was widely publicized only at the time of her death in 1992.

THEORETICAL SIGNIFICANCE. The criterion of significance also requires that theoretical significance be established. Theoretical significance is evident when the middle-range theory addresses a phenomenon of interest to a discipline by extending or filling gaps in an existing theory about that phenomenon. The phenomena of interest to the discipline of nursing, for example, are considered by many to be person, environment, health, and nursing (Fawcett, 1984, 1995). "Person" refers to the recipient of nursing. "Environment" refers to the significant others and the surroundings of the nursing recipient, as well as to the setting in which nursing occurs. "Environment" also can refer to all of the cultural, social, political, and economic conditions that are associated with the nursing recipient's health (Kleffel, 1991). "Health" refers to the recipient's state of well-being at the time that nursing occurs, which can range from high-level wellness to terminal illness. "Nursing" refers to the definition of nursing, the actions taken by nurses on behalf of or in conjunction with the recipient, and the goals or outcomes of nursing actions. Accordingly, broad categories of theories that are considered significant to the discipline of nursing focus on:

- The life process, well-being, and optimal functioning of human beings, sick or well
- The patterning of human behavior in interaction with the environment in normal life events and critical life situations
- The actions or processes by which positive changes in health status are effected
- The wholeness or health of human beings in continuous interaction with their environments
  (Donaldson and Crowley, 1978; Gortner, 1980)

APPLICATION OF THE CRITERION OF SIGNIFICANCE. In theory-generating research, the significance criterion is applied to the middle-range theory that emerged from the data analysis; in theory-testing research, the criterion is applied to the initial middle-range theory that was tested, as well as to the version that was retained after testing. The research document is examined closely to determine the extent to which the investigator justified social and theoretical significance.

Internal Consistency of the Theory

The internal consistency criterion encompasses three major requirements: semantic clarity, semantic consistency, and structural consistency.

SEMANTIC CLARITY. The internal consistency criterion requires concepts to reflect semantic clarity, that is, to be clearly defined. Semantic clarity is more likely to occur when both constitutive and operational definitions are given for each concept making up the middle-range theory than when no definitions are given or when just one type of definition is stated. The inclusion of both constitutive and operational definitions in a research document enhances semantic clarity especially when the same term can take several meanings. "Quality of life," for example, can refer to and be measured by a multitude of physical and psychosocial behaviors, including but not limited to dimensions of physical symptoms, psychological state, functional ability, and social relationships (Padilla and Frank-Stromborg, 1997). More specifically, quality of life can refer to individuals' subjective evaluation of their lives in relation to their goals, expectations, standards, and concerns, within a cultural, social, and environmental context (World Health Organization, 1993). Quality of life also can refer to an objective value assigned by a patient, a patient's family, a health care provider, policy maker, or other person to the patient's duration of life (Patrick and Erickson, 1993). The dimensions of quality of life can be operationalized by many different items on many different instruments. In particular, physical symptoms can be measured by items ranging from energy to visual disturbances. Items measuring psychological state can range from feeling sad, nervous, and hopeless, to cognitive function, to satisfaction with life. Functional ability items can encompass the capacity to engage in diverse activities of daily living, such as eating, shopping, and working. Items measuring social relationships can include support from family, friends, and coworkers, sexual intimacy, and family happiness.

Semantic clarity also is more likely to occur when concepts are not redundant. Dubin (1978) proposed the four rules listed below for the use of concepts (units) that, if followed, reduce the possibility of concept redundancy. The various types of units are described in Chapter 2 (see pp. 37–38).

1. Enumerative units may be used alone in a theory in any logically consistent manner. Associative, relational, or statistical units also may be used alone in a theory.
2. Enumerative units and associative units may be used together in a theory without any restriction other than logical consistency.
3. Relational units may not be combined in the same theory with enumerative or associative units that are themselves component parts of the relational unit. Redundancies can occur easily when the relational unit is based on a combination, such as a composite score. Consider the example of "maternal-infant communication." A redundancy would occur if the composite score that reflects the relational unit "maternal-infant communication" was correlated with the score for either of the two associative units "maternal communication" or "infant communication."
4. A statistical unit, which reflects a collective, may not be combined with any enumerative, associative, or relational unit that describes individual members of the same collective. For example, suppose it is known from Ryan's (1996) study of community-based elderly people that, on average, cognitive functioning scores decrease 5 points with every increase of 1 point in depression scores. The knowledge based on the collective "community-based elderly people" cannot be used to predict the depression score of any one community-based elderly woman or man or any one elderly woman or man who is hospitalized or in a nursing home.

SEMANTIC CONSISTENCY. The internal consistency criterion requires concepts to reflect semantic consistency, that is, consistent use of the same term and the same definition for a concept throughout the narrative presentation of the middle-range theory. This means that different words or phrases should not be used for the same concept and that different explicit or implicit constitutive and operational definitions should not be used for a concept in any one theory. For example, the terms "functional ability" and "functional status" should not be used interchangeably in the same theory. That is because "functional ability" refers to the person's capacity to perform activities, whereas "functional status" refers to the level at which the person actually is performing the activities. Thus, "functional ability" is an antecedent to "functional status" (Richmond, McCorkle, Tulman, and Fawcett, 1997).

Semantic clarity and consistency are related. In particular, clarity is obscured if the concept label is inconsistent, and consistency is difficult to determine if the meaning of the concept is unclear (Chinn and Kramer, 1995).

STRUCTURAL CONSISTENCY. The internal consistency criterion requires propositions to reflect structural consistency. One flaw in the structural consistency of a middle-range theory occurs when the operational definition for a concept identifies an empirical indicator that is not an appropriate measure of that concept as it is constitutively defined. For example, suppose that anxiety is constitutively defined as an individual's feeling of distress or panic. Suppose also that anxiety is operationally defined as the number of heart beats per minute recorded on a cardiac monitor. In this constructed example, the constitutive and operational definitions clearly are not consistent. Thus, structural consistency is evident only when the operational definition is consistent with the constitutive definition of a concept.

Moreover, flaws in the structural consistency of a theory can result in incomplete sets of propositions. Incompleteness, which is also called discontinuity, occurs in deductive proposition sets when some propositions are not explicit. For example, consider a theory asserting only that (1) the greater the hardiness, the less the job stress, and (2) the greater the job stress, the less the burnout. This theory is incomplete because the linkage between hardiness and burnout is not stated explicitly, even though that linkage can be deduced from the propositions that are given (Collins, 1996). Here, structural consistency would be evident if all propositions in a deductive set are explicit.

Flaws in structural consistency also can result in redundant propositions. Redundancy occurs when one axiom can be deduced from another and, therefore, is not independent. Consider a theory stating that (1) depression is a manifestation of stress, (2) stress results in high employee turnover rates, and (3) depression results in high employee turnover rates. Propositions 2 and 3 are redundant because stress and depression are equivalent concepts in this theory. The redundancy can be corrected by eliminating either Proposition 2 or 3. Structural consistency is evident when there are no redundancies.

Furthermore, flaws in structural consistency can result in violations of inductive or deductive reasoning. Thus, structural consistency may be evident when inductive and deductive proposition sets are related to each other in accordance with the appropriate rules of logic. Adherence to the rules of logic cannot, however, guarantee structural consistency. That is because a conclusion arrived at by means of induction can exceed the available observations or a logically deduced theorem can be reached from a faulty premise. Thus, when an inductive structure is evident, the strength of the evidence offered for the conclusion should be evaluated. More specifically, the observations should be evaluated to determine if they represent sufficient, unbiased, and relevant evidence for the conclusion (Crossley and Wilson, 1979). Moreover, when a deductive structure of axioms and theorems is evident, the adequacy of the axioms must be judged. In other words, the axioms, which are regarded as givens, must be evaluated to determine if each one has sufficient support to be regarded as adequate (Hardy, 1988).

Mixing of inductive and deductive reasoning almost always obscures the structural consistency of a theory and, therefore, should be avoided. An exception is retroduction, or abduction, a theory-development strategy that combines inductive and deductive methods in a logical and sequential manner (Hanson, 1958). Retroduction is an iterative process that begins by inducing a general proposition from several fairly specific ones. The process continues by deducing new, more specific propositions from the new general proposition.

APPLICATION OF THE CRITERION OF INTERNAL CONSISTENCY. In theory-generating research, the internal consistency criterion is applied to the theory that was generated, as presented in the report of the completed research. In theory-testing research, the criterion is applied to the middle-range theory that will be or was tested, as well as to the version that was retained after testing. In the case of theory-testing research, the repeated application of the criterion permits a comparison of the completeness of proposition sets before and after evidence is obtained.

Parsimony of the Theory

The parsimony criterion, sometimes referred to as Occam's razor or Lloyd Morgan's canon, requires a middle-range theory to be stated in the most economical way possible. This means that the fewer the concepts and propositions needed to describe, explain, or predict a phenomenon, the better. Stated in other words, the simplest theory that accounts for the most known observations is the best theory (Payton, 1994).

Marx (1976) explained that parsimony has a historical basis. He stated, "Scientists have learned that the more [theoretical statements] that are involved— or the more complex a theory is—the greater likelihood there is of error. And once a serious error creeps in, the whole theoretical superstructure may be fatally weakened" (p. 251).

Parsimonious theories that are developed by inductive reasoning include a minimum number of concepts and propositions to describe a phenomenon. Parsimonious theories that are developed by deductive reasoning include a minimum number of independent axioms from which theorems can be derived. The minimum number of axioms is reached when each axiom makes a unique contribution to the theory and is essential to the deductive structure.

The parsimony criterion is not, however, to be confused with oversimplification of the phenomenon. Parsimony that does not capture the essential features of a phenomenon is false economy. Skinner's theory stating that reinforcement accounts for all changes in behavior is considered by many psychologists to be an example of parsimony achieved by oversimplification (Goodson and Morgan, 1976).

Thus, a theory should be evaluated to determine whether the most parsimonious statement clarifies rather than obscures the phenomenon, and whether it effectively deals with all of the data about the phenomenon (Cronbach, 1975).

APPLICATION OF THE CRITERION OF PARSIMONY. Like the preceding two criteria, the parsimony criterion is applied to the results of theory-generating research. In theory-testing research, the criterion is applied to the theory that will be or was tested, as well as to the version that was retained after testing. The repeated application in the case of theory-testing research permits a judgment regarding enhanced or decreased parsimony, especially when some propositions have been rejected or when the addition of new concepts and propositions is recommended.

Testability of the Theory

The testability criterion requires the concepts and propositions of a middle-range theory to be empirically observable. A theory is testable if its concepts can be observed empirically, if its propositions can be measured, and if its derived hypotheses can be falsified.

OBSERVABILITY OF CONCEPTS. Concepts are empirically observable if they are connected to empirical indicators by operational definitions. Concepts that lack operational definitions must be connected to those that are operationally defined. The investigator has the freedom, as Marx and Cronan-Hillix (1987) pointed out, "to use some terms that have no direct relationship to empirical observations, as long as other logically related terms in the theory are tied to observation" (p. 299).

MEASURABILITY OF PROPOSITIONS. Propositions are measurable when they are stated as hypotheses. More precisely, propositions are measurable when empirical indicators are substituted for concept names in the hypotheses and when the hypothesis asserts a conjecture that can be tested statistically. When a hypothesis states a relation between empirical indicators, all assertions about that relation must be measurable. For example, if a hypothesis states that empirical indicator X' is asymmetrically and negatively related to empirical indicator Y', such that when the score of X' increases one unit, the score of Y' decreases five units, the symmetry, direction, and magnitude of change in scores all must be empirically measurable.

It is important to note that changes in practice may preclude testing certain propositions, especially those contained in predictive theories that assert a difference between an experimental treatment and "usual practice," when the form of "usual practice" is in the midst of change or has recently changed. For example, Lusk (1997) pointed out that, by 1987, an experimental work site health promotion program had been implemented in so many of one company's plants that plants that might serve as sites for a control treatment were not available.

FALSIFICATION OF HYPOTHESES. Popper (1965) maintained that the goal of theory testing is to refute or falsify hypotheses. A similar goal is evident in the philosophical position known as scientific realism (Schumacher and Gortner, 1992). Scientific progress is hindered by a hypothesis that cannot be falsified because it cannot be modified or replaced by another hypothesis. Conversely, a falsifiable hypothesis can be improved or replaced by a better one. A falsifiable hypothesis is sufficiently precise that incompatible empirical results can be easily identified. For example, the hypothesis stating that all postmenopausal women score low, medium, or high on a test of cardiovascular disease risk factors cannot be refuted because it does not rule out any logically or practically possible findings. In contrast, the hypothesis stating that all postmenopausal women score high on the risk-factors test can be refuted because it asserts that postmenopausal women will not have moderate or low scores on the test.

The requirements for testability can be summarized by reference to a masterpiece of satire written by Shearing (1973). He claimed that because theories frequently are presented in an untestable form in research documents, investigators might as well learn to make theories untestable. To that end, he then offered the following guidelines:

1. Make certain that no empirically refutable statements can be deduced from the theory. This can be done in the following ways:
   a. Provide no operational definitions for any of the concepts in the theory.
   b. Provide no propositions in the theory.
   c. If propositions are stated, ensure that the relations between concepts remain as unclear as possible.
2. Ensure that the theory is internally inconsistent.

The converse of each of these guidelines is, of course, needed to meet the testability criterion.

ALTERNATIVE REQUIREMENTS FOR TESTABILITY. Testability is frequently regarded as the primary characteristic of a scientifically useful middle-range theory. Marx (1976) maintained, "If there is no way of testing a theory it is scientifically worthless, no matter how plausible, imaginative, or innovative it may be" (p. 249). Elaborating, Marx and Cronan-Hillix (1987) explained that if the hypotheses derived from a theory do not assert testable expectations about one or more concepts, empirical observations cannot affect the theory. And, "if empirical observations cannot affect it, then the theory fails the most critical test of all: it is not testable, and in that sense it is not a scientific theory at all" (p. 307).

This view of testability is, admittedly, a strict one that is in keeping with the classic view of operationism (Bridgman, 1927). One alternative is a criterion stating that testability does not have to be direct. This criterion is appropriate in areas of inquiry in which active manipulation of concepts usually is not feasible, such as astronomy and archaeology. Another alternative is a criterion requiring theories to be potentially testable. That criterion is particularly appropriate for theories that are generated by means of interpretive research methods, such as phenomenology, ethnography, and grounded theory. That is because the empirical indicators needed to observe the theory concepts may not be available, yet it is thought that they can be developed. For example, Duffy (1984) used grounded theory methodology to generate the descriptive classification theory of transcending options. Subsequently, Duffy (1994) identified empirical indicators to measure the various concepts of the theory and conducted correlational research to test the associations between those concepts.

Still another alternative is a criterion requiring theories to be testable through imaginary or thought experiments rather than by empirical means. This criterion is appropriate when a theory cannot be empirically tested because of the time or cost involved, the unavailability of empirical indicators, technical impossibility, or ethical prohibitions. For example, although technological limitations have prevented the empirical testing of some parts of Einstein's theory of relativity, the theory has been tested by means of thought experiments that involved mathematical equations and arguments based on logic (Cohen, Sarill, and Vishveshwara, 1982). Similarly, theories about the effects of the impact of a comet on a planet had been tested for 30 years by only thought experiments involving mathematical equations and computer simulations, before astronomers were able to observe the actual impact of Comet Shoemaker-Levy 9 on Jupiter (Levy, Shoemaker, and Shoemaker, 1995).

Empirical testability is not, of course, an appropriate criterion for theories developed by such nonempirical methods as some philosophical inquiries, and it may not be an appropriate criterion for some types of historical research. Rather, these methods include their own rules for theory testing.

APPLICATION OF THE CRITERION OF TESTABILITY.   Like the preceding three criteria, the testability criterion is applied to the results of theory-generating research. Here the question is whether the concepts and propositions could be empirically tested in future studies. In contrast, in the case of theory-testing research, the application of this criterion is limited to the theory that was tested. In other words, judgments are confined to the empirical testability of the concepts and propositions that the investigator planned to study.

STEP THREE: EVALUATION OF THE RESEARCH DESIGN

Theory directs every aspect of research. Thus, the third step in the evaluation of a conceptual-theoretical-empirical structure focuses on the congruence between the middle-range theory and the empirical research methods. The criterion is operational adequacy.

Operational Adequacy

The operational adequacy criterion requires the empirical research methods used to generate or test a middle-range theory to be congruent with the theory. Every aspect of the methodology, including the sample, instruments, data-collection procedures, and data-analysis techniques, must be evaluated to determine whether the theory is appropriately operationalized. In particular, inasmuch as each aspect of methodology represents a methodological theory, such as sampling theory or statistical theory (Slife and Williams, 1995), the congruence between those methodological theories and the substantive theory that was generated or tested must be evaluated.

THE SAMPLE. The sample should be appropriate for the middle-range theory that was generated or tested and for the research procedures. More specifically, the sample should represent the population for which the theory is being developed. That is so, whether the sample is made up of human beings, animals, events, or documents. In theory-generating studies using interpretative methods, nonprobability or convenience sampling, which is frequently called theoretical sampling, is appropriate. In theory-generating studies using quantitative methods and in theory-testing studies, probability sampling that includes random selection and/or assignment of subjects is more appropriate. Regardless of the sampling procedure, however, representativeness of the sample, which is dictated by the theory, is the most important point to consider. As Serlin (1987) pointed out, "[The substantive] theory must guide the selection of a sampling procedure, and [the] theory must determine in what ways the sample should be representative" (p. 366).

The size of the sample also must be considered. Adequacy of sample size, both before and after a study has been conducted, can be determined by power analysis, which takes into consideration the size of the sample, the alpha significance criterion, the estimated population effect size, and the power of the statistical test (Cohen, 1988). Sample size is important regardless of the type of research. Indeed, although some proponents of interpretative research methods regard the size of the sample as unimportant, Sandelowski (1995) has argued that a very small sample may not support a claim of informational redundancy or theoretical saturation, whereas a very large sample may interfere with the deep, case-oriented analysis that is characteristic of interpretative methods.

THE INSTRUMENTS. The research instruments, or empirical indicators, should be appropriate for eliciting the data needed to generate or test the middle-range theory of interest to the investigator. Each instrument should be a valid measure of the intended concept as constitutively defined in a given study. This point cannot be overemphasized, because many concepts have different constitutive definitions, as well as different operational definitions. For example, the Katz Index of Activities of Daily Living is a valid measure of functional ability when constitutively defined as the capacity or ability to bath, dress, toilet, transfer, and feed oneself (Katz, 1983). The Katz Index, however, is not a valid measure of functional ability when functional ability is constitutively defined as the extent of assistance required for performance of usual daily activities and social-role activities. The latter constitutive definition is operationalized by the Enforced Social Dependency Scale (Benoliel, McCorkle, and Young, 1980), which contains items that measure the extent to which an individual requires assistance with such activities as eating, dressing, traveling, bathing, and working. Thus, the constitutive definition of each concept must be carefully considered when evaluating the validity of any research instrument. In addition, the protocols for experimental and control treatments in predictive theory-testing experimental research must be valid and must be sufficiently different to permit the detection of any differences in outcomes (Egan, Snyder, and Burns, 1992).

Each instrument also should be a reliable measure for the population of interest and for the specific research participants. A questionnaire that has demonstrated internal consistency reliability for one sample may not be reliable with another sample even when drawn from the same population. That is because measurement error, variability of scores, and other forces affecting the reliability of an instrument can vary from sample to sample.

THE PROCEDURE FOR DATA COLLECTION. The data collection procedure should be appropriate for the middle-range theory that the researcher wishes to generate or test and for the type of research conducted. For example, if a theory predicts differences between two distinct groups on a particular measure, the research procedure must include collection of data that will permit a comparison between the groups.

Each type of middle-range theory (descriptive, explanatory, predictive) is developed by a particular type of research that has its own set of procedural standards and safeguards for investigators and research participants. Detailed discussions of descriptive, correlational, and experimental research methods are presented in several good research texts, including those by Babbie (1990, 1998), Cook and Campbell (1979), Kerlinger (1986), Moody (1990), and Polit and Hungler (1995).

THE DATA-ANALYSIS TECHNIQUES. The data-analysis techniques should be appropriate for the middle-range theory being developed. Indeed, "statistics and theory inform each other" (Serlin, 1987, p. 371). Descriptive theory development may employ such summary statistics as frequency counts, percentages, medians, means, and ranges. Explanatory theory development requires a measure of association, such as the correlation coefficient. Predictive theory development usually requires a measure of differences, such as analysis of variance. The data-analysis techniques also should be appropriate for the kind of data obtained. Narrative data usually are analyzed by means of some version of content analysis. If desired, narrative data can be transformed to numerical scores by assigning numbers to categories and themes and then can be analyzed statistically. Numerical data usually are subjected to nonparametric or parametric statistics. The selection of a particular nonparametric or parametric statistic depends on the measurement scale of the numerical data (nominal, ordinal, interval, or ratio).

APPLICATION OF THE CRITERION OF OPERATIONAL ADEQUACY. In theory-generating research, the operational adequacy criterion is applied to the results. In theory-testing research, the application of this criterion is limited to the version of the theory that will be or was tested. The judgment, therefore, focuses on the extent to which the empirical indicators are appropriate proxies for the concepts, and the data-collection procedure and data-analysis techniques are the appropriate methods to measure the assertions of the theory propositions. The most important point to consider when applying the criterion of operational adequacy is the fit between the conceptual model, the middle-range theory, and the empirical research methods used to generate or test the theory. Accordingly, research built on an implicit conceptual model and an implicit theory is no more than a hobby (Serlin, 1987).

STEP FOUR: EVALUATION OF THE RESEARCH FINDINGS

Research findings direct middle-range theory development. Therefore, the fourth step in the evaluation of a conceptual-theoretical-empirical structure emphasizes the influence of study results on middle-range theory generation or refinement. The criterion is empirical adequacy.

Empirical Adequacy

The empirical-adequacy criterion requires theoretical claims to be congruent with empirical evidence derived from research. In theory-generating research, the concepts and propositions that emerge from the data analysis should clearly reflect the raw data. In theory-testing research, the interpretation of tests of hypotheses is especially important. The logic of scientific inference dictates that if the empirical data do not conform to the hypothesized expectation, it is appropriate to conclude that the hypothesis is false. Conversely, if the empirical data conform to the expectation stated by the hypothesis, then it is appropriate to tentatively accept the hypothesis as empirically adequate.

The logical form that permits rejection of a hypothesis when empirical findings do not conform to expectations, called *modus tollens*, states that a single negative instance is sufficient to falsify a hypothesis. The logical form is:

If A then C
Not C
Therefore, not A
(Crossley and Wilson, 1979, p. 271).

Acceptance of a hypothesis as adequate when findings conform to expectations, called the *fallacy of affirming the consequent*, takes the following logical form:

If A then C
C
Therefore A
(Crossley and Wilson, 1979, p. 272).

The argument is fallacious because "the positive result does not give unequivocal support to the . . . hypothesis" (Phillips, 1987, pp. 14–15). Indeed, it is always possible that exceptions can occur. Thus, the argument underscores the logical flaw that occurs when extraneous concepts that could have influenced the results are ignored. For example, if study findings reveal a significant difference in fatigue between a group that engaged in moderate walking exercise and a group that did not, one must ask whether extraneous concepts, such as the age, ordinary activity, and pretest physical health of the participants, could account for the findings (Mock et al., 1997). Of course, extraneous concepts also could account for negative findings. Consequently, the empirical adequacy of hypotheses and the theories from which they are derived always is based on probability rather than certainty.

Consideration of the empirical adequacy of a theory must take into account all assertions made about all of the propositions that make up the theory. If, for example, propositions assert the direction and strength of relations, the hypothesized direction (negative, positive) and strength (weak, moderate, strong) must be evident at the required level of statistical significance. If the statistical test yields a nonsignificant level of probability, the correct conclusion is that the relation probably does not exist. It is not correct to say, for example, that the relation is positive but nonsignificant.

It is important to point out that a theory that turns out to be empirically inadequate can be just as informative as one that is empirically adequate. Indeed, it is equally important to learn what is and is not so. Knowing what is not so actually advances theory development by eliminating a false line of reasoning before much time and effort are invested in that line of reasoning. Thus, as Marx and Cronan-Hillix (1987) pointed out, "a theory should be sensitive to empirical findings. If a theory makes bad predictions, the theory should be changed. Here the point is that even a bad prediction is better than no prediction at all, for the bad prediction may point toward improvements" (p. 307).

Hart's (1995) test of an explanatory theory of the relations of number of pregnancies, weeks of gestation, prenatal risk designation, self-care agency, basic prenatal care (PNC) actions, and foundation for dependent-care agency (DCA) to pregnancy outcomes is an example of the informative nature of an empirically inadequate theory. The theory, which was derived from Orem's (1991) Self-Care Framework, and contains several contingent relations, was tested with a random sample of 127 pregnant women. As can be seen in Figure 3–2, the data did not support the existence of several of the contingent relations that were part of the original theory. The new theory clearly is much more parsimonious and focuses attention on the relations of just a few concepts to pregnancy outcomes.

ALTERNATIVE METHODOLOGICAL AND SUBSTANTIVE EXPLANATIONS. Regardless of the empirical adequacy of a theory, competing or alternative explanations for empirical findings must be taken into account. Two alternative explanations that always must be considered are methodological. One explanation is that the findings were produced by the research design, such as the sample of observations or measurements actually made out of all those that could have been made. In addition, in the case of tests of predictive theories, the experimental research design may not provide a sufficiently strong "dose" of the treatment to produce the expected effect (Brooten and Naylor, 1995; Cook and Shadish, 1994). The other explanation is that

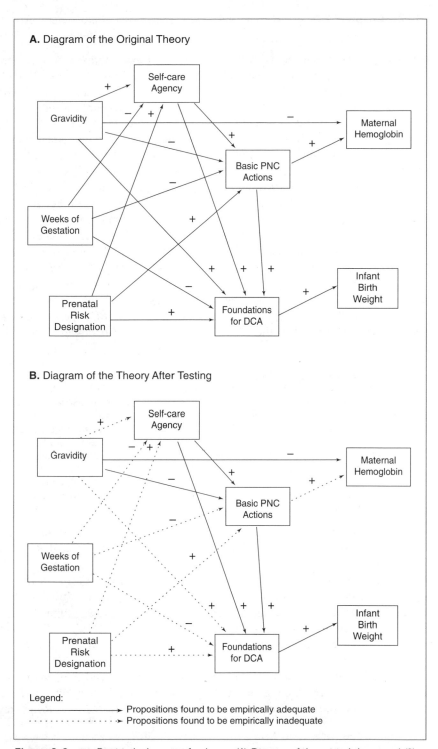

A. Diagram of the Original Theory

B. Diagram of the Theory After Testing

Legend:

⟶ Propositions found to be empirically adequate

····▸ Propositions found to be empirically inadequate

Figure 3–2 ■ Empirical adequacy of a theory. (A) Diagram of the original theory and (B) diagram of the theory after testing. (Diagrams from Hart, 1995, pp. 121, 125, with permission.)

the findings were produced by many small errors of measurement, such as perceptual and coding errors associated with participants' and investigators' uses of the research instruments.

Other explanations are substantive; they attempt to account for the study findings by recommending the elimination of some concepts, the addition of other concepts, and/or different linkages between concepts. A substantive explanation may also include the recommendation of an entirely different theory to account for the findings.

Alternative methodological and substantive explanations are given in Ryan's (1996) research report. Ryan tested an explanatory theory of the relations of loneliness, social support, and depression to cognitive functioning, which was derived from Roy's Adaptation Model (Roy and Andrews, 1991), in a sample of 74 community-based ambulatory elderly women and men. She found that the data did not provide support for any of the hypotheses that were tested. More specifically, she found that, contrary to hypothesized expectations, there was no evidence of a relation between cognitive functioning and loneliness, social support, or depression.

One methodological explanation for the lack of support for the hypotheses focused on the congruence of the instruments with Roy's Adaptation Model. Ryan explained:

> ■ Because no significant relationships were found between the main [theory concepts], a review of the fit between the [conceptual] framework and the instruments that were used in the study is indicated. Although both the social support and depression scales were designed and constructed by nurses, they were based on psychological theories, as was the loneliness scale. The instruments therefore reflect the use of non-nursing conceptual systems. The possibility must be considered that these non-nursing conceptualizations of loneliness, social support, and depression as measured by the instruments in this study were not congruent with that of Roy. If this is the case, it is further evidence of the need for the discipline of nursing to design and construct measurement tools that are based on nursing concepts and that reflect nursing [conceptual] models. (p. 112)

Another methodological explanation focused on the variability in scores for the instrument used to measure cognitive functioning. Ryan reported that "the lowest score on the [Mini Mental Status Examination] was 22 (one person) and the mean score was 29 (out of a possible 30); therefore, there was little variability in cognitive [functioning]" (p. 113). This explanation reflects the statistical artifact that low variability in the score for one concept in a relational proposition is associated with a correlation coefficient of low magnitude. In Ryan's study, the magnitude of the correlation coefficients was exceptionally low, ranging from $r = .03$ to $r = .06$.

One substantive explanation offered by Ryan emphasized the need to incorporate another concept into the theory. More specifically, this explanation focused on the need to take the participants' educational level into account. Ryan stated:

> ■ One other factor may have contributed to the lack of significant findings in this study. Substantial evidence exists in the literature supporting the positive relationship between educational levels and higher cognitive functioning. (p. 113)

Another substantive explanation focused on the need to test a different theory. Ryan based this explanation on additional findings from the study. She stated:

■ The number of significant ancillary findings relating to the study variables is important. Subjective ratings of health, the impact that chronic health conditions have on quality of life, and satisfaction with living arrangements emphasize some of the primary issues that have a large impact on the quality of life of older adults residing in the community. . . . [There is a need] to evaluate the client's coping behaviors in relation to the individual's perception of health, satisfaction with living arrangements, depression, social support, and the ability to perform activities of daily living. (p. 113)

COMPETING HYPOTHESES. A theory can be a barrier or act as blinders to an investigator by structuring observations to the extent that data that do not conform to expectations may be ignored (Chinn and Kramer, 1995). This limitation of any theory can be overcome by posing competing hypotheses derived from alternative theories to determine which theory fits best with the data.

Indeed, Platt (1964) maintained that every theory-testing study should include multiple competing hypotheses derived from alternative theories. He claimed that this approach eliminates errors in interpreting findings that are due to the researcher's intellectual or emotional investment in one particular theory. A test of the two most likely substantive theories about a phenomenon is called a crucial experiment. It requires the investigator "to construct, for any two competing theories, conditions in which they yield different observable results" (Popper, 1965, p. 174). A crucial experiment is a culminating experiment that follows considerable work to refine methods and techniques that narrow down the question asked to an either/or situation. If research findings indicate that the hypothesis derived from one theory is not rejected but the alternative hypothesis *is* rejected, then the appropriate interpretation is that the first theory is very adequate and the second theory is false.

These experiments are possible only when rigid external control is possible, such as in physics and chemistry laboratories, but rare in situations involving human beings in natural settings. Runciman (1983) pointed out that crucial experiments actually are elusive in the natural sciences and even more elusive in the social sciences because of the difficulty of conducting true experiments with human beings. Moreover, Marx and Cronan-Hillix (1987) pointed out that any one experiment probably is not sufficient to provide a clear-cut answer to the question of which of two theories is the adequate one, and that such a question may be too simplistic. Nevertheless, the notion of crucial experiments is useful if it leads to informative research.

A hypothetical example of a crucial experiment involving humans can be constructed by comparing two alternative predictive theories accounting for reduction of exceptionally high levels of psychological distress associated with radiation therapy. Suppose that one theory proposes that concrete, objective information about radiation therapy, given prior to the start of treatment, reduces the psychological distress associated with the radiation therapy (Johnson, Fieler, Wlasowicz, Mitchell, and Jones, 1997). Suppose also that the most likely alternative to the information theory is a theory postulating that the presence of a supportive person reduces psychological distress associated with the radiation therapy. The information theory implies that the presence of a supportive person has an insignificant effect on reduction of distress, and the supportive person theory implies that information has an insignificant effect. If research findings demonstrate that the presence of the supportive person had no statistically significant effect on distress reduction and if information given prior to the radiation therapy reduced distress at a statistically significant level, then the appropriate interpretation is that the supportive person theory is false and the information theory is the best available theory. Another version of a crucial experiment using the supportive person and information theories would be to compare the effects of a combination of the two theories with each theory alone.

Although crucial experiments are very rare, critical tests of two or more competing theories have been conducted with human beings in clinical situations. For example, Yarcheski, Mahon, and Yarcheski (1997) tested two alternative explanatory theories of positive health practices in adolescents. One explanatory theory proposed that age, gender, self-esteem, social support, and future time perspective were related to adolescents' positive health practices. The other explanatory theory proposed that age, gender, self-esteem, social support, and perceived health status were related to adolescents' positive health practices. The special contribution of this critical test was the examination of the differential contributions of future time perspective and perceived health status to adolescents' positive health practices.

Although a crucial experiment or a critical test of competing theories can improve the empirical adequacy of a theory, that theory should not be regarded as truth. Indeed, inasmuch as the assertions made by a theory proposition can never be proved, no theory should be considered final or absolute, for it is always possible that additional tests of the theory will yield different findings or that other theories will provide a better fit with the data (Judd, Smith, and Kidder, 1991). Tests of the explanatory theory of planned behavior (Ajzen, 1991), which was linked with Neuman's (1995) Systems Model, serve as an example. A diagram of the original theory proposed by Ajzen is given in Figure 2–1, p. 30. As can be seen in Figure 3–3, three tests of the theory for the situation of cigarette smoking intention revealed different findings for African-American, Puerto Rican, and non-Hispanic white teenage females (Hanson, 1995, 1997).

The aim of research, then, is not to determine the absolute truth of theories, but rather to determine the degree of confidence warranted by the best empirical evidence. If confidence is high, the theory may be retained and should be subjected to continued testing. If, however, confidence is low, the researcher must be prepared to abandon the theory and search for a better theory (Serlin, 1987).

Taken together, the requirements of the empirical adequacy criterion stipulate that conclusions do not go beyond what was demonstrated by the data. Possible conclusions are (1) the data are inaccurate and cannot be relied upon for theory development, (2) the data are accurate but the theory is faulty and should be abandoned or must be modified, (3) the data are accurate and the theory should be regarded as empirically adequate, and (4) the data are accurate but have no relevance to the theory (Downs, 1984).

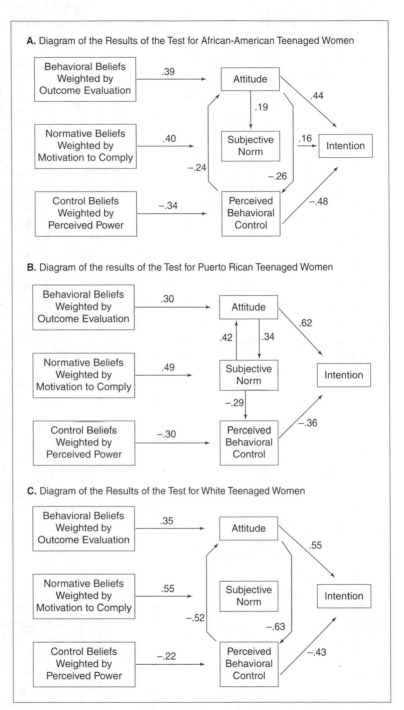

Figure 3–3 ■ Three tests of the Theory of Planned Behavior. (A) Diagram of the results of the test for African-American teenaged women (B) diagram of the results of the test for Puerto Rican teenaged women, and (C) diagram of the results of the test for white teenaged women. (Diagrams from Hanson, 1997, pp. 159–160, with permission.

APPLICATION OF THE CRITERION OF EMPIRICAL ADEQUACY. In theory-generating research, the empirical adequacy criterion is once again applied to the results that yield the new theory. In theory-testing research, this criterion is applied to a comparison of the version of the theory that was tested and the version that was retained after testing. The repeated application of the criterion in the case of theory testing yields an informative judgment about what was proposed versus what was actually found.

It is unlikely that any one test of a hypothesis or theory will provide the definitive evidence needed to establish empirical adequacy. More to the point, perhaps, is that researchers are reluctant to abandon a theory after just one test that does not yield supporting evidence. Moreover, researchers do not always subject theories to repeated tests if the initial test yields supporting evidence. Yet decisions about empirical adequacy should take the findings of several related studies into account. Formal procedures for integrating the results of related studies are discussed in detail in Chapter 4. Suffice it to say here that the more tests of a theory that yield supporting evidence, the more empirically adequate the theory.

STEP FIVE: EVALUATION OF THE UTILITY OF THE THEORY FOR PRACTICE

The fifth step in the evaluation of a conceptual-theoretical-empirical structure focuses on the implications of the middle-range theory for practice. The criterion is pragmatic adequacy.

Pragmatic Adequacy

The pragmatic adequacy criterion requires the middle-range theories of professional disciplines such as nursing, medicine, social work, education, law, and engineering to be useful in practice. Indeed, as Kerlinger (1979) pointed out, "the most important influence on practice is theory" (p. 296). Despite their importance, theories have an indirect rather than a direct influence on practice. The indirect influence is best appreciated when it is understood that theories, per se, cannot be applied in practical situations. Instead, such innovative actions as assessment formats and intervention protocols are derived from the theories and used in practice.

Furthermore, the indirect influence of theories on practice is slow to occur because no theory actually tells clinicians what to do. Rather, a theory gradually influences thinking and doing over the long periods of time required to first disseminate the theory and then to change fixed sets of beliefs (Funk, Tornquist, and Champagne, 1995).

RELATION OF A THEORY TO A CLINICAL SITUATION. The pragmatic adequacy criterion requires the theory to be related to the particular area of practice for which a theory is sought. That means that the theory is applicable to a particular clinical specialty, particular problems, and/or particular ages or developmental phases. Although that may seem self-evident, it is not unusual to find that an innovative action is based on a theory that is unrelated to the relevant clinical problem and patient population. Suppose, for example, that a clinician wants to use an intervention that will reduce the anxiety experienced by women who are about to undergo breast cancer surgery. Suppose also that the intervention protocol was based on a theory dealing with the anxiety individuals experience prior to taking an achievement test. In this constructed example, the theory deals not with anxiety associated with breast cancer surgery, but rather with test anxiety. In contrast, suppose that the protocol was based on a theory of anxiety experienced by men who are about to undergo prostate cancer surgery. Here, one question would be whether the anxiety associated with cancer surgery is the same for women as it is for men. Another question would be whether the site of the cancer has an influence on anxiety.

FEASIBILITY. The pragmatic adequacy criterion further requires the implementation of an innovative action in a particular practice setting to be feasible. Feasibility is determined by an evaluation of the resources needed to establish a new way of doing things, including the time needed to learn and implement the innovation, the number, type, and expertise of personnel required for its implementation, and the cost of in-service education, salaries, equipment, and testing procedures. Furthermore, the willingness of those who control financial resources to pay for the innovation must be determined.

CONGRUENCE WITH RECIPIENTS' EXPECTATIONS. The pragmatic adequacy criterion also requires innovative actions to be congruent with the recipients' expectations of practice. If the actions do not meet existing expectations, they should be abandoned or attention should be given to helping recipients to develop new expectations. Indeed, "current . . . practice is not entirely what it might become and [thus recipients] might come to expect a different form of practice, given the opportunity to experience it" (Johnson, 1974, p. 376).

LEGAL CONTROL. In addition, the pragmatic adequacy criterion requires the practitioner to have legal control over the implementation of the innovation and the measurement of its effectiveness. Such control may be problematic, in that, because of resistance of others, practitioners are not always able to carry out legally sanctioned responsibilities. Sources of resistance against implementation of nursing innovations, for example, include attempts by physicians to control nursing practice, financial barriers imposed by clinical agency administrators and third-party payers, and skepticism by other health professionals about the ability of nurses to carry out the proposed interventions (Funk et al., 1995). The cooperation and collaboration of others may, therefore, have to be secured. Implementation of a medication education program, for example, may be opposed by physicians who are concerned that patients will be upset by information about side effects or even develop certain side effects due to their expectation that those side effects actually will occur. Implementation of the educational program also may be opposed by health system administrators who are concerned about the cost of the resources needed to implement the program.

SOCIAL MEANINGFULNESS. Finally, the pragmatic adequacy criterion requires the innovative actions to be socially meaningful, that is, to address major social problems and to lead to favorable outcomes for recipients of the action. Major social problems include universal situations such as care of the poor as well as more time-bound situations such as epidemics of a disease for which a treatment has not yet been developed. Examples of favorable outcomes include reduced incidence of patient complications, improved patient health status, reduced rates of student attrition or staff turnover, and increased patient, student, and staff satisfaction. Repeated tests of innovations in practical situations provide the evidence needed to determine whether the innovations result in favorable outcomes. Quantitative analyses of outcomes should consider not only statistical significance, but also clinical or practical significance. Statistical significance is, of course, determined by the alpha or p value. An important point to keep in mind here is that "statistical significance does not guarantee clinical significance and more to the point, *the magnitude of the* p *value (.05, .01, .001, .00029, or whatever) is no guide to clinical significance*" (Slakter, Wu, and Suzuki-Slakter, 1991, p. 249). Rather, clinical significance is determined by the magnitude of the outcome, which can be calculated as an effect size that can be classified as a small, medium, or large relation between concepts or difference between groups (Cohen, 1988).

The importance of statistical *and* clinical significance is exemplified by an integrative review of studies testing predictive theories of the effects of various medical and nursing interventions on adult cardiac patients' quality of life (Kinney, Burfitt, Stullenbarger, Rees, and DeBolt, 1996). The findings of the quantitative integrative review revealed that the experimental group participants experienced a 15% benefit from the intervention over the control group. Although the difference between the quality of life scores of the experimental and control groups was statistically significant in many of the studies, the investigators pointed out that the clinical significance of such a relatively small benefit is unclear and requires further investigation.

The importance of statistical *and* clinical significance also is exemplified by a test of a predictive theory addressing the accuracy of tympanic membrane and glass mercury thermometers in afebrile pregnant women (Yeo, Hayashi, Wan, and Dubler, 1995). The investigators reported that the correlation coefficient between the two types of thermometers was of relatively low magnitude but statistically significant ($r = .38$, $p = .01$). Given what they characterized as "reasonable agreement" between the tympanic membrane thermometer (TMT) and glass mercury thermometer measurements, the investigators recommended use of the TMT with pregnant women because the "cost effectiveness of TMTs is better than or similar to electronic oral or rectal thermometers. The price of TMTs for professional use varies depending on brand, ranging from $300 to $378 per unit. [Moreover] the ease and speed of use of the TMTs may save nurses' time" (p. 723).

OUTCOMES OF EVALUATION OF PRAGMATIC ADEQUACY. The outcome of evaluation of pragmatic adequacy is a thorough understanding of the theoretical and empirical base for various clinical practices, including methods of observation, assessment, and intervention. As can be seen in Figure 3–4, the evaluation of prag-matic adequacy leads to identification of what needs to be studied as well as the ef-ficacy of what has been studied (Hunt, 1981).

Evaluation of a descriptive or explanatory theory frequently leads to a recom-mendation to develop predictive theories about interventions that address a clinical problem. In that case, a relevant clinical practice has not yet been developed. For example, the findings of a Roy's Adaptation Model-based descriptive study designed to generate a descriptive naming theory of responses to vaginal birth after cesarean birth (VBAC) led to the following recommendation regarding clinical practice:

> ■ The results of the current study indicate a need for a high quality of nursing and obstetric care for all women. Emphasis should be placed on interventions di-rected toward the physiologic and interdependence modes of adaptation, oper-ationalized clinically by relief of pain and provision of support and information. The exploratory nature of the study and the small sample preclude the identifi-cation of more definitive implications for nursing practice. Additional research with a larger sample is recommended. (Fawcett, Tulman, and Spedden, 1994, p. 258)

In contrast, when a predictive theory has been tested and found to be empiri-cally adequate, the recommendation may be for additional research, adoption of a new practice, a trial of a new practice in the clinical setting, or discontinuation of a current practice (Fig. 3–4). Many reports of tests of predictive theories end with recommendations for additional research. Such recommendations indicate that the theory does not yet meet the pragmatic adequacy criterion. For example, the results of a test of a predictive theory about three methods of monitoring blood pressure—indirect bell component of stethoscope method, indirect diaphragm component of stethoscope method, and direct arterial method—led to a recommendation for ad-ditional research prior to incorporating one particular method into clinical practice (Norman, Gadaleta, and Griffin, 1991). Moreover, the investigators recommended that a single method be used for baseline and subsequent monitoring of blood pres-

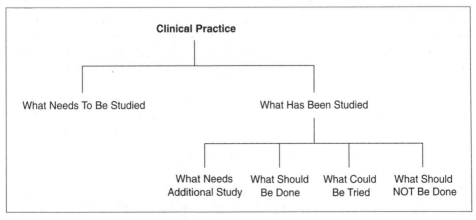

Figure 3–4 ■ Outcomes of evaluation of pragmatic adequacy.

sure. They based their recommendations on possible sources of bias introduced by their study design.

The findings of other tests of predictive theories indicate that the experimental intervention should be adopted. A test of a predictive theory addressing the accuracy of tympanic membrane and glass mercury thermometers in afebrile pregnant women exemplifies this situation. The investigators concluded that TMTs "are acceptable for use with pregnant women because of reasonable agreement between the new measurement [i.e., TMT] and an established measurement (i.e., glass mercury thermometers)" (Yeo et al., 1995, p. 723).

The recommendation for adoption of a clinical practice may be qualified by a further recommendation to conduct a trial of the intervention under controlled real-world clinical conditions and systematically evaluate the outcomes. Fourteen nursing practices identified by the staff of the Conduct and Utilization of Research in Nursing (CURN) Project exemplify this situation (Horsley, Crane, Crabtree, and Wood, 1983). One such practice is mutual goal setting by patient and nurse, which has been found to enhance goal achievement and increase patient and nursing staff satisfaction (Horsley, Crane, Haller, and Reynolds, 1982).

Conversely, some reports of tests of predictive theories end with a recommendation to discontinue a practice. The results of a test of a maternal attachment theory that specified a particular sequence of handling newborn infants supported the discontinuation of a widely used method of assessing maternal attachment. More specifically, the investigator maintained, "The results of this study cast some doubt on the validity of fingers-palms-arms-trunk as a parameter for clinically assessing maternal attachment for either vaginally or cesarean-delivered women. The continued use of the fingers-palms-arms-trunk sequence as a nursing clinical assessment tool . . . is therefore not a valid clinical practice" (Tulman, 1986, p. 299).

PRAGMATIC ADEQUACY AND POLICIES. The outcome of evaluation of pragmatic adequacy not only is a thorough understanding of the theoretical and empirical base for various clinical practices but also is a catalyst for the development of clinical and public policies. Indeed, Cohen and associates (1996) underscored the importance of translating empirically and pragmatically adequate theories into policies for the public's good. Clinical policies typically are presented in the form of clinical practice guidelines, such as those developed and disseminated by the Agency for Health Care Policy and Research (e.g., Agency for Health Care Policy and Research, 1992, 1994). Public policies typically are presented in the form of legislation or the benefits offered by a business. For example, the findings of tests of descriptive and explanatory theories addressing the functional status of childbearing women need to be translated into legislation and organizational benefits that address the length and timing of maternity leave (Tulman and Fawcett, 1991).

SELECTING THE BEST THEORY. Sometimes the actions derived from more than one equally adequate theory are found to be useful in a particular situation. In this admittedly rare case, the theory that leads to the most effective actions should be selected. Hardy (1988) offered the following guidelines for selection of the best theory:

1. Select the theory that deals most adequately with the variables of concern to the clinician.
2. Select the theory whose central variables can be altered or modified by the clinician to bring about the desired change.
3. Select the theory whose application leads.to desired changes that are strong enough or significant enough to make it worthwhile to implement a plan of action based on the theory.

APPLICATION OF THE CRITERION OF PRAGMATIC ADEQUACY. In theory-generating research, the pragmatic adequacy criterion is applied to the long-range potential of the study results; in theory-testing research, it is confined to the version of the theory that was retained after analysis of the study findings.

STEP SIX: EVALUATION OF THE CONCEPTUAL MODEL

The sixth and final step in the evaluation of a conceptual-theoretical-empirical structure focuses on the credibility of the conceptual model that guided the middle-range theory development effort. The criterion is credibility.

Credibility

Credibility determination is necessary to avoid the danger of uncritical acceptance and adoption of conceptual models, which could easily lead to their use as ideologies. Indeed, critical reviews of the empirical evidence regarding the credibility of each conceptual model must be encouraged and acceptance of work that is "fashionable, well-trodden or simply available in the nursing library" must be avoided (Grinnell, 1992, p. 57).

The ultimate aim of credibility determination is to ascertain which conceptual models are appropriate for use in which situations and with which populations. Inasmuch as the abstract and general nature of a conceptual model precludes direct empirical testing, instead the propositions of the conceptual model are tested indirectly through the empirical testing of the corresponding propositions of middle-range theories that are derived from or linked with the model. In theory-generating research, the judgment about credibility may be limited to the utility of the conceptual model to guide the selection of empirical research methods and the success of those methods in generating a new theory. In addition, if the concepts of the conceptual model served as a priori categories for data analysis, the judgment about credibility can be extended beyond the utility of empirical research methods to the comprehensiveness of the conceptual model content. For example, Breckenridge (1997) used five concepts from Neuman's Systems Model as the a priori categories for a secondary content analysis of interview transcripts. She reported that all of the interview data could be categorized within those five concepts, namely "physiological variables," "psychological variables," "sociocultural variables," "developmental variables," and "spiritual variables." In this case, Neuman's Systems Model can be regarded as credible. Suppose, however, that the data could be categorized within only three of the concepts, or that some of the data could be categorized within the five concepts but other data did not reflect any of the concepts, or even that the interview data did not reflect any of the five concepts. In any of those cases, the credibility of Neuman's Systems Model would have to be questioned.

In theory-testing research, if the theory is found to be empirically adequate, it is likely that the conceptual model is credible. For example, a test of a predictive theory of the effects of walking exercise on physical functioning, exercise level, emotional distress, and symptom experience of women with breast cancer who were receiving chemotherapy yielded evidence of its empirical adequacy. Since the study was guided by Roy's Adaptation Model, the investigators concluded that the model was credible (Mock et al., 1997).

If, however, the research findings do not support the empirical adequacy of the theory, the credibility of the conceptual model must be questioned. For example, a test of a predictive theory of the effects of cancer support groups on symptom distress, emotional distress, functional status, and quality of relationship with a significant other revealed that the theory was not empirically adequate. Since the theory was directly derived from Roy's Adaptation Model, the investigators concluded that the study findings "raise questions about the credibility of the [model] and its utility for research dealing with the effects of social support and education on adaptation to breast cancer" (Samarel, Fawcett, and Tulman, 1997, p. 24).

The two examples given here illustrate the difficulty in reaching a definitive decision regarding the credibility of any one conceptual model. The need for integrative reviews of all studies guided by a particular conceptual model is obvious. The topic of integrative reviews is discussed in detail in Chapter 4.

Application of the Criterion of Credibility

The credibility criterion can be applied only if the criteria of specification adequacy and linkage adequacy have been met (see pp. 86–88). If those criteria have been met, determination of credibility may proceed by comparing the research results with the concepts and propositions of the conceptual model.

CONCLUSION

The merit of research frequently is said to be based on the logical consistency among the theoretical, design, and analysis components of an investigation. The criteria for evaluation of a conceptual-theoretical-empirical structure presented in this chapter direct attention to those three components of a research document, as well as to the conceptual basis for the research and the research results. All criteria are summarized in Table 3–1. Use of the criteria should enhance understanding of the relation between conceptual models, theories, and research. Examples of use of the criteria for evaluation of conceptual-theoretical-empirical structures for descriptive, correlational, and experimental research are presented in the Appendices.

Table 3-1 ■ STEPS IN THE EVALUATION OF A CONCEPTUAL-THEORETICAL-EMPIRICAL STRUCTURE

Step One: Evaluation of the Conceptual-Theoretical-Empirical Linkages
Specification adequacy is evident.
- A conceptual model is explicitly identified as the underlying guide for the theory-generating or theory-testing research.
- The conceptual model is discussed in sufficient breadth and depth so that the relation of the model to the middle-range theory and the empirical research methods is clear.

Linkage adequacy is evident.
- The linkages between the conceptual model concepts and propositions and the middle-range theory concepts and propositions are stated explicitly.
- The methodology reflects the conceptual model.
  —The study subjects are drawn from a population that is appropriate for the focus of the conceptual model.
  —The instruments are appropriate measures of phenomena encompassed by the conceptual model.
  —The study design clearly reflects the focus of the conceptual model.
  —The statistical techniques are in keeping with the focus of the conceptual model.

Step Two: Evaluation of the Theory
The theory is *significant.*
- The theory addresses a phenomenon of interest to society.
- The theory addresses a phenomenon of interest to a discipline by extending or filling a gap in an existing theory.

The theory is *internally consistent.*
- The concepts reflect semantic clarity and consistency.
- No concepts are redundant.
- The propositions reflect structural consistency.
- There are no incomplete or redundant sets of propositions.
- The observations substantiate the conclusions of an inductively developed theory.
- The premises of a deductively developed theory are valid.

The theory is *parsimonious.*
- The theory is stated clearly and concisely.

The theory is *testable.*
- The concepts can be empirically observed.
- The propositions can be measured.
- The derived hypotheses can be falsified.

Step Three: Evaluation of the Research Design
Operational adequacy is evident.
- The sample is representative of the population of interest.
- The empirical indicators are valid and reliable.
- The research procedure is appropriate.
- The procedures for data analysis are appropriate.

Step Four: Evaluation of the Research Findings
Evidence regarding the *empirical adequacy* of the theory is given.   •
- Theoretical claims are congruent with empirical evidence.
- Alternative methodological and substantive theories are considered.

Step Five: Evaluation of the Utility of the Theory for Practice
Evidence regarding the *pragmatic adequacy* of the theory is given.
- The theory is related to the practical problem of interest.
- It is feasible to implement innovative actions derived from the theory.
- The innovative actions are congruent with recipients' expectations.
- The practitioner has legal control over the implementation of the innovation and the measurement of its effectiveness.
- The innovative actions lead to favorable outcomes.
- The theory serves as a catalyst for the development of clinical practice guidelines and public policies.

Step Six: Evaluation of the Conceptual Model
Evidence regarding the *credibility* of the conceptual model is given.
- Discussion of research results includes conclusions regarding the credibility of the conceptual model.

References

Agency for Health Care Policy and Research, Public Health Service, U.S. Department of Health and Human Services. (1992). *Pressure ulcers in adults. Prediction and prevention. Clinical practice guideline, number 3.* (AHCPR Publication No. 92-0047). Rockville, MD: Author.

Agency for Health Care Policy and Research, Public Health Service, U.S. Department of Health and Human Services. (1994). *Treatment of pressure ulcers. Clinical practice guideline, number 15.* (AHCPR Publication No. 94-0527). Rockville, MD: Author.

Babbie, E. (1998). *The practice of social research* (8th ed.). Belmont, CA: Wadsworth.

Babbie, E. R. (1990). *Survey research methods* (2nd ed.). Belmont, CA: Wadsworth.

Benoliel, J.Q., McCorkle, R.M., & Young, K. (1980). Development of a social dependency scale. *Research in Nursing and Health, 3,* 3–10.

Bottomley, A. (1997). Cancer support groups— are they effective? *European Journal of Cancer Care, 6,* 11–17.

Breckenridge, D.M. (1997). Decisions regarding dialysis treatment modality: A holistic perspective. *Holistic Nursing Practice, 12*(1), 54–61.

Bridgman, P.W. (1927). *The logic of modern physics.* New York: Macmillan.

Brooten, D., & Naylor, M.D. (1995). Nurses' effect on changing patient outcomes. *Image: Journal of Nursing Scholarship, 27,* 95–99.

Chalmers, I., Enkin, M., & Keirse, M.J.N.C. (1989). *Effective care in pregnancy and childbirth.* New York: Oxford University Press.

Chinn, P.L., & Kramer, M.K. (1995). *Theory and nursing. A systematic approach* (4th ed.). St. Louis: Mosby YearBook.

Cohen, J. (1988). *Statistical power analysis for the behavioral sciences* (2nd ed.). Hillsdale, NJ: Lawrence Erlbaum.

Cohen, J.M., Sarill, W.J., & Vishveshwara, C.V. (1982). An example of induced centrifugal force in general relativity. *Nature, 298*(5877), 829.

Cohen, S.S., Mason, D.J., Kovner, C., Leavitt, J.K., Pulcini, J., & Sochalski, J. (1996). Stages of nursing's political development: Where we've been and where we ought to go. *Nursing Outlook, 44,* 259–266.

Collins, M.A. (1996). The relation of work stress, hardiness, and burnout among full-time hospital staff nurses. *Journal of Nursing Staff Development, 12,* 81–85.

Cook, T.D., & Campbell, D.T. (1979). *Quasi-experimentation: Design and analysis issues for field settings.* Boston: Houghton Mifflin.

Cook, T.D., & Shadish, W.R. (1994). Social experiments: Some developments over the past fifteen years. *Annual Review of Psychology, 45,* 545–580.

Cronbach, L. (1975). Beyond the two disciplines of scientific psychology. *American Psychologist, 3,* 116–127.

Crossley, D.J., & Wilson, P.A. (1979). *How to argue: An introduction to logical thinking.* New York: Random House.

Donaldson, S.K., & Crowley, D.M. (1978). The discipline of nursing. *Nursing Outlook, 26,* 113–120.

Downs, F.S. (1984). *A sourcebook of nursing research* (3rd ed.). Philadelphia: F.A. Davis.

Dubin, R. (1978). *Theory building* (rev. ed.). New York: The Free Press.

Duffy, M.E. (1984). Transcending options: Creating a milieu for practicing high level wellness. *Health Care for Women International, 5,* 145–161.

Duffy, M.E. (1994). Testing the theory of transcending options: Health behaviors of single parents. *Scholarly Inquiry for Nursing Practice, 8,* 191–202.

Egan, E.C., Snyder, M., & Burns, K.R. (1992). Intervention studies in nursing: Is the effect due to the independent variable? *Nursing Outlook, 40,* 187–190.

Fawcett, J. (1984). The metaparadigm of nursing: Current status and future refinements. *Image: Journal of Nursing Scholarship, 16,* 84–87.

Fawcett, J. (1995). *Analysis and evaluation of conceptual models of nursing* (3rd ed.). Philadelphia: F.A. Davis.

Fawcett, J., Tulman, L., & Spedden, J.P. (1994). Responses to vaginal birth after cesarean section. *Journal of Obstetric, Gynecologic, and Neonatal Nursing, 23,* 253–259.

Feeg, V.D. (1989). From the editor: Is theory application merely an intellectual exercise? *Pediatric Nursing, 15,* 450.

Funk, S.G., Tornquist, E.M., & Champagne, M.T. (1995). Barriers and facilitators of research utilization. *Nursing Clinics of North America, 30,* 395–407.

Goodson, F.E., & Morgan, G.A. (1976). Evaluation of theory. In M.H. Marx & F.E. Goodson (Eds.), *Theories in contemporary psychology* (2nd ed., pp. 286–299). New York: Macmillan.

Gortner, S.R. (1980). Nursing science in transition. *Nursing Research, 29,* 180–183.

Grinnell, F. (1992). Theories without thought? *Nursing Times, 88*(22), 57.

Hanson, M.J.S. (1995). *Beliefs, attitudes, sub-*

jective norms, perceived behavioral control, and cigarette smoking in white, African-American, and Puerto Rican-American teenage women. Unpublished doctoral dissertation, University of Pennsylvania.

Hanson, M.J.S. (1997). The theory of planned behavior applied to cigarette smoking in African-American, Puerto Rican, and non-Hispanic white teenage females. *Nursing Research, 46,* 155–162.

Hanson, N.R. (1958). *Patterns of discovery.* New York: Cambridge University Press.

Hardy, M.E. (1988). Perspectives on science. In M.E. Hardy & M.E. Conway (Eds.), *Role theory. Perspectives for health professionals* (2nd ed., pp. 1–27). Norwalk, CT: Appleton and Lange.

Hart, M.A. (1995). Orem's self-care deficit theory: Research with pregnant women. *Nursing Science Quarterly, 8,* 120–126.

Horsley, J.A., Crane, J., Crabtree, M.K., & Wood, D.J. (1983). *Using research to improve nursing practice: A guide.* New York: Grune and Stratton.

Horsley, J.A., Crane, J., Haller, K.B., & Reynolds, M.A. (1982). *Mutual goal setting in patient care.* New York: Grune and Stratton.

Hunt, J. (1981). Indicators for nursing practice: The use of research findings. *Journal of Advanced Nursing, 6,* 189–194.

Johnson, D.E. (1974). Development of theory: A requisite for nursing as a primary health profession. *Nursing Research, 23,* 372–377.

Johnson, J.E., Fieler, V.K., Wlasowicz, G.S., Mitchell, M.L., & Jones, L.S. (1997). The effects of nursing care guided by self-regulation theory on coping with radiation therapy. *Oncology Nursing Forum, 24,* 1041–1050.

Johnson, S.H. (1982). Developing an article using the nursing model. *Dimensions of Critical Care Nursing, 1,* 57–58.

Judd, C.M., Smith, E.R., & Kidder, L.H., (1991). *Research methods in social relations* (6th ed.). New York: Holt, Rinehart and Winston.

Katz, S. (1983). Assessing self-maintenance: Activities of daily living, mobility, and instrumental activities of daily living. *Journal of the American Geriatrlc Society, 31,* 721–727.

Kerlinger, F.N. (1979). *Behavioral research: A conceptual approach.* New York: Holt, Rinehart and Winston.

Kerlinger, F.N. (1986). *Foundations of behavioral research* (3rd ed.). New York: Holt, Rinehart and Winston.

Kinney, M.R., Burfitt, S.N., Stullenbarger, E., Rees, B., & DeBolt, M.R. (1996). Quality of life in cardiac patient research: A meta-analysis. *Nursing Research, 45,* 173–180.

Kleffel, D. (1991). Rethinking the environment

as a domain of nursing knowledge. *Advances in Nursing Science, 14*(1), 40–51.

Levy, D.H., Shoemaker, E.M., & Shoemaker, C.S. (1995). Comet Shoemaker-Levy 9 meets Jupiter. *Scientific American, 273*(August), 84–91.

Lusk, S.L. (1997). Health promotion and disease prevention in the work site. In J.J. Fitzpatrick & J. Norbeck (Eds.), *Annual review of nursing research* (Vol. 15, pp. 187–213). New York: Springer.

Marx, M.H. (1976). Formal theory. In M.H. Marx & F.E. Goodson (Eds.), *Theories in contemporary psychology* (2nd ed., pp. 234–260). New York: Macmillan.

Marx, M.H., & Cronan-Hillix, W.A. (1987). *Systems and theories in psychology* (4th ed.). New York: McGraw-Hill.

Mock, V., Dow, K.H., Meares, C.J., Grimm, P.M., Dienemann, J.A., Haisfield-Wolfe, M.E., Quitasol, W., Mltchell, S., Chakravarthy, A., & Gage, I. (1997). Effects of exercise on fatigue, physical functioning, and emotional distress during radiation therapy for breast cancer. *Oncology Nursing Forum, 24,* 991–1000.

Moody, L.E. (1990). *Advancing nursing science through research* (Vols. 1 and 2). Newbury Park, CA: Sage.

Neff, M. (1991). President's message: The future of our profession from the eyes of today. *American Nephrology Nurses' Association Journal, 18,* 534.

Neuman, B. (1995). *The Neuman systems model* (3rd ed.). Norwalk, CT: Appleton and Lange.

Norman, E., Gadaleta, D., & Griffin, C.C. (1991). An evaluation of three blood pressure methods in a stabilized acute trauma population. *Nursing Research, 40,* 86–89.

Orem, D.E. (1991). *Nursing: Concepts of practice* (4th ed.). St. Louis: Mosby YearBook.

Padilla, G.V., & Frank-Stromborg, M. (1997). Single instruments for measuring quality of life. In M. Frank-Stromborg & S.J. Olsen (Eds.), *Instruments for clinical health-care research* (2nd ed., pp. 114–134). Boston: Jones and Bartlett.

Patrick, D.L., & Erickson, P. (1993). *Health status and health policy: Quality of life in health care evaluation and resource allocation.* New York: Oxford University Press.

Payton, O.D. (1994). *Research: The validation of clinical practice* (3rd ed.). Philadelphia, F.A. Davis.

Phillips, D.C. (1987). *Philosophy, science and social inquiry: Contemporary methodological controversies in social science and related applied fields of research.* New York: Pergamon Press.

Platt, J.R. (1964). Strong inference. *Science, 146,* 347–353.

Polit, D.F., & Hungler, B.P. (1995). *Nursing research: Principles and methods* (5th ed.). Philadelphia: Lippincott.

Popper, K.R. (1965). *Conjectures and refutations: The growth of scientific knowledge.* New York: Harper and Row.

Richmond, T., McCorkle, R., Tulman, L., & Fawcett, J. (1997). Measuring function. In M. Frank-Stromborg & S.J. Olsen (Eds.), *Instruments for clinical health-care research* (2nd ed., pp. 75–85). Boston: Jones and Bartlett.

Roy, C., & Andrews, H.A. (1991). *The Roy adaptation model. The definitive statement.* Norwalk, CT: Appleton and Lange.

Runciman, W.G. (1983). *A treatise on social theory. Volume 1: The methodology of social theory.* New York: Cambridge University Press.

Ryan, M.C. (1996). Loneliness, social support and depression as interactive variables with cognitive status: Testing Roy's model. *Nursing Science Quarterly, 9,* 107–114.

Samarel, N., Fawcett, J., & Tulman, L. (1997). Effect of support groups with coaching on adaptation to early stage breast cancer. *Research in Nursing and Health, 20,* 15–26.

Sandelowski, M. (1995). Sample size in qualitative research. *Research in Nursing and Health, 18,* 179–183.

Schumacher, K.L., & Gortner, S.R. (1992). (Mis)conceptions and reconceptions about traditional science. *Advances in Nursing Science, 14*(4), 1–11.

Serlin, R.C. (1987). Hypothesis testing, theory building, and the philosophy of science. *Journal of Counseling Psychology, 34,* 365–371.

Shearing, C.D. (1973). How to make theories untestable: A guide to theorists. *The American Sociologist, 8,* 33–37.

Silva, M.C. (1987). Conceptual models of nursing. In J.J. Fitzpatrick & R.L. Taunton (Eds.), *Annual review of nursing research* (Vol. 5, pp. 229–246). New York: Springer.

Slakter, M.J., Wu, Y-W.B., & Suzuki-Slakter, N.S. (1991). *, **, and ***; Statistical nonsense at the .00000 level. *Nursing Research, 40,* 248–249.

Slife, B.D., & Williams, R.N. (1995). *What's behind the research? Discovering hidden assumptions in the behavioral sciences.* Thousand Oaks, CA: Sage.

Tulman, L.J. (1986). Initial handling of newborn infants by vaginally and cesarean-delivered mothers. *Nursing Research, 35,* 296–299.

Tulman, L., & Fawcett, J. (1991). Factors influencing recovery from childbirth. In J.S. Hyde & M.J. Essex (Eds.), *Parental leave and child care: Setting a research and policy agenda* (pp. 294–303). Philadelphia: Temple University Press.

World Health Organization. (1993). *WHO QOL study protocol: The development of the World Health Organization Quality of Life assessment instrument* (Publication MNH/PSF/93/9). Geneva, Switzerland: Division of Mental Health, World Health Organization.

Yarcheski, A., Mahon, N.E., & Yarcheski, T.J. (1997). Alternative models of positive health practices in adolescents. *Nursing Research, 46,* 85–92.

Yeo, S., Hayashi, R.H., Wan, J.Y., & Dubler, B. (1995). Tympanic versus rectal thermometry in pregnant women. *Journal of Obstetric, Gynecologic, and Neonatal Nursing, 24,* 719–724.

Additional Readings

Acton, G.J., Irvin, B.L., & Hopkins, B.A. (1991). Theory-testing research: Building the science. *Advances in Nursing Science, 14*(1), 52–61.

Bircumshaw, D. (1990). The utilization of research findings in clinical practice. *Journal of Advanced Nursing, 15,* 1272–1280.

Blalock, H.M., Jr. (1969). *Theory construction: From verbal to mathematical formulations.* Englewood Cliffs, NJ: Prentice-Hall.

Bower, B. (1997). Null science: Psychology's statistical status quo draws fire. *Science News, 151,* 356–357.

Cohen, J. (1990). Things I have learned (so far). *American Psychologist, 45,* 1304–1312.

Cronenwett, L.R. (1995). Effective methods for disseminating research findings to nurses in

practice. *Nursing Clinics of North America, 30,* 429–438.

Diesing, P. (1971). *Patterns of discovery in the social sciences.* New York: Aldine, Atherton.

Duffy, M.E. (1988). The research appraisal checklist: Appraising nursing research reports. In O.L. Strickland & C.F. Waltz (Eds.), *Measurement of nursing outcomes. Vol. 2. Measuring nursing performance: Practice, education, and research* (pp. 420–437). New York: Springer.

Grady, P. (1997). NINR and the nursing research community: The next 10 years . . . The next century. *Nursing Outlook, 45,* 43.

Haller, K.B., Reynolds, M.A., & Horsley, J.A. (1979). Developing research-based innovation protocols: Process, criteria, and issues. *Research in Nursing and Health, 2*, 45–51.

Hinds, P.S., Scandrett-Hibden, S., & McAulay, L.S. (1990). Further assessment of a method to estimate reliability and validity of qualitative research findings. *Journal of Advanced Nursing, 15*, 430–435.

Hinshaw, A.S. (1979). Planning for logical consistency among three research structures. *Western Journal of Nursing Research, 1*, 250–253.

Hinshaw, A.S. (1997). International nursing research priorities. *Journal of Professional Nursing, 13*, 68.

Knafl, K.A., & Howard, M.J. (1984). Interpreting and reporting qualitative research. *Research in Nursing and Health, 7*, 17–24.

Knapp, T.R. (1996). The overemphasis on power analysis. *Nursing Research, 45*, 379–381.

Kuhn, T.S. (1981). A function for thought experiments. In I. Hacking (Ed.), *Scientific revolutions* (pp. 6–27). New York: Oxford University Press.

Merton, R.K. (1957). *Social theory and social structure* (rev. ed.). New York: The Free Press.

Nunnally, J.C., & Bernstein, I.H. (1994). *Psychometric theory* (3rd ed.). New York: McGraw-Hill.

Popper, K.R. (1968). *The logic of scientific discovery*. New York: Harper and Row.

Silva, M.C., (1986). Research testing nursing theory: State of the art. *Advances in Nursing Science, 9*(1), 1–11.

Suppe, F. (1977). Afterword. In F. Suppe (Ed.), *The structure of scientific theories* (2nd ed., pp. 615–730). Chicago: University of Illinois Press.

Walker, L.O., & Avant, K.C. (1995). *Strategies for theory construction in nursing* (3rd ed.). Norwalk, CT: Appleton and Lange.

4 Preparing Integrative Reviews of Research Findings

■ When more than one study has been conducted on the same phenomenon, some procedure for integrating the findings is needed so that conclusions regarding the weight of the evidence for and/or against the theory that was generated or tested, as well as the parent conceptual model, can be reached. Integrative reviews of research findings supply the requisite evidence by providing crucial information about the existence of nonrelational propositions, and the existence, direction, and strength of relational propositions.

This chapter extends the discussion of the empirical adequacy of middle-range theories and the credibility of conceptual models that began in Chapter 3. In this chapter, formal procedures that can be used to integrate the findings of empirical research, and to estimate the magnitude of relations between concepts, are described. However, this chapter is not meant to be a thorough treatise on integrative reviews; therefore, readers are referred to the references and the additional readings listed at the end of this chapter.

PURPOSES OF INTEGRATIVE RESEARCH REVIEWS

The purpose of integrative research reviews is to determine the collective evidence across a series of studies about a phenomenon. In particular, the integration of research findings plays a pivotal role in the refutation or refinement of the middle-range theories and conceptual models that enhance understanding of phenomena and guide clinical practice. More specifically, the results of an integrative review represent the evidence that is, as Hunter and Schmidt (1990) pointed out, "indispensable for theory construction" (p. 40). Furthermore, the results of an integrative review supply the evidence that clinicians need to determine the "risks, benefits, and efficacy of clinical interventions" (Murphy, 1997, p. 1).

Consider, for example, a theory about the relation between the quality of the home environment provided by parents and the temperament of their prematurely born infant (see Holditch-Davis and Miles, 1997). Suppose that a review of several studies revealed no evidence of a relation between the quality of the home environment and premature infant temperament. In this case, the evidence indicates that the theory is not empirically or pragmatically adequate and the parent conceptual model, in turn, is not credible. Thus, further research is not warranted. Conversely, suppose that a review of the findings of many studies with diverse samples revealed consistent support for a strong relation between the quality of the home environment and premature infant temperament. In that case, further research addressing that relation also is not warranted. This is because the evidence indicates that the theory is empirically and pragmatically adequate and that the conceptual model from which the theory was derived is, in turn, credible. Suppose, however, that the relation was found to be strong in some studies but weak in others. In this case, the available evidence indicates that the original theory is not empirically or pragmatically adequate and the parent conceptual model may not be credible. Further research would, therefore, be needed to refine the theory and the conceptual model prior to its adoption in clinical practice, possibly by exploring the influence of one or more other concepts suggested by the conceptual model on the theoretical relation between home environment and premature infant temperament.

The procedures described in this chapter should be used to evaluate the cumulative evidence that will permit conclusions about the empirical adequacy and pragmatic adequacy of middle-range theories and the credibility of conceptual models. In particular, these procedures should be used when reviewing literature prior to undertaking a new study, making recommendations for future research, and preparing state-of-the-art manuscripts that present a critique and integration of existing studies, as well as recommending research-based clinical practice guidelines and public policies (Conn and Armer, 1996; Cooper, 1989).

The procedures for integrative reviews typically are applied to correlational and experimental studies dealing with two or more concepts. They also may be employed to integrate descriptive studies dealing with only one concept (Broome, 1993). The various approaches to concept analysis are, in fact, variations of integrative reviews that focus on a single concept (Rodgers and Knafl, 1993). In addition, descriptive research employing interpretative methods that yield qualitative data may be the subject of integrative reviews. Indeed, Sandelowski (1997) maintained that much more effort should be directed toward integrating the findings of research that employs interpretative methods. Moreover, studies of the psychometric properties of an empirical indicator for a concept may be the subject of an integrative review (e.g., Ottenbacher, Hsu, Granger, and Fiedler, 1996).

In short, integrative reviews are crucial to the advancement of knowledge. Moreover, they are essential to decision making about the continuation of current educational programs, nursing interventions, and medical treatments, or about the implementation of new programs, interventions, and treatments. Indeed, the evidence compiled in integrative reviews of research frequently is sought by governmental and private sector decision makers (Grady, 1997).

STEPS OF INTEGRATING RESEARCH FINDINGS

The integration of research findings encompasses three steps. The first step is the retrieval of studies that address a particular concept or concepts, within the context of one or more theories and conceptual models. The second step is the classification of studies according to the merit of research methodology and the type of findings, and the third step is the qualitative and/or quantitative integration of the findings of the studies. Some type of work sheet should be used to systematically record the studies retrieved and their classification. An example of a work sheet is given in Figure 4–1.

STEP ONE: RETRIEVAL OF STUDIES

The first step of an integrative review is the retrieval of relevant research. Integrative reviews should include all reports of pertinent studies that can be retrieved. Therefore, reviewers should use several sources and diverse retrieval strategies to locate studies.

Sources of Studies

The primary sources of studies are the journals, books, and monographs in the reviewer's personal library, along with publications found in university or other libraries. Other studies can be located in the reference lists of research reports already obtained, as well as in research documents obtained from state and federal government printing offices and in published bibliographies about a particular concept, theory, or conceptual model.

Other sources of studies include the reviewer's own research, reports given to the reviewer by students and faculty colleagues, master's theses and doctoral dissertations, and conference proceedings. Still another source of studies is the reviewer's own research network, or what Price (1966) called the "invisible college." The core of a research network is made up of highly influential, well-established investigators who communicate frequently with each other about their ongoing studies. Research networks also include less established investigators who may communicate with one or more of the core members, as well as with each other.

INDEXING AND ABSTRACTING SERVICES. Retrieval of relevant studies is facilitated by use of indexing and abstracting services. Printed and/or on-line computer

Citation Author(s)/ Year	Name of Conceptual Model	Name of Theory/ Concepts	Simple Size/ Characteristics	Instruments	Results	Effect Size	Quality of Study

Figure 4–1 ■ Work sheet for integrative research reviews.

versions of these services are available at university libraries, and many services are now available via personal computers with telecommunications capability. One limitation of print- or computer-based literature searches is that most data bases contain only published reports; another is the time lag between completion of a study and the appearance of the publication citation in the data base (Cooper, 1989). Access to unpublished research can be facilitated by use of data bases such as the Computer Retrieval of Information on Scientific Projects (CRISP), which contains citations of biomedical research supported by the United States Public Health Service, and Sigma Theta Tau International's on-line Registry of Nursing Research, which contains citations of ongoing and completed nursing research.

RETRIEVAL OF UNPUBLISHED STUDIES. A limitation of any integrative review is the inability to retrieve completed research that has never been presented at a conference or submitted for publication. Rosenthal (1979, 1991) pointed out that an estimated 95% of all the empirical research actually conducted remains in investigators' file drawers. That is because many investigators believe that reports of research with statistically nonsignificant (e.g., $p > .05$) results will not be accepted for publication. Furthermore, investigators whose findings conflict with a theory previously thought to be empirically adequate or a conceptual model regarded as credible may be reluctant to submit their reports because they believe that journal reviewers will reject such research (Cooper, 1989). In addition, novice researchers may not submit for publication papers presented at conferences, in the mistaken belief that the presentation and possible publication of an abstract in the proceedings is sufficient. Moreover, a great deal of thesis and dissertation research may not be submitted for publication, because of the investigators' lack of continued interest in their studies.

INCLUSION OF FLAWED STUDIES. Some research remains unpublished because it suffers from serious theoretical and/or methodological flaws. Conversely, some studies that suffer from serious theoretical or methodological flaws *are* published. The inclusion of flawed studies in an integrative review, whether published or unpublished, is a cause for concern because it is widely believed that such research yields inflated estimates of the strength of relations. This belief has been supported by the findings of some integrative reviews. For example, Brown (1992) found evidence of stronger effects for diabetes patient education programs in unpublished studies and in published studies with less rigorous designs.

Not all unpublished studies with or without flaws or published studies with flaws, however, yield inflated estimates of the strength of relations. For example, Heater, Becker, and Olson (1988) found no evidence of a statistically significant difference in the strength of relations in published versus unpublished studies in their integrative review of nursing interventions. Moreover, Kinney, Burfitt, Stullenbarger, Rees, and DeBolt (1996) found evidence of stronger relations in the better studies of the quality of life of cardiac patients.

Thus, although the inclusion of unpublished studies and published studies with flaws certainly will lead to a more comprehensive integrative review, it is unclear whether these studies will lead to a more accurate appraisal of the empirical adequacy of theories and the credibility of conceptual models. Therefore, reviewers should take into account the quality of each study as well as its publication status when reporting the findings of integrative research reviews.

RETRIEVAL COST AND TIME. The sources searched and the number and types of studies included in an integrative review may be limited by the reviewer's funding and time available for the project (Broome, 1993). The cost of an integrative review includes charges for on-line computer searches and photocopying, as well as the price of each thesis and dissertation obtained from University Microfilms. Additional costs are the salaries of the reviewer and the research assistants.

Furthermore, integrative reviews require a considerable amount of time to retrieve all of the studies, identify the most relevant studies, analyze and evaluate each study, and write the review. Publishers' or funding agency deadlines, as well as the reviewer's other commitments, may place a limit on the time available for the review. Therefore, reviewers should make every effort to secure adequate funding for the project and to begin the review many months prior to the deadline.

THREATS TO THE VALIDITY OF INTEGRATIVE REVIEWS. The validity of many integrative reviews is compromised by the reviewer's failure to consider the conceptual and theoretical basis of each study. Different conceptual models, of course, address different phenomena and, therefore, lead to different theories. Consequently, a decision must be made to limit the review to only one perspective or to justify the decision to include studies that reflect diverse conceptual and theoretical perspectives.

For example, the Boston-Based Adaptation Research Nursing Society (1998) prepared an integrative review of 25 years of research limited to studies that were explicitly derived from Roy's Adaptation Model (Roy & Andrews, 1991). Furthermore, in her integrative review of research related to the theory of uncertainty in acute illness, Mishel (1997) explicitly excluded the literature dealing with Selder's (1989) life transition theory because the latter theory does not specifically address acute illness. In contrast, Goeppinger and Lorig (1997) included four different theories—community development, self-efficacy, learned helplessness, and diffusion of innovations—in their integrative review of studies of community-based arthritis patient education. They explained that those theories "have strongly influenced the development, testing, and dissemination of the major community-based arthritis patient education interventions designed by nurse-researchers" (p. 113), and went on to compare study findings on the basis of the theory used.

Furthermore, a conceptual model can serve as the organizing framework for studies that are retrieved, even if the individual studies were not explicitly derived from that conceptual model. For example, Fetzer and Vogelsang (1995) used Orem's (1991) Self-Care Framework to guide their integrative review of ambulatory postanesthesia nursing research on patient outcomes. They explained, "Ambulatory postanesthesia nursing operates within two of Orem's basic nursing systems: partly compensatory and supportive-educative. Research findings should validate nursing assessment, actions, and interventions that promote self-care using these two systems thereby optimizing patient outcomes" (p. 250).

Another threat to the validity of an integrative review is the inability to identify all relevant studies (Cooper, 1989). This threat can be overcome by including as many sources of studies as is feasible to ensure that no avoidable bias exists. One avoidable bias would be the exclusion of a relevant indexing and abstracting service. For example, reviewers of health-related research should use both the *Cumulative Index to Nursing and Allied Health Literature* (CINAHL, on-line) and *Index Medicus* (MEDLINE, on-line), because the two data bases do not include exactly the same journals. A related avoidable bias would be the exclusion of dissertation research in the review, especially because the citations for many dissertations can easily be retrieved from the print or on-line versions of *Dissertation Abstracts International.* Another avoidable bias is an arbitrary restraint on the number of years included in an integrative review (e.g., the past 5 years) when it is widely known that the research has been ongoing for many years.

A reviewer may, of course, appropriately limit studies to be retrieved by specifying inclusion criteria. Goeppinger and Lorig (1996), for example, listed three inclusion criteria. One criterion was that the study had to examine the clinical outcomes of arthritis patient education. The second criterion was that the study had to include adults ages 18 and older with a confirmed diagnosis of osteoarthritis, rheumatoid arthritis, systemic lupus erythematosus, fibromyalgia, or a combination of those diseases, and that the unit of analysis was an aggregate, that is, populations of individual patients. The third criterion was that the studies were community-based, that is, the educational programs were led by community residents and were held in such community settings as churches, schools, and libraries.

Still another threat to validity is that the target population may not be adequately represented (Cooper, 1989). Reviewers cannot, of course, control the selection of samples by the primary investigators, but they can describe the missing elements of the target population and draw careful and precise conclusions regarding generalization of the findings of the integrative review. For example, Beck (1996a) noted that the generalizability of the integrative review finding of a moderate relation between postpartum depression and infant temperament was limited by lack of inclusion of samples of health professionals who could have provided objective measures of postpartum depression and infant temperament.

DOCUMENTING RETRIEVAL STRATEGIES. Unless the reviewer can provide a sound rationale for the exclusion of one or more sources of studies, all sources of research should be tapped. Moreover, all decisions regarding retrieval strategies should be documented in writing as the review progresses and should be justified (Broome, 1993). Documentation should include all sources utilized, along with the inclusive years and key words for each data base employed.

ASSESSING THE ADEQUACY OF RETRIEVAL. The adequacy of the number of studies retrieved can be determined by calculating a fail-safe number. This descriptive statistic represents the minimum number of unretrieved studies that might yield evidence of no relation between the concepts of interest, and which would be needed to overturn the findings of the integrative review. Stated in other words, the fail-safe number answers the question, "How many comparisons [or studies] totaling to a null hypothesis confirmation would have to be added to the results of the retrieved comparisons [studies] in order to change the conclusion that a relation exists?" (Cooper, 1989, p. 97). The formula for the fail-safe number is:

$$N_{FS.05} = \left(\frac{\sum\limits_{i=1}^{N} z_i}{1.645} \right)^2 - N$$

where

■ $N_{FS.05}$ = the number of additional null-summing comparisons needed to raise the combined probability to just above $p < .05$;

■ 1.645 = the standard normal deviate associated with $p < .05$ (one-tailed);

■ Z_i = the standard normal deviate for the ith comparison; and

■ N = the total number of comparisons in the integrative review.

(Cooper, 1989, p. 97)

The fail-safe number can be used in combination with a calculation to determine the reasonable level of tolerance for unretrieved studies. The tolerance formula is:

$$5K + 10$$

where

■ K = the number of comparisons or studies included in the integrative review.

(Rosenthal, 1991, p. 106)

For example, Beck (1996a) reported a fail-safe number of 809 unpublished studies. She went on to apply the tolerance formula to the 17 studies included in her integrative review and concluded that the fail-safe number of 809 exceeded the 95 unpublished studies that would need to be retrieved to overturn her finding of a moderate relation between postpartum depression and infant temperament. Although Beck did not provide sufficient data to show the calculation for the fail-safe number, the tolerance formula calculation can be shown. The calculation is:

$$5(17) + 10 = 85 + 10 = 95$$

The validity of the fail-safe number, according to Cooper (1989), is restricted by the assumption that the unretrieved studies would yield a cumulative finding of no relation between concepts. Cooper explained that the assumption is challenged by the possibility that the unretrieved studies actually would add support to the findings of the integrative review or would conflict in the opposite direction with those findings, rather than yielding a cumulative finding of no relation.

STEP TWO: CLASSIFICATION OF RESEARCH

The second step of research integration requires evaluation of the scientific merit of each study included in an integrative review, as well as assessment of the findings. The following discussion draws from but extends the contents of Chapter 3 of this book.

Evaluation of Scientific Merit

Evaluation of the scientific merit of each study should begin with rating the quality of the linkage of the conceptual model used to guide the study with the middle-range theory that was generated or tested and the empirical research methods. As noted throughout this book, the conceptual model should be explicitly identified. In addition, the conceptual model should be discussed in sufficient breadth and depth so that the links between its concepts and propositions, the middle-range theory concepts and propositions, and the empirical research methods are clear. Furthermore, consideration should be given to the logic of the linkages.

Evaluation of the scientific merit of each study continues with rating its operational adequacy. As discussed in Chapter 3, the operational adequacy criterion requires the empirical research methods to be congruent with the middle-range theory, and ultimately, with the parent conceptual model. Particular attention should be given to evaluation of the rigor of the research methods in terms of threats to internal and external validity. Comprehensive and now classic discussions of threats to validity are available in Cook and Campbell (1979) and Bracht and Glass (1968).

In addition, study characteristics that may reflect scientific merit should be assessed (Smith and Stullenbarger, 1991). Characteristics typically assessed include publication status (e.g., unpublished, published in a peer-reviewed journal, published in a book as a result of an invitation by the book editor, or dissertation), and funding status (e.g., no funding, intramural funding, or extramural funding).

Other typically assessed study characteristics may or may not have a bearing on scientific merit. These include authorship (e.g., single author or multiple authors), as well as the status and expertise of the first author (e.g., student or faculty member; rank or experience).

Broome (1993) pointed out that the evaluation of scientific merit reflects the amount of information provided in the research report, which is, at least in part, governed by journal or book chapter page limitations. Furthermore, Broome cautioned reviewers to avoid unintentionally inflating ratings by inferring what is not stated explicitly in the report, which is a special concern when the reviewer is already an expert in the research area.

METHODS OF CLASSIFYING SCIENTIFIC MERIT. The outcome of evaluation of the scientific merit of each study is its classification as more or less flawed. One method of classification is a continuum of scores ranging from "few flaws" to "many flaws." The continuum could include a "no flaws" pole, although it is unlikely that such a study ever could be conducted. Beck (1996a), for example, used a scoring continuum of 29 points—with higher scores indicating greater scientific merit—in her integrative review of studies of the relation between postpartum depression and infant temperament.

Another method of classifying scientific merit is a dichotomy, such as "good" and "bad" studies. For example, Brown (1992) used a dichotomous classification of "high quality" and "low quality" in her integrative review of the studies of diabetes patient education. Brown developed the dichotomy by means of a median split of the score for each study on a 21-point rating scale.

Cooper (1989) recommended relying on the conclusions reached by integrating the findings of "good" studies if overall results are different from those of "bad" studies. If no differences are evident, however, the "bad" studies should be retained because the additional data may facilitate refinement of a theory by providing clues to the generalizability of the theory and to intervening or extraneous variables. Rosenthal (1991) added, "The fundamental method of coping with bad studies, or more accurately, variations in the quality of research, is by differential weighting of studies. Dropping studies is merely the special case of zero weighting" (p. 130).

Assessment of Research Findings

Assessment of the findings of studies included in an integrative review is accomplished by classifying the results of each study as supportive or nonsupportive of the middle-range theory. That is, the theory is classified as empirically adequate or inadequate. In addition, the conceptual model should be classified as credible or not credible.

If relations were tested, each one can be considered separately or an overall conclusion regarding the evidence for or against the middle-range theory and the parent conceptual model can be drawn. The traditional criterion for tentative acceptance or rejection of hypotheses about relations is the statistical significance level. The level is most frequently set at $p < .05$, although a more or less stringent level may be used. When the criterion of statistical significance is used, each relation can be classified as statistically significant or nonsignificant. The direction of the relation (positive or negative), if known, also should be noted.

Each study also should be assessed for the magnitude of the findings. The observed incidence of a phenomenon, the strength of relations, and the extent of differences between treatment groups are examples of magnitude. The value of the additional information obtained when magnitude is taken into account is illustrated by a study of temperature measurement. Cusson, Madonia, and Taekman (1997) found that the temperature of the environment affects infants' temperatures at different body sites. In particular, they found a statistically significant elevation in tympanic membrane temperature compared with rectal, inguinal, and axillary temperatures when the infants were in a radiant warmer or in an incubator. They pointed out that although the temperature difference was statistically significant, "the clinical significance of this difference is less dramatic, particularly in the radiant warmer environment. However, in the incubator, the difference between tympanic and rectal temperature was 0.5°C and between tympanic and axillary, 0.9°C. Differences of this magnitude could result in alterations in clinical management" (p. 205). Cusson et al. went on to report that although the differences by site of temperature measurement across the environments of radiant warmer, incubator, and bassinet were statistically significant, "all of [these] differences were less than 0.5°C and thus not clinically significant" (p. 206).

Coding the Research

All information about each study should be entered into a database that reflects a code book developed by the reviewer (Broome, 1993; Cooper, 1989). The code book may require repeated revisions as the reviewer becomes increasingly familiar with the type of information that can be extracted from the studies and adds additional information about retrieval strategies. The various drafts of the code book should be used to code information about several studies prior to undertaking the coding of all studies to be used in the review.

Interrater reliability should be determined for the coding of the studies. The meaning of every item in the code book should be fully described, and raters should be given an opportunity to practice the coding (Cooper, 1989). Reviewers frequently report interrater reliability as the percentage of agreement and indicate that consensus was obtained on any disagreements between the raters. For example, Beck (1996a) reported that 100% agreement was achieved on most variables in the code book but that just 87% agreement was achieved on two other variables. She went on to report that "All disagreements were discussed until a consensus was obtained between the two raters" (p. 226). The Kappa coefficient or a Pearson product moment coefficient of correlation also can be used to calculate interrater reliability (Cooper, 1989; Rosenthal, 19981).

STEP THREE: INTEGRATION OF FINDINGS

The third step of research integration is the actual integration of the findings of the separate studies. The qualitative approach to integration is a narrative evaluation of related studies that leads to relatively subjective conclusions about the empirical adequacy and the pragmatic adequacy of a middle-range theory and the credibility of its parent conceptual model. The quantitative approach to integration uses statistical techniques that lead to relatively objective conclusions about the empirical and pragmatic adequacy of theories and the credibility of conceptual models.

Qualitative Integration of Research Findings

The typical review of research using a qualitative approach to integration of research findings includes a detailed narrative description of each study and its findings. The qualitative approach to research integration should be a true integration of related studies. Thus, this type of integrative review should not be limited to a serial or chronological listing of studies. Rather, the review should be a logical arrangement of ideas about the proposition or propositions of interest (Haller, 1992). For example, a study report may contain findings dealing with two propositions. Therefore, the relevant finding should be cited when discussing one proposition (e.g., $x_1 \rightarrow y$) and the other relevant finding should be cited later in the review when discussing the other proposition (e.g., $x_2 \rightarrow y$).

The literature review section of grant applications for new research and reports of completed research, including dissertations, most commonly is reported as a qualitative integration of related research. Conclusions regarding the empirical and pragmatic adequacy of the theory and the parent conceptual model typically reflect the reviewer's subjective impressions of the evidence rather than use of formal procedures of integration. An example of the qualitative approach to integration of research is Bauer's (1994) review of studies dealing with relations between psychosocial variables and immune function in people with cancer. She concluded that such psychosocial variables as coping style and social support were related to immune function and survival, and that behavioral interventions had a beneficial effect on overall survival and immunocompetence. Bauer did not, however, report any formal procedure that led to those conclusions.

The typical qualitative approach to integration of the findings of related studies is strengthened by use of a formal procedure to assess the empirical and pragmatic adequacy of a theory (Stinchcombe, 1968) and the credibility of a conceptual model. This procedure is based on the assumption that the studies are of equal scientific merit. One situation in Stinchcombe's procedure is the interpretation of multiple tests of the propositions of a theory that used the same empirical research methods with similar samples. If the findings for all of the tests of propositions are statistically significant in the hypothesized direction and reach the expected magnitude, then the appropriate interpretation is that the theory is more empirically and pragmatically adequate and the parent conceptual model is more credible than it would be with just one test.

The above situation is exemplified by tests of a theory of adaptation to chronic illness (Pollock, 1989, 1993), which was derived from Roy's (1984) Adaptation Model. A series of studies that tested the theory revealed support for the hypothesized relation between health-related hardiness and components of psychosocial adaptation in a total of 597 chronically ill adults divided into four diagnostic groups—rheumatoid arthritis, insulin-dependent diabetes, multiple sclerosis, and hypertension. The appropriate interpretation of the findings from those studies of chronically ill adults is that the theory is more empirically and pragmatically adequate and Roy's model is more credible than the theory and the model would be if only one diagnostic group had been included.

A second situation in Stinchcombe's procedure is the interpretation of multiple tests of a theory that used the same or similar empirical research methods with different samples or populations. If all findings of all tests of the propositions are statistically significant in the hypothesized direction and reach the expected magnitude, the appropriate interpretation is that the theory is much more empirically and pragmatically adequate and the parent conceptual model is much more credible.

Pollock's (1989) research with healthy adults illustrates the second situation. In that study, Pollock found that hardiness was again related to a component of psychosocial adaptation. When the findings of this study of well adults are combined with those of the studies of chronically ill adults, the appropriate interpretation is that the theory is much more empirically and pragmatically adequate and Roy's model is much more credible than the theory and the model were when only chronically ill adults were used as subjects.

In contrast to situations in which findings support the theory, consider those in which findings reject the theory. A theory may be considered empirically and pragmatically inadequate, and a conceptual model may be considered not credible, when any one test yields statistically nonsignificant findings. Researchers, however, rarely abandon a theory or a conceptual model after just one test. Nonetheless, if additional tests of equal scientific merit consistently reveal nonsignificant findings, the appropriate interpretation must be that the theory is not empirically or pragmatically adequate and the conceptual model is not credible. This situation is exemplified by repeated empirical tests that failed to yield support for the propositions comprising a theory of similarity in wives' and husbands' pregnancy-related experiences (Fawcett, 1989), which was derived from a conceptual model of the family based on Rogers' (1970) Life Process Model.

Stinchcombe's (1968) procedure is helpful when the findings of several studies of equal scientific merit are similar. When studies are of unequal merit and/or when findings conflict, a quantitative approach to integration is required.

Quantitative Integration of Research Findings

The two major approaches to the quantitative integration of research findings are the voting method and meta-analysis.

THE VOTING METHOD. The voting method, also referred to as the vote count or the box count, is the weaker of the two formal quantitative procedures used for integration of the findings of related studies. The voting method involves a simple tally of study findings as significantly positive (i.e., in the hypothesized direction), significantly negative (i.e., in the direction opposite to that hypothesized), or not statistically significant. The modal category is considered the winner and is assumed to be the best estimate of the empirical and pragmatic adequacy of the theory (Light and Smith, 1971) and the credibility of the parent conceptual model.

The voting method is based on the assumption that the nonmodal categories of findings are due either to chance alone or to undetected methodological errors. If studies differ in scientific merit, weights may be assigned to account for the differences in quality. Although exactly what weight to assign each study is a very complex question that requires further investigation (Hunter and Schmidt, 1990), suggestions include sample size or degrees of freedom, estimated quality of the study, internal validity, or "real-life representativeness (ecological validity)" (Rosenthal, 1991, p. 93).

Cooper (1989) recommended moving beyond reliance on the modal category of the voting method to use of the sign test to determine if the tally of results indicates that the hypothesized direction occurs more frequently than chance would suggest. He explained, "If the null hypothesis is true—that is, if no relation between the variables under consideration exists in the population sampled by any study—we would expect the number of findings in each direction to be equal" (p. 92). The formula for the sign test is:

$$Z_{vc} = \frac{(N_p) - (\frac{1}{2} \times N_t)}{\frac{1}{2}\sqrt{N_t}}$$

where

■ Z_{vc} = the Z-score for the overall series of comparisons;

■ N_p = is the number of positive findings; and

■ N_t = the total number of comparisons (positive plus negative findings).

(Cooper, 1989, p. 92)

The significance of Z_{vc} is determined by reference to a table of standard normal deviates.

The voting method and sign test are illustrated by the following example, drawn from Lusk's (1997) integrative review of the effects of work site health promotion and disease prevention programs. Lusk reported that 68 of 73 published studies demonstrated that diverse health promotion and disease prevention programs had positive effects on participants' health or resulted in cost savings for the employers. Application of the sign test to these results yielded a statistically significant $Z_{vc} = 7.37$, $p < .0002$, two-tailed. The calculation used to obtain this value is as follows:

$$\frac{68 - \frac{1}{2}(73)}{\frac{1}{2}\sqrt{73}} = \frac{31.5}{} = 7.37$$

These results support the empirical and pragmatic adequacy of the theories and the credibility of the conceptual models that guided the health promotion and disease prevention programs.

META-ANALYSIS. The techniques of meta-analysis are regarded as strong formal quantitative procedures. The term meta-analysis refers to "nothing more than the attitude of data analysis applied to quantitative summaries of individual [studies]" (Glass, McGaw, and Smith, 1981, p. 21). One technique combines the significance tests obtained from two or more independent studies. The other technique is the average effect size for a group of related studies.

Combining significance tests. The technique of combining significance tests can be accomplished in several ways, including adding logs of p levels, adding p levels, adding ts, adding Zs, adding weighted Zs, testing the mean p, and testing the mean Z (Rosenthal, 1991). This meta-analytic technique permits conclusions to be drawn about the empirical and pragmatic adequacy of a theory and the credibility of a conceptual model on the basis of the statistical significance of propositions that were tested.

The technique of combining significance tests is based on the assumption that the studies are essentially replicates of each other. Rosenthal (1991) outlined the advantages and limitations of each method of combining significance tests. He pointed out that the method of adding p levels, for example, requires exact probability values. Furthermore, although Rosenthal regarded this method as "useful and ingenious," he noted that it is "limited to small sets of studies, [because] it requires that the sum of the p levels not exceed unity [1.0] by very much" (p. 92). The formula for adding p levels is:

$$P = \frac{(\Sigma p)^N}{}$$

where

■ P = the overall significance level;

■ p = the exact probability for each study; and

■ N = the number of studies.

(Rosenthal, 1991, p. 90)

Carlson and colleagues (1996) used the method of adding p levels in their meta-analysis of the effects of occupational therapy for individuals 60 years and older. They reported an overall significance level of $P < .001$ across all 15 studies included in the meta-analysis. They also reported overall significance levels of $P < .05$ for 6 studies that included physical health outcomes, $P < .001$ for 10 studies that included psychosocial well-being outcomes, and $P < .001$ for 6 studies that included functional status outcomes. Carlson and colleagues did not provide the data to show the calculations for the combined P values. A constructed example, however, can be used. Suppose that three studies of the effect of support groups on adaptation to prostate cancer yielded P values of .03, .05, and .07 for the outcome of mood state. Here, the overall significance level, P, is calculated as follows:

$$\frac{(.03 + .05 + .07)^3}{(1)(2)(3)} = \frac{.15^3}{6} = \frac{.003375}{6} = .0006$$

Although the various methods of combining significance tests provide procedures for resolving conflicting findings, most methods do not take into account the merit of each study. An exception is the method of adding weighted Zs, which requires assignment of a weight reflecting scientific merit to the Z obtained in each study. As noted earlier in the section on the voting method, possible weights include the sample size or degrees of freedom, study quality, internal validity, or ecological validity (Rosenthal, 1991).

Furthermore, the voting method and combined significance tests have the same limitations as a single probability level—they depend on sample size and indicate only that the observed results occurred more or less by chance. Nothing is known about the magnitude of the findings across studies.

Average effect size. The magnitude of the findings of a group of studies can be determined by means of the meta-analytic technique of average effect size (Glass et al., 1981). Effect size is a standardized numerical index of the magnitude of a research finding, including the observed incidence of a phenomenon, the strength of relations, or the extent of differences between treatment groups. The technique of average effect size also takes into account the direction of research findings by attaching a plus [+] or minus [−] sign to each effect size used to calculate the average. Statistical significance also can be addressed with the average effect size technique by calculating a confidence interval. If the 95% confidence interval, for example, does not contain zero, it may be concluded that the findings of interest are statistically significant at the $p < .05$ level (Cooper, 1989). Thus, this meta-analytic technique permits conclusions to be drawn about the empirical and pragmatic adequacy of a middle-range theory and the credibility of a conceptual model on the basis of the magnitude, direction, and statistical significance of propositions that were tested.

Although investigators rarely include the effect size for statistics in their research reports, sometimes it can be calculated from the available statistical information. For example, the effect size for the correlation coefficient is the actual correlation coefficient, r. This metric usually is reported in correlational studies, although it is rarely labeled as the effect size. Formulas for the effect sizes for many other statistics are given in Cohen (1988), Cooper (1989), Hunter and Schmidt (1990), and Rosenthal (1991), among others. For example, one effect size metric for the difference between two groups, the d metric, can be obtained by the formula:

$$d = \frac{(X_1 - X_2)}{SD}$$

where

■ X_1 = the mean of one group (e.g., experimental group);

■ X_2 = the mean of the other group (e.g., control group); and

■ SD = the average standard deviation of the two groups.

(Cooper, 1985, p. 101)

Cooper pointed out that this formula for d is based on the assumption that the standard deviations for the two groups are approximately equal. If the assumption is not valid, d can be computed by using the standard deviation of one of the groups, typically the control group, if that standard deviation is available.

The technique of average effect size involves computation of an arithmetic mean for the effect sizes of two or more studies. The findings of the separate studies must be converted to a common effect size metric (e.g., r or d) and then averaged. Moreover, when the r metric is used, each effect size first must be transformed to Fisher's z_r, which is accomplished using the table of r to z_r transformations found in many statistics books and reprinted in Cooper (1989). A formula for the computation of the average effect size using the r metric is:

$$z_{av} = \frac{\sum_{i=1}^{N} (n_i - 3) z_i}{\sum_{i=1}^{N} (n_i - 3)}$$

where

- ■ z_{av} = the average effect size;

- ■ N = the total number of studies or comparisons;

- ■ n_i = the total sample size for the ith comparison; and

- ■ z_i = the Fisher's z_r value for the ith comparison.

(Cooper, 1989, p. 108)

When the d metric is used, one approach is to weight the effect size by the inverse of its variance to obtain an unbiased effect size estimate (Cooper, 1989), and then calculate the mean of the weighted effect sizes using the following formula:

$$d_{av} = \frac{\sum_{i=1}^{N} d_i w_i}{\sum_{i=1}^{N} w_i}$$

where

- ■ d_{av} = the average weighted effect size;

- ■ d_i = the effect size for the ith comparison;

- ■ w_i = the inverse of the variance associated with each effect size; and

- ■ N = the number of comparisons.

(Cooper, 1989, p. 108)

The interpretation of a single effect size or the average effect size is relative in that it depends on the size of other effects within a particular research area. A comprehensive discussion of the interpretation of various effect sizes is presented by Glass et al. (1981). Moreover, Cohen (1988) developed general guidelines for "small," "medium," and "large" effect sizes for different metrics that take into account the typical magnitude of findings from behavioral sciences research. For example, $r = .1$ is considered a small effect size; $r = .3$, a medium effect size; and $r = .5$, a large effect size. In contrast, $d = .2$ is considered a small effect size; $d = .5$, a medium effect size; and $d = .8$, a large effect size.

Rosenthal and Rubin (1982) have refined the interpretation of effect size with their binomial effect size display (BESD). The BESD is a measure of the rate of improvement (e.g., success rate, survival rate, cure rate, accuracy rate, selection rate) of a treatment, procedure, or predictor variable, and can be used to determine the pragmatic adequacy of the findings of one study or a group of studies. It is calculated by the formula:

$$.50 \pm \frac{r}{2}$$

where

■ r = the effect size expressed as a correlation coefficient;

■ + = the sign used for the experimental group; and

■ − = the sign used for the control group.

(Rosenthal, 1991, p. 134)

The BESD can be used with any effect size metric by converting the metric to r. Conversion formulas are given by Rosenthal (1991). One formula for the conversion of the effect size metric d to r is:

$$r = \frac{d}{\rule{2cm}{0.4pt}}$$

■ (Rosenthal, 1991, p. 20)

This formula is used when the total population from which the sample for one group has been drawn is equal or equal in principal to the total population from which the sample for the other group has been drawn, which is the case in most experimental studies. Application of the BESD formula for the average effect size in a meta-analysis of the effects of occupational therapy on functional status, physical health, and psychosocial well-being revealed an outcome success rate of 37% for the control group compared with an outcome success rate of 63% for the experimental groups, based on an average effect size of $d = +.54$ (Carlson et al., 1996). The calculations for the BESD reported by Carlson et al. require conversion of the effect size d to r, followed by application of the BESD formula. The calculations are as follows:

$$r = \frac{.54}{\rule{2cm}{0.4pt}} = \frac{.54}{\rule{1.5cm}{0.4pt}} = .26$$

$$.50 - \frac{.26}{\rule{1cm}{0.4pt}} = .50 - .13 = .37 \; [37\%]$$

$$.50 + \frac{.26}{\rule{1cm}{0.4pt}} = .50 + .13 = .63 \; [63\%]$$

The average effect size technique permits conflicting findings to be resolved because effect sizes that are in the hypothesized direction are averaged with those in the opposite direction. Furthermore, variations in substantive, methodological, and other study characteristics can be taken into account by comparing the average effect sizes of more flawed versus less flawed studies, published versus unpublished studies, recent versus older studies, and any other comparisons of interest to the reviewer. In addition, substantive characteristics can be considered, such as subject age or gender. If such characteristics are found to be associated with the effect size, a theory about the relations between the concepts of interest may have to be modified to account for the characteristic.

Beck's (1996a) meta-analysis of the effects of postpartum depression on infant temperament is an example of the technique of average effect size. Beck reported unweighted and weighted effect sizes using the r metric. The average effect size was $r = .36$ when effects were unweighted; $r = .31$, when weighted by sample size; and $r = .35$, when weighted by a quality of study score. Using Cohen's (1988) standards for the r metric, Beck noted that the obtained average effect sizes indicated a positive relation of moderate strength between postpartum depression and infant temperament. Beck reported that the 95% confidence interval ranged from .261 to .369, which indicated a statistically significant relation between postpartum depression and infant temperament. The BESD was not reported.

Beck also explored the relation of substantive and methodological study characteristics to effect size. The substantive characteristics were mother's and infant's ages, as well as mother's parity, marital status, ethnicity, education, socioeconomic status, and employment status. The methodological characteristics were date and type of publication (journal, book, dissertation), source (computer, journal issue, or dissertation search), number of authors, funding, country, sampling technique, sample size, research design, data collection method, statistics used, type of measurement for postpartum depression and infant temperament, and instruments used. None of the substantive characteristics and just two of the methodological characteristics were negatively related to effect size: year of publication, $r = -.65, p = .006$; and sample size, $r = -.81, p = .0004$.

Initial interpretation of the findings of Beck's (1996a) meta-analysis indicate that the theory of a relation between postpartum depression and infant temperament is empirically adequate. Judgment regarding pragmatic adequacy depends on whether a relation of moderate strength is regarded as large enough to warrant the development and testing of interventions that might reduce postpartum depression. The evidence also supports the credibility of the conceptual model that guided the studies. That conceptual model was not explicitly identified by Beck, although she alluded to a different conceptual perspective in the discussion of the findings.

More specifically, Beck claimed that the interpretation of the moderate relation between postpartum depression and infant temperament was problematic because infant temperament ratings were done by the mothers. She pointed out that a multimethod rating strategy using an objective observer as well as the mother would be more appropriate. In addition, Beck noted that the instruments used to measure postpartum depression may not have been sufficiently sensitive to detect the minor episodes of depression that have been observed in new mothers. Beck also noted that few longitudinal studies have been conducted. All of these issues suggest that Beck would use a different conceptual model and associated empirical research methods to guide development of her own theory of postpartum depression and infant temperament, one that would lead to longitudinal research using multiple raters of infant temperament and instruments that are sensitive to both minor and major postpartum depression.

Given Beck's conceptual and methodological concerns, it is likely that she would conclude that the theory of a relation between postpartum depression and infant temperament as tested in the studies that she included in the meta-analysis is *not* empirically adequate and its parent conceptual model is *not* credible. The difference between the initial interpretation and Beck's possible interpretation underscores the influence of a conceptual model and its associated empirical research methods on conclusions about data.

Uses of meta-analysis. Meta-analysis typically is used to determine the average effect of an experimental treatment. Indeed, most of the literature on meta-analysis focuses on experimental research. For example, Moody (1990) explained that meta-analysis is used when findings regarding the effects of interventions conflict across studies, when data from a series of experimental studies could be used to test a theory, when lingering questions about interventions could be answered by a statistical summary of results across studies, or when the need for additional research on an intervention is controversial.

In recent years, considerable attention has been given to the applicability of meta-analysis for descriptive and correlational research as well (e.g., Hunter and Schmidt, 1990; Reynolds, Timmerman, Anderson, and Stevenson, 1992). Wilkie and her associates (1990), for example, conducted a meta-analysis of descriptive studies to determine normative values on the McGill Pain Questionnaire (MPQ). They noted that the information obtained from the meta-analysis "is crucial to help pain researchers make informed decisions about using the MPQ" (p. 36). Beck's (1996a) meta-analysis of the relation between postpartum depression and infant temperament is an example of meta-analysis applied to correlational research.

COMPUTERS AND INTEGRATIVE REVIEWS. Integrative reviews may be facilitated by the use of computer software programs for management of the literature that serves as the data base for the review. The archs© computer program was designed to store and manage the literature, graphically depict relations between concepts, and identify gaps and conflicts in the findings of related studies (Graves, 1990; Sigma Theta Tau International, 1997). Furthermore, computer programs for meta-analysis are given in Mullen and Rosenthal (1985) and Hunter and Schmidt (1990). Moreover, Mullen and Rosenthal (1985) and Mullen (1989) developed computer software programs for management of the meta-analysis data base and calculation of effect sizes. Mullen's (1989) program is described in detail by Beck (1996b).

Comparison of Qualitative and Quantitative Integrative Reviews

Integrative reviews of research that employ quantitative methods generally are more informative than qualitative narrative reviews because the quantitative reviews include an estimate of the magnitude of the findings, such as the observed incidence of a phenomenon, the strength of a relation, or the extent of the difference between treatment groups. A comparison of the steps involved in qualitative and quantitative integrative reviews is shown in Figure 4–2.

McCain and Lynn's (1990) meta-analysis of 15 of the 29 studies of patient teaching included in Wilson-Barnett and Oborne's (1983) qualitative narrative review illustrates the increase in information obtained in a quantitative review. Wilson-Barnett and Oborne concluded that patient teaching has a beneficial effect. McCain and Lynn's meta-analysis of the 15 studies that provided sufficient data for calculation of effect sizes revealed a weighted average effect size of $d = +.50$. Their finding indicated that "there was indeed a clear benefit of patient teaching: The score of the average individual in the experimental group exceeded that of 69% of the individuals in the control group" (McCain and Lynn, 1990, p. 352).

McCain and Lynn (1990) also calculated average effect sizes for various categories of studies. The categories, which were based on the goals of teaching, and their respective average effect sizes were as follows: improving knowledge, $d = +.54$; improving compliance, nonsignificant effect size; improving physical well-

Identify concept(s)
Formulate questions to be answered by the review
Search the literature
Extract relevant information*

Qualitative Approach	Quantitative Approach
Describe the literature	Calculate effect sizes
Critically evaluate the literature	Examine relations between methodological and substantive variables
Integrate the results in a narrative format	Integrate the results by reporting the average effect size

State future research and practice implications

* See Figure 4-1, work sheet for integrative research reviews.

Figure 4–2 ■ Integrative reviews of research: comparison of qualitative and quantitative approaches. (Adapted from Broome, 1993, p. 197, with permission.)

being, $d = +.43$; improving psychological well-being, $d = +.59$; and improving self-care, $d = +.55$. These effect size calculations revealed that teaching was not effective in one of the teaching goal categories, whereas the results of the narrative review indicated that teaching was effective in all five teaching goal categories.

CONCLUSION

Investigators usually conclude their research reports by recommending that the study be replicated or that the research be extended to determine the generalizability of findings or to discover more about the nature of theoretical propositions. Although researchers tend to believe that "more is better," there are times when a research area should be abandoned because the underlying theory is not empirically adequate and the conceptual model is not credible, or the magnitude of findings is so small that no matter how many studies are conducted, pragmatic adequacy will never be established.

A research area also should be abandoned when the evidence from several studies supports the empirical adequacy of the theory and the credibility of the conceptual model. In this case, little if any knowledge is to be gained by continuing the research. Thus, the use of the procedures for integrating research findings presented in this chapter should help scholars to determine the empirical adequacy and the pragmatic adequacy of middle-range theories and the credibility of conceptual models and decide if more research is, indeed, warranted.

References

Bauer, S.M. (1994). Psychoneuroimmunology and cancer: An integrated review. *Journal of Advanced Nursing, 19*, 1114–1120.

Beck, C.T. (1996a). A meta-analysis of the relationship between postpartum depression and infant temperament. *Nursing Research, 45*, 225–230.

Beck, C.T. (1996b). The practical computer: Use of a meta-analytic data base management system. *Nursing Research, 45*, 181–184.

Boston-Based Adaptation Research Nursing Society. (1998). *Roy adaptation model-based research: 25 years of contributions to nursing science.* Indianapolis: Sigma Theta Tau International Center Nursing Press.

Bracht, G.H., & Glass, G.V. (1968). The external validity of experiments. *American Educational Research Journal, 5*, 437–474.

Broome, M.E. (1993). Integrative literature reviews in the development of concepts. In B.L. Rodgers & K.A. Knafl (Eds.), *Concept development in nursing: Foundations, techniques, and applications* (pp. 193–215). Philadelphia: Saunders.

Brown, S.A. (1992). Meta-analysis of diabetes patient education research: Variations in intervention effects across studies. *Research in Nursing and Health, 15*, 409–419.

Carlson, M., Fanchiang, S.-P., Zemke, R., & Clark, F. (1996). A meta-analysis of the effectiveness of occupational therapy for older persons. *American Journal of Occupational Therapy, 50*, 89–98.

Cohen, J. (1988). *Statistical power analysis for the behavioral sciences* (2nd ed.). Hillsdale, NJ: Lawrence Erlbaum.

Conn, V.S., & Armer, J.M. (1996). Meta-analysis and public policy: Opportunity for nursing impact. *Nursing Outlook, 44*, 267–271.

Cook, T.D., & Campbell, D.T. (1979). *Quasi-experimentation. Design and analysis issues for field settings.* Boston: Houghton Mifflin.

Cooper, H.M. (1989). *Integrating research: A guide for literature reviews* (2nd ed.). Newbury Park, CA: Sage.

Cusson, R.M., Madonia, J.A., & Taekman, J.B. (1997). The effect of environment on body site temperature in full-term neonates. *Nursing Research, 46*, 202–207.

Fawcett, J. (1989). Spouses' experiences during pregnancy and the postpartum. *Image: Journal of Nursing Scholarship, 21*, 149–152.

Fetzer, S.J., & Vogelsang, J. (1995). An integrative review of ambulatory postanesthesia nursing patient outcome research: 1982–1993. *Journal of Postanesthesia Nursing*, *10*, 249–258.

Glass, G.V., McGaw, B., & Smith, M.L. (1981). *Meta-analysis in social research.* Beverly Hills: Sage.

Goeppinger, J., & Lorig, K. (1997). Interventions to reduce the impact of chronic disease: Community-based arthritis patient education. In J.J. Fitzpatrick & J. Norbeck (Eds.), *Annual review of nursing research* (Vol. 15, pp. 101–122). New York: Springer.

Grady, P.A. (1997). News from NINR. *Nursing Outlook*, *45*, 113.

Graves, J.R. (1990). A research-knowledge systems (ARKS [archs©]) for storing, managing, and modelling knowledge from the scientific literature of nursing. *Advances in Nursing Science*, *13*(2), 34–45.

Haller, K.B. (1992). Solving puzzles [Editorial]. *Journal of Obstetric, Gynecologic, and Neonatal Nursing*, *21*, 444.

Heater, B.S., Becker, A.M., & Olson, R.K. (1988). Nursing interventions and patient outcomes: A meta-analysis of studies. *Nursing Research*, *37*, 303–307.

Holditch-Davis, D., & Miles, M.S. (1997). Parenting the prematurely born infant. In J.J. Fitzpatrick & J. Norbeck (Eds.), *Annual review of nursing research* (Vol. 15, pp. 3–34). New York: Springer.

Hunter, J.E., & Schmidt, F.L. (1990). *Methods of meta-analysis. Correcting error and bias in research findings.* Newbury Park, CA: Sage.

Kinney, M.R., Burfitt, S.N., Stullenbarger, E., Rees, B., & DeBolt, M.R. (1996). Quality of life in cardiac patient research: A meta-analysis. *Nursing Research*, *45*, 173–180.

Light, R.J., & Smith, P.V. (1971). Accumulating evidence: Procedures for resolving contradictions among different research studies. *Harvard Educational Review*, *41*, 429–471.

Lusk, S.L. (1997). Health promotion and disease prevention in the work site. In J.J. Fitzpatrick & J. Norbeck (Eds.), *Annual review of nursing research* (Vol. 15, pp. 187–213). New York: Springer.

McCain, N.L., & Lynn, M.R. (1990). Meta-analysis of a narrative review. Studies evaluating patient teaching. *Western Journal of Nursing Research*, *12*, 347–358.

Mishel, M.H. (1997). Uncertainty in acute illness. In J.J. Fitzpatrick & J. Norbeck (Eds.), *Annual review of nursing research* (Vol. 15, pp. 57–80). New York: Springer.

Moody, L.E. (1990). Meta-analysis: Qualitative and quantitative methods. In L.E. Moody (Ed.), *Advancing nursing science through research* (Vol. 2, pp. 70–110). Newbury Park, CA: Sage.

Mullen, B. (1989). *Advanced BASIC meta-analysis.* Hillsdale, NJ: Lawrence Erlbaum.

Mullen, B., & Rosenthal, R. (1985). *BASIC meta-analysis: Procedures and programs.* Hillsdale, NJ: Lawrence Erlbaum.

Murphy, P.A. (1997). Evidence-based care: A new paradigm for clinical practice [Editorial]. *Journal of Nurse-Midwifery*, *42*, 1–3.

Orem, D.E. (1985). *Nursing: Concepts of practice.* (3rd ed.) New York: McGraw-Hill.

Ottenbacher, K.J., Hsu, Y., Granger, C.V., & Fiedler, R.C. (1996). The reliability of the Functional Independence Measure: A quantitative review. *Archives of Physical Medicine and Rehabilitation*, *77*, 1226–1232.

Pollock, S.E. (1989). The hardiness characteristic: A motivating factor in adaptation. *Advances in Nursing Science*, *11*(2), 53–62.

Pollock, S.E. (1993). Adaptation to chronic illness: A program of research for testing nursing theory. *Nursing Science Quarterly*, *6*, 86–92.

Price, D. (1966). Collaboration in an invisible college. *American Psychologist*, *21*, 1011–1018.

Reynolds, N.R., Timmerman, G., Anderson, J., & Stevenson, J.S. (1992). Meta-analysis for descriptive research. *Research in Nursing and Health*, *15*, 467–475.

Rodgers, B.L., 7 Knafl, K.A. (Eds.), *Concept development in nursing: Foundations, techniques, and applications.* Philadelphia: Saunders.

Rogers. M.E. (1970). *An introduction to the theoretical basis of nursing.* Philadelphia: F.A. Davis.

Rosenthal, R. (1979). The "file drawer problem" and tolerance for null results. *Psychological Bulletin*, *86*, 638–641.

Rosenthal, R. (1991). *Meta-analytic procedures for social research* (rev. ed). Beverly Hills: Sage.

Rosenthal, R., & Rubin, D.B. (1982). A simple, general purpose display of magnitude of experimental effect. *Journal of Educational Psychology*, *74*, 166–169.

Roy, C. (1984). *Introduction to nursing: An adaptation model* (2nd ed.). Englewood Cliffs, NJ: Prentice-Hall.

Roy, C., & Andrews, H.A. (1991). *The Roy adaptation model: The definitive statement.* Norwalk, CT: Appleton and Lange.

Sandelowski, M. (1997). "To be of use": Enhancing the utility of qualitative research. *Nursing Outlook*, *45*, 125–132.

Selder, F. (1989). Life transition theory: The resolution of uncertainty. *Nursing and Health Care*, *10*, 437–451.

Sigma Theta Tau International. (1997). New technology will impact nursing research, education, practice. *Nursing Excellence, June,* 2.

Smith, M.C., & Stullenbarger, E. (1991). A prototype for integrative review and meta-analysis of nursing research. *Journal of Advanced Nursing, 16,* 1272–1283.

Stinchcombe, A.L. (1968). *Constructing social theories.* New York: Harcourt, Brace and World.

Wilkie, D.J., Savedra, M.C., Holzemer, W.L., Tesler, M.D., & Paul, S.M. (1990). Use of the McGill Pain Questionnaire to measure pain: A meta-analysis. *Nursing Research, 39,* 36–41.

Wilson-Barnett, J., & Oborne, J. (1983). Studies evaluating patient teaching: Implications for practice. *International Journal of Nursing Studies, 20,* 33–44.

Additional Readings

Bailar, J.C. (1995). The practice of meta-analysis. *Journal of Clinical Epidemiology, 48,* 149–157.

Bangert-Drowns, R.L. (1986). Review of developments in meta-analytic method. *Psychological Bulletin, 99,* 388–399.

Beck, C.T. (1995). Meta-analysis: Overview and application to clinical nursing practice. *Journal of Obstetric, Gynecologic, and Neonatal Nursing, 24,* 131–135.

Brown, S.A. (1991). Measurement of quality of primary studies for meta-analysis. *Nursing Research, 40,* 352–355.

Bryant, F., & Wortman, P.M. (1984). Methodological issues in meta-analysis of quasi-experiments. *New Directions in Program Evaluation, 24,* 25–42.

Cook, T.D., Cooper, H., Cordray, D.S., Hartmann, H., Hedges, L.V., Light, R.J., Louis, T.A., & Mosteller, F. (Eds.). (1992). *Meta-analysis for explanation.* New York: Russell Sage Foundation.

Cook, T.D., & Leviton, L.C. (1980). Reviewing the literature: A comparison of traditional methods with meta-analysis. *Journal of Personality, 48,* 449–472.

Dykeman, M.C., & Loukissa, D. (1993). The science of unitary human beings: An integrative review. *Nursing Science Quarterly, 6,* 179–188.

Engle, V.F., & Graney, M.J. (1990). Meta-analysis for the refinement of gerontological nursing research and theory. *Journal of Gerontological Nursing, 16*(9), 12–15.

Hedges, L.V., & Olkin, I. (1985). *Statistical methods for meta-analysis.* Orlando, FL: Academic Press.

Hedges, L.V., Shymansky, J.A., & Woodworth, G. (1989). *A practical guide to modern methods of meta-analysis.* Washington, DC: National Science Teachers Association.

Jackson, G.B. (1980). Methods for integrative reviews. *Review of Educational Research, 50,* 438–460.

Jensen, L.A., & Allen, M.N. (1994). A synthesis of qualitative research on wellness-illness. *Qualitative Health Research, 4,* 349–369.

Lynn, M.R. (1989). Meta-analysis: Appropriate tool for the integration of nursing research? *Nursing Research, 38,* 302–305.

Mosteller, F. (1994). *Meta-analysis for medicine: Applications and methods.* Boston: Harvard School of Public Health.

Noblit, G.W., & Hare, R.D. (1988). *Meta-ethnography: Synthesizing qualitative studies.* Newbury Park, CA: Sage.

Pillemer, D.B., & Light, R.J. (1980). Synthesizing outcomes: How to use research evidence from many studies. *Harvard Educational Review, 50,* 176–195.

Sandelowski, M., Docherty, S., & Emden, C. (1997). Qualitative meta-synthesis: Issues and techniques. *Research in Nursing and Health, 20,* 365–371.

Sampselle, C.M., Burns, P.A., Dougherty, M.C., Newman, D.K., Thomas, K.K., & Wyman, J.F. (1997). Continence for women: Evidence-based practice. *Journal of Obstetric, Gynecologic, and Neonatal Nursing, 26,* 375–385.

Stock, W.A., Okun, M.A., Haring, M.J., Miller, W., Kinney, C., & Ceurvorst, R.W. (1982). Rigor in data synthesis: A case study of reliability in meta-analysis. *Educational Researcher, 11*(6), 10–14, 20.

Vrabec, N.J. (1997). Literature review of social support and caregiver burden, 1980 to 1995. *Image: Journal of Nursing Scholarship, 29,* 383–388.

Wolf, F. (1986). *Meta-analysis: Quantitative methods for research synthesis.* Newbury Park, CA: Sage.

5 Writing Research Proposals and Reports

■ The analysis of conceptual-theoretical-empirical (C-T-E) structures and the technique of C-T-E formalization, the criteria for evaluation of C-T-E structures, and the methods of integrating research findings, presented in Chapters 2 to 4, can be used not only to analyze and evaluate existing research documents but also to prepare those documents. This chapter presents guidelines for the preparation of research documents that emphasize the close connections between conceptual models, middle-range theories, and empirical research methods. Examples from existing research documents are used to illustrate the guidelines. The chapter concludes with specific suggestions that should facilitate the writing of proposals for research and reports of the completed research.

GUIDELINES FOR RESEARCH PROPOSALS AND REPORTS

The guidelines for writing research proposals and reports are summarized in Table 5–1. The guidelines address the customary sections of a research document. In the case of a research proposal, the usual sections consist of the introduction to the research problem, including the conceptual and theoretical components of the C-T-E structure, and the method, which encompasses all parts of the empirical component of the C-T-E structure. In the case of reports of completed research, the usual sections consist of the introduction to the research problem, the method, the results, and the discussion of results. These guidelines can be used to prepare applications for research funds, journal articles, books or book chapters, monographs, dissertations, theses, and other documents such as papers for doctoral degree qualifying and preliminary examinations. Readers are, however, cautioned to refer to the specific

---

Table 5–1   ■   **GUIDELINES FOR WRITING RESEARCH PROPOSALS AND REPORTS**

For All Research Documents

Abstract
The abstract presents a concise summary of the conceptual-theoretical-empirical structure.
* State the purpose of the research.
* Identify the conceptual model that guides the research.
* For theory-testing research, identify the theory that will be or was tested.
* Describe the research design and methods.
* For reports of completed research, summarize and interpret the research results.

Introduction
The introduction establishes the need for theory-generating or theory-testing research to investigate a particular physical, psychological, social, or behavioral problem. The introduction also identifies the frame of reference for the research.
* Summarize the social significance of the research by explaining how the study addresses a research priority or social policy issue.
* Summarize the theoretical significance of the research by explaining how the study extends or fills gaps in existing theories about a phenomenon of interest to a discipline.
* State the purpose or specific aims of the study.
* Describe the background for the study.
    —Summarize the conceptual model that guides the study.
    —Describe the linkages between the conceptual model, the theory concepts and propositions, and the empirical research methods.
    —For theory-testing research, describe the theory that will be or was tested.
    —Provide a critical review of relevant theoretical and empirical literature, including pilot or preliminary studies conducted by the investigator.
    —For theory-testing research, provide constitutive definitions for the concepts of the theory to be tested.
    —For theory-testing research, provide evidence regarding any propositions that are to be tested.
    —For theory-testing research, state the research hypotheses.
    —For research proposals, link the proposed study to long-range goals in a program of research.

Method
The method section includes a description of the sample, instruments, procedure, and data-analysis plan.
* Describe the sample.
    —Describe the source of the data (individuals, groups, animals, documents).
    —Identify the number of participants and report the power analysis calculations.
    —Explain how participants will be or were recruited.
    —Give anticipated or actual refusal and attrition rates.
    —Identify restrictions on the sample and relevant characteristics that set the limits on generalizability of study findings.
    —Explain how informed consent will be or was obtained.
* Identify each instrument used.
    —Identify the theory concept measured by each instrument.
    —Describe the psychometric properties of each instrument, including validity and reliability for the study sample.
    —Describe the items on each instrument and the scale used to rate the items.
    —Identify the range of possible scores and explain how the scores are interpreted.
    —For experimental research, describe the experimental and control treatment protocols.
* Describe the procedures used to collect the data.
    —Identify the data collectors.
    —Identify the setting and time required for data collection.
    —For experimental research, describe the experimental and control conditions.
    —State the order of administration of the instruments.
    —For research proposals, provide a timetable for the conduct of all phases of the study, from training of personnel to preparation of the final report.

Table 5–1 ■ GUIDELINES FOR WRITING RESEARCH PROPOSALS AND REPORTS (Continued)

—For research proposals, provide a detailed protocol for protection of human or animal subjects.
• Describe the data-analysis plan.
—Identify the strategies for data processing and the statistical techniques for analysis of the data.

For Reports of Completed Research

Results
The results section presents the findings of data analysis. This section is structured according to specific aims, purposes, or hypotheses.
• For theory-generating research, identify and describe the concepts and propositions of the theory that emerged from the analysis of data.
• For theory-testing research, provide descriptive statistics for study variables and the results of inferential statistical tests of hypotheses.
• For theory-testing research, draw a definitive conclusion regarding support or lack of support for each hypothesis.

Discussion
The discussion section presents the investigator's interpretation of the results. This section also is structured according to specific aims, purposes, or hypotheses.
• Draw conclusions with regard to the empirical adequacy of the theory and the credibility of the conceptual model.
• Provide alternative methodological and/or substantive explanations.
• Identify implications for future research.
• Discuss pragmatic adequacy, including implications for formulation of practice guidelines and public policies.

---

directions for preparation of research documents provided by each funding agency, journal or book publisher, or university.

Tables and figures can be used throughout a proposal for research or a report of completed research to convey a large amount of information succinctly. Guidelines for constructing tables and figures are given in Table 5–2.

Examples taken from two funded research grant proposals and several published research reports are used to illustrate the guidelines given in Tables 5–1 and 5–2. Complete references are available in the original documents for the literature cited in the examples. All examples focus on the generation or testing of middle-range theories that were derived from or linked with explicit conceptual models.

THE ABSTRACT

The abstract for any research document presents a concise summary of the C-T-E structure. All abstracts should include a statement of the purpose of the research and identify the conceptual model that guides the research. The statement of the research purpose may include a sentence that identifies the social or theoretical significance of the research. In abstracts of theory-testing research, the theory that will be or was tested also is identified. In addition, abstracts frequently include a brief description of the empirical research methods, including the number and particularly important characteristics of the sample and, if space permits, the instruments used and the data-analysis techniques employed. Reports of completed re-

---

Table 5–2 ■ **GUIDELINES FOR CONSTRUCTING TABLES AND FIGURES**

Tables
Use a table to summarize a large amount of numerical data or text in a small amount of space. Limit the number of tables, reserving them only for information that would be difficult or cumbersome to read if presented in narrative form.
• Provide a number and a succinct, informative title for every table.
• Refer to every table and highlight the most relevant information in the narrative.
• Provide headings for all rows and columns of the table.
• Provide enough information for the table to be understandable without reference to the narrative.
• Identify all units of measurement for numerical values.
• Explain all abbreviations that are not standard statistical abbreviations.
• Use the minimum number of decimal places for appropriate precision in the particular unit of measurement.
• Be consistent in the use of rounded numbers and decimal places.
• Present probability values within a column of the table or use asterisks for different probability values in a footnote to the table.
• Use single words, short phrases, or succinct sentences for text-based tables.

Figures
Use a figure to convey an overall pattern of numerical data or linkages between concepts at the same level or different levels of abstraction. Figures include charts, line or bar graphs, circle or pie graphs, scatter plots, photographs, drawings, diagrams of conceptual-theoretical-empirical structures, diagrams of constitutive definitions for multidimensional concepts, and diagrams of relational propositions. Limit the number of figures, reserving them only for information that can be presented best in pictorial form.
• Provide a number and a succinct, informative title for every figure.
• Refer to every figure and highlight the most relevant information in the narrative.
• Provide enough information for the figure to be understandable without reference to the narrative.
• Identify all units of measurement for numerical values.
• Explain all abbreviations that are not standard statistical abbreviations.
• Use different symbols or types of shading to represent different times, groups, or experimental and control treatments.
• Use captions to explain data.

---

search include a succinct summary of the results and the investigator's interpretation of those results. In abstracts for theory-generating research reports, the result is the theory that emerged from the analysis of the data, including its concepts and their dimensions. In abstracts for theory-testing research reports, the results are the findings of statistical tests.

The exact format of an abstract is specified by the agency, organization, publisher, or university to whom the document will be submitted. Some agencies, organizations, and journal publishers require a structured abstract with explicit headings, whereas others specify an unstructured format. Virtually all agencies, organizations, publishers, and universities place an upper limit on the number of words to be contained in an abstract.

The following example of an abstract was taken from a funded research proposal. The experimental research, which was guided by Roy's Adaptation Model (Roy and Andrews, 1991), was designed to test a predictive theory of the effects of different types of social support and education on emotional and interpersonal adaptation to breast cancer.

■ Example: **ABSTRACT FROM A RESEARCH PROPOSAL**

The purpose of the proposed three-group controlled clinical trial with repeated measures is to test the effectiveness of an intervention designed to promote emotional and interpersonal adaptation to the diagnosis and treatment of breast cancer. The study design and the selection of the outcome variables were guided by our recently completed research on short-term group support, Roy's Adaptation Model, the research literature describing the impact of breast cancer diagnosis and treatment sequelae, and the research literature on social support and education related to adaptation to cancer. The proposed study extends our recently completed research investigating the effects of short-term (8 weeks) group support beginning at 1 to 3 months postdiagnosis on adaptation to breast cancer diagnosis and treatment.

A combined 13-month program of individual and group social support and education will be provided to women newly diagnosed with non-metastatic breast cancer. The individual support and education component will be provided via telephone; the group support component, by group meetings of subjects and facilitators. Subjects ($N = 174$) will be randomized, by cohort, into three study treatment groups: the experimental treatment group will receive combined individual social support and education via telephone along with group social support; control treatment group 1 will receive individual social support and education only via telephone; and control treatment group 2 will receive education only through mailed information manuals. The adaptation outcomes are mood disturbance, cancer–related worry, well-being, quality of relationship with significant other, and loneliness. A cost analysis will be used to calculate the economic costs of each study treatment and to compare breast cancer–related direct and indirect costs, from time of entry into the study, of the three study treatment groups.

Although numerous interventions currently are available, there is no evidence that any of these interventions meet the changing emotional and interpersonal needs of women during their entire first year following diagnosis. The experimental treatment in the proposed project is designed to meet the evolving emotional and interpersonal needs of women following diagnosis, during and following the termination of adjuvant treatment, and continuing through the 1-year "anniversary" of the diagnosis. An intervention that can meet the needs of the one in nine women who will be diagnosed with breast cancer, thus assisting them with adaptation, has potentially significant clinical implications. Although the proposed study focuses on women with breast cancer, the experimental treatment has the potential to enhance adaptation in patients with various types and stages of malignant disease. The experimental treatment also may enhance adaptation to other chronic diseases. (Samarel, Fawcett, and Tulman, 1995–1997)

The next example of an abstract was taken from the final report of a federally funded study. The correlational research was designed to test an explanatory theory of correlates of functional status in childbearing women. The theory was derived from Roy's Adaptation Model (Andrews and Roy, 1986).

■ Example: **ABSTRACT FROM A FINAL REPORT OF FUNDED RESEARCH**

The prospective panel study was designed to measure changes in functional status and determine the relationship and relative importance of selected health, individual psychosocial, family, and demographic variables to functional status during pregnancy and the postpartum period. Functional status during pregnancy was defined as the extent to which the pregnant woman continues her usual personal-care, household, social and community, child-care, and occupational activities. Postpartum functional status was defined as the woman's readiness to assume infant-care responsibilities and resume usual personal-care, household, social and community, child-care, and occupational activities.

A sample of 250 low-risk English-speaking married women was recruited from obstetrical and nurse-midwifery practices during the first trimester of pregnancy. The women were followed until 6 months after delivery, with data collected at the end of each trimester of pregnancy and at 3 weeks, 6 weeks, 3 months, and 6 months postpartum using questionnaires and semi-structured interview schedules administered in subjects' homes by trained research assistants. Of the 250 women enrolled in the study, 233 completed the study through pregnancy; 226 completed the study through the 6-month postpartum visit for an attrition rate of 9.6% over the course of the year during which the subjects were followed.

Overall functional status increased from the first to the second trimesters, and then declined during the third trimester. During the postpartum period, functional status improved from 3 weeks to 6 weeks, from 6 weeks to 3 months, and from 3 months to 6 months. During the third trimester of pregnancy, less than half of the women (46.7%) reported full functional status. At 6 weeks postpartum, the medical end of the postpartum period, barely half of the women (56.6%) had regained their usual prepregnancy levels of functional status.

During pregnancy, the health variables of physical energy, number of physical symptoms, presence of complications, medical restrictions, and parity were related to level of functional status. In addition, the individual psychosocial variables of acceptance of pregnancy, fear of pain, helplessness, and loss of control during labor, identification with the motherhood role, preparation for labor, and anxiety were related to functional status. Moreover, the demographic variables of income and education also were related to functional status. However, family variables were found not to be related to the women's functional status during pregnancy.

During the postpartum period, the number of physical symptoms, physical energy, type of delivery, presence of complications during labor and delivery, and parity were the health variables that were related to functional status. Furthermore, the individual psychosocial variables of satisfaction with the parental role, maternal competence, and anxiety were related to functional status. Moreover, the family variables of infant fussiness and quality of the marital relationship were related to functional status, and the demographic variables of age, income, and employment status were related to functional status.

When all of the variables found to be related to functional status were simultaneously analyzed, health variables accounted for the largest amount of the variance, followed by individual psychosocial variables for pregnancy. At 3 and 6 weeks and 3 months postpartum, health variables continued to account for the largest amount of the variance. However, at 6 months postpartum, individual psychosocial variables accounted for the largest amount of the variance.

This study was limited to women who were low-risk at the time of enrollment during the mid to later part of the first trimester of pregnancy. Further research is warranted into changes in functional status in high-risk women and the mates of both high- and low-risk women to obtain a more complete picture of the childbearing population as well as to explore similarities and differences between the high- and low-risk groups. Knowledge of alterations in maternal and paternal functional status during the childbearing period among high-risk and low-risk couples would provide an empirical base for formulating clinical interventions to facilitate their performance of usual social role activities during pregnancy and the postpartum period, as well as a data-based social policy regarding parental leave. (Tulman and Fawcett, 1994)

The following example is a structured abstract taken from a journal article reporting the results of theory-generating research. The research, which was based on Neuman's (1995) Systems Model and Degner and Beaton's (1987) life-death decisions in health care framework, generated a theory of the why, how, and by whom of dialysis treatment modality decision making.

▪ Example: **STRUCTURED ABSTRACT FOR THEORY-GENERATING RESEARCH IN A JOURNAL ARTICLE**

Objective: The purpose of this qualitative study was to elicit patients' perceptions of why, how, and by whom their dialysis treatment modality—hemodialysis or continuous ambulatory peritoneal dialysis (CAPD)—was chosen.

Design: The study design utilized a naturalistic method of inquiry employing a qualitative approach. The research was guided by the life-death decisions in health care framework developed by Degner and Beaton and the Neuman Systems Model.

Sample/Setting: Twenty-two informants were recruited from inpatient and outpatient renal dialysis units at a large urban tertiary care center on the east coast of the United States.

Methods: Data were collected by individual, focused, semistructured in-depth interviews.

Results: A grounded theory, "Patient's Choice of a Treatment Modality versus Selection of Patient's Treatment Modality," emerged from the data provided by the informants. The theory consisted of 11 themes that addressed the why, how, and by whom of decision making: self decision; access rationing decision; significant other decision; to live decision; physiologically dictated decision; expert decision; to-be-cared-for decision; independence versus dependence decision; no patient choice in making decision; patient preference/choice; and switching modalities due to patient preference/choice.

Conclusion: The themes reflected two patterns of decision making: the patient and/or significant other chose the treatment modality, and the treatment modality was selected because of clinical or practical circumstances. (Breckenridge, 1997b, p. 313)

The next example of a structured abstract was taken from a journal article reporting the results of correlational research designed to test an explanatory theory of the relation of spirituality, perceived social support, and death anxiety to nurses' willingness to care for AIDS patients. The theory was derived from Rogers' (1992) Science of Unitary Human Beings.

■ Example: **STRUCTURED ABSTRACT FOR THEORY-TESTING RESEARCH IN A JOURNAL ARTICLE**

Objective: Use Rogers' (1992) framework of the science of unitary human beings to examine relationships among spirituality, perceived social support, death anxiety, and nurses' willingness to care for AIDS patients.

Design: Descriptive, correlational.

Population, Sample, Setting: Population, female RNs in New York City metropolitan area who care for patients with AIDS. Convenience sample of 220 RNs who worked in eight hospitals either on AIDS-dedicated units ($n = 88$), or medical-surgical scatterbed units ($n = 132$) with a daily AIDS patient census of between 5 to 50%. Data were collected in 1992.

Measures: Spiritual Orientation Inventory, the Personal Resource Questionnaire-85, the Templer Death Anxiety Scale, and the Willingness to Care for AIDS Patients Instrument.

Methods: Pearson product-moment correlations and hierarchical multiple regression analyses to test hypotheses.

Findings: Willingness to care for AIDS patients was positively correlated with spirituality and perceived social support, and negatively correlated with death anxiety. Death anxiety moderated the relationship between spirituality and willingness to care. In total, 17% of the variance in nurses' willingness to care for AIDS patients was explained. Additional regression analyses indicated that group membership as either an AIDS-dedicated nurse or medical-surgical nurse did not moderate or change hypothesized relationships.

Conclusion: Because group membership explained 22% of the variance in willingness to care, the data indicate that group culture or professional identity should be further examined as predictors of nurses' willingness to care for AIDS patients.

Clinical Implications: Social support at work from administrators and colleagues, as well as the support from patients themselves is important to nurses and should be fostered. (Sherman, 1996, p. 205)

The next example is an unstructured abstract, which was taken from a journal article reporting the results of theory-generating research. The ethnographic study, which was based on Orem's (1991) Self-Care Framework, generated a descriptive naming theory of Mexican-American people's meanings and expressions of pain and associated self-care and dependent-care actions. Specification of the conceptual model that guided the research has been added to the abstract in [brackets] to illustrate how this important information could be incorporated. The conceptual model was identified explicitly within the introductory section of the full research report.

■ Example: **UNSTRUCTURED ABSTRACT FOR THEORY-GENERATING RESEARCH IN A JOURNAL ARTICLE**

The experience of pain within specific cultural groups has not been well studied. The purpose of this ethnographic study [which was guided by Orem's Self-Care Framework] was to discover Mexican-American meanings, expressions, and care associated with pain. Data were obtained from 20 key and 14 general informants and analyzed using thematic and pattern analysis. Themes identified included: pain as [an] encompassing experience of suffering; the obligation to bear pain and to endure it stoically; and the primacy of caring for others. Based on study findings, a beginning description of the cultural context is provided from which pain as experienced by Mexican-Americans can be understood and from which culturally competent nursing care can be designed. (Villarruel, 1995, p. 427)

The following example of an unstructured abstract was taken from a journal article reporting a correlational study designed to test an explanatory theory of correlates of grief responses. The research was guided by Roy's Adaptation Model (Roy and Andrews, 1991).

■ Example: **UNSTRUCTURED ABSTRACT FOR THEORY-TESTING RESEARCH IN A JOURNAL ARTICLE**

This ex post facto descriptive correlational design study of widows during their second year of bereavement utilizes Roy's adaptation model as a guiding framework. Contextual stimuli (social support, social network, income/education, spiritual beliefs) were related to the cognator function (coping process), which was related to adaptation outcome (grief response). Significant moderate positive relationships were found between social support and coping process, and between social network and coping process. A significant relationship also was found between coping process and grief

> response. The path model accounted for 18% [of the] explained variance. (Robinson, 1995, p. 158)

INTRODUCTION TO THE RESEARCH PROBLEM

The introduction section of a research document provides an overview of the problem. This section establishes the need for the research and identifies the frame of reference that guides it. The introduction has three major subsections: a brief description of a physical, psychological, social, or behavioral problem that requires investigation, a statement of the purpose of the research, and the background literature.

Description of the Research Problem

The research problem subsection should present a compelling reason for the research. It is *not* sufficient to state that no research dealing with the topic has been conducted (Downs, 1994). Rather, the social significance and the theoretical significance of the research are described. The social significance of the research can be established by identifying the magnitude or prevalence of a problem or by explaining how the research addresses a socially sanctioned priority or social policy issue. The theoretical significance of the research can be established by delineating what is already known about the problem and explaining how the current research extends or fills gaps in existing theories about a phenomenon of interest to a discipline.

The following examples illustrate the description of the social and theoretical significance of research. The first example illustrates how social significance can be described by identifying the magnitude of a social problem. The second example illustrates how theoretical significance can be established by a brief review of current research and identification of the gap in existing theories. The excerpts were taken from a journal article reporting the results of correlational research designed to test an explanatory theory of the relation of various concepts representing basic conditioning factors to the adjustment responses of children and their mothers to the children's cancer. The theory was directly derived from Orem's (1995) Self-Care Framework.

■ Example: **DESCRIPTION OF THE SOCIAL SIGNIFICANCE OF A STUDY**

The American Cancer Society (1997) estimates that approximately 1,382,400 new cases of cancer will be diagnosed in the United States in 1997. Of these cases, an estimated 8,000 will be children. In the past, receiving a diagnosis of cancer meant impending death, but approximately 71% of children affected with cancer today will survive. (Moore and Mosher, 1997, p. 519)

■ Example: **DESCRIPTION OF THE THEORETICAL SIGNIFICANCE OF A STUDY**

It is only now, because the majority of children are surviving, that the long-term effects of cancer and its therapy are being identified. Physiologic effects such as cardiac, neurologic, pulmonary, and endocrine abnormalities related to therapy have been discovered, as well as second malignancies. The psychosocial adjustment of survivors, however, is less well-documented. In the nursing literature, researchers have focused almost exclusively on the physiologic rather than psychosocial effects of cancer. (Moore and Mosher, 1997, p. 519)

Purpose of the Research

The subsection containing the statement of the research purpose might come at the end of the introduction, or it could be the very first sentence of the research document. The research purpose is stated precisely and concisely. Proposals for or reports of completed theory-generating research identify the topic to be studied. In theory-testing research, the statement of the research purpose typically identifies the main concepts and propositions of the theory.

The purpose of the study may be stated as a list of aims, in narrative form, or in the form of research questions. The typical format for research proposals is a list of specific aims, whereas a narrative or question format frequently is seen in reports of completed research. The statement of the research purpose also may identify the kind of research.

The following example illustrates the statement of the research purpose in the form of specific aims. The excerpt was taken from a funded proposal for an experimental study designed to test a predictive theory of the effects of different types of social support and education on emotional and interpersonal adaptation to breast cancer. The theory was based on Roy's Adaptation Model (Roy and Andrews, 1991).

■ Example: **PURPOSE OF THE STUDY STATED AS AIMS**

The specific aims of the proposed study, which is derived from Roy's Adaptation Model (Roy and Andrews, 1991), are to:

1. Test the effects of an experimental intervention consisting of extended duration (13-month) Individual and group social support and education by describing and comparing emotional and interpersonal adaptation among three groups of women with breast cancer: (1) those who receive an experimental treatment combination of individual and group social support and education; (2) those who receive a control treatment of individual social support and education only; and (3) those who receive a control treatment of education only.

2. Determine the subjects' perceptions of their adaptation to breast cancer by identifying their perceptions of breast cancer; and their descrip-

> tion of the effect of study participation on their emotional and inter-
> personal adaptation.
> 3. Analyze the direct (the sum of the intervention and breast cancer–
> related health care costs from time of entry into the study) and indi-
> rect breast cancer–related economic costs for the experimental and
> control treatments. (Samarel et al, 1995–1997)

The next two examples illustrate the statement of the research purpose in narrative form. The first example was taken from a journal article reporting the results
of descriptive research that employed the ethnographic method to generate a descriptive naming theory of Mexican-American people's meanings and expressions
of pain and associated self-care and dependent-care actions. The research was guided
by Orem's (1991) Self-Care Framework.

■ Example: **PURPOSE OF THEORY-GENERATING RESEARCH
STATED IN NARRATIVE FORM**

> The purpose of this ethnographic investigation was to discover Mexican-
> American meanings and expressions of pain and to describe associated self-
> care and dependent-care actions. (Villarruel, 1995, p. 428)

The second example was taken from a journal article reporting the results of
experimental research designed to test a predictive theory of the effects of special
"boomerang" pillows on respiratory vital capacity. The theory was based on Levine's
Conservation Model (Schaefer and Pond, 1991).

■ Example: **PURPOSE OF THEORY-TESTING RESEARCH
STATED IN NARRATIVE FORM**

> The purpose of this study was to determine whether the use of
> boomerang pillows as compared with conventional or straight pillows de-
> creased the respiratory capacity. (Roberts, Brittin, Cook, and deClifford,
> 1994, p. 158)

The next two examples illustrate the statement of the research purpose in question form. The first example was taken from a journal article reporting the results
of descriptive research designed to generate a descriptive naming theory of the incidence of pressure ulcers in an acute care hospital, a rehabilitation hospital, a skilled
care nursing home, a hospital-based home health agency, and a hospice agency. The
second example was taken from a journal article reporting the results of experimental research designed to test a predictive theory of the effectiveness of a pressure ulcer prevention or early intervention program on the prevalence of pressure
ulcers in a rehabilitation hospital. Both theories were based on Levine's Conservation
Model.

■ Example: **PURPOSE OF THEORY-GENERATING RESEARCH STATED AS A RESEARCH QUESTION**

This prospective, concurrent, descriptive study was guided by four research questions:

1. What is the incidence of pressure ulcers acquired after admission to each of the five patient care settings?
2. What are the specificity and sensitivity of the Braden Scale for predicting pressure sore risk in each of the five patient care settings?
3. What is the Braden Scale score for each of the five patient care settings that best predicts [pressure ulcer] risk?
4. What factors are predictive of pressure ulcer development after admission to each of the five patient care settings? (Langemo, Olson, Hunter, Hanson, Burd, and Cathcart-Silberberg, 1991, p. 26)

■ Example: **PURPOSE OF THEORY-TESTING RESEARCH STATED AS A RESEARCH QUESTION**

This study focused on the following question: What is the effectiveness of a pressure ulcer prevention or early intervention program in reducing the prevalence of pressure ulcers in a rehabilitation setting? (Hunter et al., 1995, p. 251)

Background

The background subsection includes a description of the conceptual model that guides the research. The need to explicitly identify the conceptual model that guides the research is underscored by the fact that this component of a research proposal is included in the criteria used to evaluate research grant proposals submitted to the National Institutes of Health (Grant, 1997).

The background subsection also includes a critical and integrative review of relevant theoretical and empirical literature. Using the analogy of pieces of a jigsaw puzzle, Haller (1992) explained that "Good literature reviews organize pieces of knowledge in a meaningful way, allowing us to see the big picture and stimulating us to take further action" (p. 444). The literature review for most research documents should not, however, include all that is known about the research problem and related methodology. Rather, this subsection should include only those citations that provide the rationale for the kind of research conducted and for any hypotheses proposed (Brooks-Brunn, 1991). Indeed, Downs (1994) recommended the citation of no more than four references for each point in the literature review. She explained:

■ Readers will believe a thorough literature search was done without an exhaustive list of all the studies available on the subject. Use the most recent and credible work as evidence. Unless an early study contains information that is of a stature that cannot be ignored, use only the most recent evidence for support.

. . . [Moreover,] a literature review dominated by a laundry list of citations is boring reading. It usually signals the author's inability to synthesize the content. In a good literature review, the reason the current research was undertaken and the logic behind the choice of variables is clear. . . . The importance of the work comes from the evidence in the review that discontinuities or ambiguities exist in available knowledge. (p. 323)

The exception to the guideline of no more than four references for each point is when the purpose of the research document is to present a comprehensive integrated review. Furthermore, the limitation on the number of references included in the literature review does not mean that the investigator has not read the older literature and considered the place of each previous study and competing theories in the development of a particular theory.

THEORY-GENERATING RESEARCH. In theory-generating research proposals or reports, the background subsection may be quite brief. Here the conceptual model that guides the study is summarized and linked to the research problem and empirical research methods. The typical literature review is a critical discussion of previous theoretical and empirical works that clearly underscores the lack of knowledge that supports the need for a theory-generating study.

The following example of the background subsection was taken from a journal article reporting a secondary analysis of data that was designed to generate a descriptive classification theory of dialysis modality decision making. The empirical research methods and theory were guided by Neuman's Systems Model. The excerpt illustrates the explicit identification of the conceptual model upon which the empirical research methods were based and clearly links that conceptual model to the theory that was generated. Furthermore, the literature review enhances understanding of the need for the study by presenting a brief review of related descriptive reports.

■ Example: **BACKGROUND FOR THEORY-GENERATING RESEARCH**

The conceptual framework used for the original study of clients' perceptions (Breckenridge, 1995) was based on the Neuman Systems Model (1995), which specifically asks clients to assess their own situations. In keeping with the first line of assessment of the Neuman Systems Model, the source of data in [that] study was the clients' perceptions of why, how, and by whom the decision regarding dialysis modality was made.

Qualitative research related to the life of the client with ESRD [end-stage renal disease] who is undergoing dialysis has been conducted by asking the client questions from instruments developed from the health care provider's perspective (Deniston, Carpertier-Atling, Kneisley, Hawthorne, and Port, 1989; Evans et al., 1985). Wu (1993) states that there is a great need to study life on dialysis from the client's perspective. Therefore, a qualitative study based on a conceptual model presenting the client's perspective as the phenomenon of interest is both timely and necessary.

> The Neuman Systems Model further guided this secondary analysis because it fits well with the holistic concept of optimizing a dynamic yet stable interrelationship of spirit, mind, and body in a constantly changing environment and society. Holism, a central feature of the Neuman Systems Model, is a philosophical viewpoint that directs attention to relationships and processes arising from wholeness as the person adjusts to stressors in internal and external environments. Based on a holistic systems approach both to protect the client and to promote client welfare, nursing actions must be skillfully related to the meaningful and dynamic organization of the variables making up the whole client system (Neuman, 1995).
>
> The Neuman Systems Model considers the person a system. Five variable areas are considered:
>
> 1. physiologic—bodily structure and function
> 2. psychologic—mental processes and relationships
> 3. sociocultural—combined social and cultural functions
> 4. developmental—life developmental processes
> 5. spiritual—spiritual belief influence
>
> In keeping with the Neuman Systems Model, the investigator specifically looked for data that reflected these five variable areas in this secondary analysis. (Breckenridge, 1997a, p. 55)

THEORY-TESTING RESEARCH. In theory-testing research proposals or reports of completed research, a concise summary of the conceptual model is presented and relational definitions linking the conceptual model concepts and propositions with the concepts and propositions of the middle-range theory that will be or was tested are given. A diagram of the C-T-E structure for the study also may be presented here (Table 5–2, Guidelines for Constructing Tables and Figures). The review of literature includes statements of the theory propositions and critical discussion of the evidence for each proposition. Constitutive definitions for the theory concepts may be given as each concept is introduced. Alternatively, constitutive definitions may be given when the empirical indicators are described in the method section. Relational propositions may introduce the paragraph(s) dealing with relations between particular concepts, or these propositions may be presented as the summary statements. The review of literature may conclude with a statement of the research hypotheses. The concepts and propositions of the theory that are explicated in the narrative also may be depicted in a diagram (Table 5–2, Guidelines for Constructing Tables and Figures).

The following example illustrates how a conceptual model can be linked to an existing theory and how a C-T-E structure can be discussed and displayed in a journal article. The excerpt was taken from a report of correlational research designed to test an explanatory theory of pain experienced by Mexican-American and Anglo-American women undergoing elective surgery. The theory was based on Roy's Adaptation Model (Roy and Andrews, 1991). The narrative continued with a detailed discussion of each component of the C-T-E structure.

■ Example: **BACKGROUND FOR THEORY-TESTING RESEARCH
WITH LINKAGE OF CONCEPTUAL MODEL TO
THEORY CONCEPTS AND PROPOSITIONS AND A
DIAGRAM OF THE CONCEPTUAL-THEORETICAL-
EMPIRICAL STRUCTURE**

Roy's adaptation model provided the boundaries and identified the scope of
the study. The major concepts described in Roy's model provided direction for
identifying relevant variables and in designing the study. According to the adaptation model of nursing, persons are biopsychosocial beings in constant interac-
tlon with a changing environment (Andrews and Roy, 1991). Persons cope with
the changing environment by a positive response known as adaptation. Internal
or external stimuli (focal, contextual, and residual) affect the behavior of a person. The person adapts to these stimuli through four adaptive modes: physiologic, self-concept, interdependence, and role function (Andrews and Roy, 1991).

The gate control theory of pain developed by Melzack and colleagues (1975,
1983) and research literature related to pain and culture, anxiety, social support,
self-esteem and sick role provided operational definitions of the concepts and
propositions to be tested. This theory proposes that pain is not just a physiologic response to tissue damage but that sociocultural and psychologic variables
influence the perception of pain as well. The gate control theory suggests that
many pre-existing factors, such as expectations of a culture, influence pain im-
pulses in the brain and how the person responds overtly during the pain experience. Empirical indicators for measuring each of the major variables were identified through the model and its supporting theories. Figure [5–1] demonstrates
the conceptual-theoretical-empirical structure . . . as applied to Roy's adaptation
model and the gate control theory of pain. (Calvillo and Flaskerud, 1993, p. 119)

The next example illustrates how conceptual model concepts and propositions
can be used to derive an explanatory theory, including the specification of the relational propositions of that theory. The excerpt was taken from the report of correlational research designed to test an explanatory theory of the relation of severity
of illness, hardiness, perceived control over visitation, and state anxiety to length
of stay (LOS) in an intensive care unit (ICU). The theory was derived from Roy's
Adaptation Model (Roy and Andrews, 1991). The excerpt illustrates the specification of relational propositions and hypotheses, stated in concept names. In addition,
the concepts and propositions of the theory are depicted in a diagram.

■ Example: **BACKGROUND FOR THEORY-TESTING RESEARCH,
WITH LINKAGE OF CONCEPTUAL MODEL TO
THEORY, SPECIFICATION OF RELATIONAL
PROPOSITIONS AND HYPOTHESES, AND A DIAGRAM
OF THE THEORY CONCEPTS AND PROPOSITIONS**

The interdependence mode is the category of human responses identified by Roy and Andrews (1991) that focuses on interactions related to the

Major Concepts of the Adaptation Model

	Environmental Stimuli Independent Variables			Adaptive Modes: Limits of Adaptation Dependent Variables			
Adaptation Model Concepts	Focal	Contextual	Residual	Physiological	Self-Concept	Role Function	Interdependence
Gate Control Theory Concepts	Noxious Stimulus	Psychological Emotional Factors	Sociocultural Factors	Regulation of Senses: Pain	Self-Consistency and Self-Esteem	Sick Role	Support System
Empirical Indicators	Elective Cholecystectomy	1. State-Trait Anxiety Scale 2. Anxiety Analog Scale	1. Sample Selection Criteria 2. Sociodemographic Items 3. Acculturation Scale	1. McGill Pain Questionnaire 2. Total Number of Pain Medications 3. Blood Pressure, Pulse, and Respirations 4. Pain Evaluation by Nurse (PPI) 5. Total Amount of Pain Medication Taken	1. Self-Esteem Inventory 2. Sense of Coherence Scale	1. Activities of Daily Living Scale 2. Length of Hospital Stay	1. Zich's Social Support Scale 2. Number of Visitors 3. Identity of Visitors

Figure 5–1 ■ Conceptual-theoretical-empirical structure for a study. (From Calvillo and Flaskerud, 1993, p. 119, with permission.)

giving and receiving of love. The goal of the interdependence mode is achievement of affectional adequacy, that is, emotional support. Tedrow (1991) stated, "People who are ill . . . usually experience an increased need for love, respect, and affirmation" (p. 391) that can lead to improved physiologic status. Yet on admission to an ICU, critically ill patients are often separated from significant others.

[Figure 5–2 depicts the linkage of the conceptual model and theory concepts, as well as the relations between the concepts of the theory that was tested.] The focal stimulus confronting an ICU patient is severity of illness. Perceived control over visitation (PCV) is a contextual stimulus that modifies the effects of the major or focal stimulus. As a contextual stimulus, PCV modifies the effect that severity of illness exerts on length of stay (LOS). State anxiety is another contextual stimulus that modifies the effect of the focal stimulus and influences perceptions of control over visitation. Hardiness is viewed as a residual stimulus because it is an internal factor a patient brings to an ICU. Hardiness influences perceptions of control as well as LOS in the unit.

In this study, a proposition of the interdependence mode proposed by Roy and Roberts (1981) was tested. The proposition is: Freedom of communication patterns will positively influence the adequacy of seeking and receiving affection. It is assumed that the more PCV one feels, the more freedom of communication one has, which can have a positive relationship to seeking and receiving affection as reflected by physiologic mode adaptation, that is, by a decreased LOS.

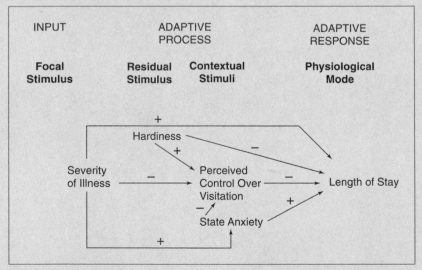

Figure 5–2 ■ Diagram of linkages between conceptual model and theory concepts and relational propositions of the theory. (From Hamner, 1996, p. 216, with permission.)

The following hypotheses were developed:

1. Severity of illness will have (a) a direct negative effect on perceived control over visitation; (b) a direct positive effect on LOS; (c) a direct positive effect on state anxiety; and (d) an indirect positive effect on LOS through PCV. That is, as severity of illness increases, PCV decreases, causing an increase in LOS.
2. PCV has a direct negative effect on LOS.
3. Hardiness will have (a) a direct positive effect on PCV; (b) a direct negative effect on LOS; and (c) an indirect negative effect on LOS through PCV. That is, as hardiness increases, PCV increases, causing a decrease in LOS.
4. State anxiety will have (a) a direct negative effect on PCV; (b) a direct positive effect on LOS; and (c) an indirect positive effect on LOS through PCV. That is, as state anxiety increases, PCV decreases, causing an increase in LOS. (Hamner, 1996, p. 215)

PRELIMINARY STUDIES. The background subsection of both theory-generating and theory-testing research documents may include discussion of pilot studies or preliminary research conducted by the investigator. The following example was taken from a funded research grant proposal for an experimental study designed to test a predictive theory of the effects of different types of social support and education on emotional and interpersonal adaptation to breast cancer. The theory was based on Roy's Adaptation Model (Roy and Andrews, 1991). The excerpt presents a description of preliminary studies undertaken by the investigators in preparation for the proposed study.

■ Example: **DESCRIPTION OF PRELIMINARY STUDIES IN A RESEARCH PROPOSAL**

We have recently completed a project designed to examine the effect of short-term (8 week) group social support and education, with and without coaching by a significant other, in an experimental study with a sample of 181 women with newly diagnosed early-stage breast cancer [Samarel, Fawcett, and Tulman, 1997]. This study, which was based on Roy's Adaptation Model (Roy and Andrews, 1991), has been funded by the American Cancer Society (#PBR-64A) and the National Institutes of Health-National Cancer Institute (KO7, Career Development Grant used for principal investigator (PI) salary support). Dr. Samarel is the PI for the study; Dr. Fawcett serves as the co-investigator (ACS) and sponsor (KO7), and Dr. Tulman is the methodology and statistics consultant. Data were collected at the time of entry into the study (baseline), at the end of the 8-week support group (posttest$_1$) and again 8 weeks later (posttest$_2$). Subjects were randomized into one experimental treatment group (receiving group social support and education with coaching, $n = 58$), and two control treatment groups (control group 1, receiving group social support and education without coaching, $n = 64$; and control group 2, no support or education, $n = 59$). In a check of randomization, statistical analyses revealed that the three groups were equivalent on demographic variables and the baseline measures of the quantitative outcome variables (symptom distress, emotional distress, functional status, and changes in the quality of the relationship with the significant other). Qualitative data from interviews, program evaluations, and follow-up questionnaires were collected to enhance quantitative posttest measures.

Mean age of the sample was 52.5 years with a range of 28–86 years. All subjects were tumor, node, metastasis (TNM) Stage I or II. Subjects entered the study at an average of 2.6 months following surgery. Of the 181 subjects, 114 (63%) had a mastectomy. Eighty-three (46%) of the 181 women received adjuvant chemotherapy during study participation. All 67 of the women who had lumpectomies received radiation therapy during study participation or had recently completed a course of radiation therapy.

Analysis of the outcome variables for the 181 subjects revealed that unmarried women in the experimental treatment and control treatment 1 groups (group social support and education, with and without coaching) experienced significantly less ($p = .043$) emotional distress, as measured by the Profile of Mood States-Linear Analogue Self-Assessment, than their counterparts who were in the control treatment 2 group (no social support or education). Furthermore, both married and unmarried subjects in the experimental treatment group experienced significantly greater ($p = .019$) improvement in their interpersonal relationships with significant others, as measured by the Relationship Change Scale, than the subjects in the two control treatment groups. Interestingly, the improvement in interpersonal relationships was even more significant ($p = .003$) for those married women participating in the experimental treatment group. These effects, however, were only observed at the end of the 8-week treatment period and were not sustained 2 months following the termination of group support. Subjects in the control treatment group 2 (no social support or education) actually experienced a decline in the quality of interpersonal relationships.

The quantitative findings with regard to the effects on emotional and interpersonal responses were further supported by our qualitative interview data from the 120 study subjects who completed interviews conducted 8 weeks after the end of the intervention. In particular, chi-square analyses of the coded interview data revealed that the experimental and control treatment 1 groups experienced a statistically significant ($p < .0001$) improvement in emotional well-being and relationships with significant others over the control treatment 2 group. These results indicated that group social support and education enhanced emotional and interpersonal adaptation to breast cancer diagnosis and treatment. There were, however, no differences between the experimental treatment and control treatment 1 groups, indicating that the addition of coaching to group social support and education had no effect. Therefore, coaching by a significant other will not be a component of the intervention in the proposed study.

There were no differences among the groups in symptom distress or functional status at either posttest period. This may be due to the fact that an intervention consisting of social support and education would more logically have a direct effect only on emotional and interpersonal responses. We have, therefore, limited the proposed study to the examination of the effects of social support and education on emotional and interpersonal responses.

Analysis of data from a second interview with 18 subjects, conducted 1 year following surgery, yielded the suggestion that an extension of social support and education prior to and beyond the 8-week experimental treatment, which started at 2.6 months postsurgery, would be beneficial. In particular, the subjects stated that support beginning within a few weeks after surgery and lasting for 1 year would have been helpful. Although subjects indicated that weekly group support helped them to adapt, they also indicated that continuing support could be less intense than the weekly group meetings and could be in the form of telephone calls to each subject. The subjects stated that such an individualized treatment would be appropriate because their needs had become less acute and, in most instances, subjects had resumed busy lifestyles which would have made attendance at weekly group-support meetings impractical.

Analyses of the data obtained from the outcome measures used in our recently completed study, along with the results of the qualitative data, indicated that some modifications in outcome variables and instruments are required to tap the full range of emotional and interpersonal responses to the diagnosis and treatment of breast cancer. We have, therefore, added instruments to measure outcomes that were evident only in themes extracted from our qualitative interview data. Those themes revealed that the subjects experienced changes in: affective mood state; feelings about the sense of purpose and satisfaction with life, or well-being; frequency and intensity of feelings of cancer–related concern or worry; and feelings of loneliness or isolation. Moreover, we have modified the content of the experimental treatment to address these outcomes in an explicit manner.

Our analysis suggested that, by 3 months after surgery, subjects had fully recovered from surgery and had resumed virtually all of their usual role activities. Our analysis further suggested that frequency and intensity of treatment–related physical symptoms were not affected by the study intervention. Functional status and symptom distress will not be used, therefore, as study outcomes in the proposed study.

A pilot ($n = 30$) for the proposed project began in late spring 1994. Using a three-group experimental design with repeated measures, we are exploring the efficacy of a treatment of longer duration (13 months) that consists of combined individual telephone and group social support and education. Outcomes for this pilot are: mood disturbance, measured by the Profile of Mood States; cancer–related worry, measured by the Visual Analogue Scale-Worry; level of well-being, measured by the Existential Well-Being Scale; quality of relationship with a significant other, measured by the Relationship Change Scale; and feelings of loneliness, measured by the UCLA Loneliness Scale-Version 3.

Mean age for this sample is 54 years with a range of 36–72 years. All subjects in this sample are TNM Stage I or II and entered the study at an average of 3.2 weeks following surgery. Of the 30 subjects, 23 had mastectomies. . . . Group means for demographic and baseline outcome measures are similar. The small sample, however, precludes testing for group equivalence. Interestingly, most of the baseline outcome measures were heavily intercorrelated. The pilot study results will help finalize effective training procedures for research assistants and refine the proposed study protocol. (Samarel et al., 1995–1997)

The next example illustrates how a preliminary pilot study can be summarized in the background subsection of a journal article reporting the completed research. The excerpt was taken from a journal article reporting the results of an experimental study designed to test a predictive theory of the effects of different types of cancer support groups (CSG) on physical, emotional, functional, and interpersonal adaptation to breast cancer. The theory was based on Roy's Adaptation Model (Roy and Andrews, 1991).

■ Example: DESCRIPTION OF A PRELIMINARY STUDY IN A JOURNAL ARTICLE

In an experimental pilot study, Samarel, Fawcett, and Tulman (1993) randomized 64 subjects to one of three treatment groups: experimental treatment, participation in a CSG with coaching; control treatment, participation in a similar CSG without coaching; and no treatment control, no CSG participation. Outcomes measured were symptom and emotional distress, functional status, and quality of relationship with a significant other. Data were collected at the time of entry into the study (baseline) and 8 weeks later, at the end of the CSGs. There was a significant overall multivariate effect of coaching on adaptation to breast cancer with evidence of a difference among the groups for symptom distress, emotional distress, and functional status. Univariate tests indicated trends toward less symptom distress for the experimental treatment group and greater functional status for the no-treatment control group, but no differences among the groups in emotional distress. The posttest scores for functional status were lower than baseline measures for all three groups, which suggests a decrease in role function for all subjects during the 8 weeks of study participation. This finding may be due to the fact that most of the women who participated in the study were concurrently receiving chemotherapy, radiation therapy, or combined chemotherapy and radiation. There were no differences between the groups in quality of the relationship with a significant other. (Samarel, Fawcett, and Tulman, 1997, p. 17)

LONG-RANGE GOALS. The background subsection of research proposals frequently ends by linking the proposed study to long-range goals in a program of research. The next example illustrates how a proposed study can be linked to the long-range goals of the research program, including the development of nursing interventions and the formulation of public policies. The excerpt was taken from a funded research grant proposal for correlational research designed to test an explanatory theory of correlates of functional status in childbearing women. The theory was based on Roy's Adaptation Model (Andrews and Roy, 1986).

> ■ Example: **DESCRIPTION OF LONG-RANGE GOALS IN A RESEARCH PROPOSAL**
>
> The proposed study will provide normative data from healthy women on the within-subjects changes in functional status from the end of the first trimester of pregnancy until 6 months postpartum. In addition, factors affecting functional status during pregnancy and after childbirth will be delineated. Furthermore, the findings of the proposed study will provide data that may be used to develop interventions that may facilitate optimal functional status during pregnancy and the postpartum period.
>
> Socioeconomically, the results of this study would supply data that could help shape legislation concerning state and national maternity leave/compensation policies. Currently, experts in the field of social policy have limited research data on functional status during pregnancy and after childbirth on which to base various proposed lengths of maternity leave (Kamerman, Kahn, and Kingston, 1983; Zigler and Frank, 1988). This critical information would place current discussions on length of maternity leave on a firm empirical basis. (Tulman and Fawcett, 1990–1993)

METHOD

The method section includes a description of the sample, instruments, procedure, and data-analysis plan. Within the limits of space, the information given should be sufficient to enable other researchers to replicate the study.

Sample

The sample subsection presents a description of the study participants, the sample size, how the participants will be or were recruited, restrictions on the sample (e.g., age range, language spoken, or medical condition), and relevant sample characteristics that set the limits on generalizability of study findings (e.g., age, education, occupation). The sample subsection also may include the anticipated or actual response rate or the number of invited individuals who actually agreed to participate in the study, as well as the attrition rate. This subsection also may include the informed-consent procedure, or that information may be given in the subsection describing data-collection procedures. The characteristics of the sample are discussed in the narrative of the final research report, and the narrative can be augmented by a table (Table 5–2, Guidelines for Constructing Tables and Figures).

A proposal for research includes the power analysis calculations to justify the number of participants to be included. The final report may include a power analysis stating the obtained power based on the actual sample size and the effect size of the study results.

The first example of the sample subsection was taken from a funded research grant proposal for an experimental study designed to test a predictive theory of the effects of different types of social support and education on emotional and interpersonal adaptation to breast cancer. The theory was based on Roy's Adaptation Model (Roy and Andrews, 1991). The excerpt includes the typical content of the sample subsection, as well as the procedure for random assignment of the participants to the experimental and control treatment groups.

■ Example: **DESCRIPTION OF THE SAMPLE IN A RESEARCH PROPOSAL**

Profile. All subjects will be English-speaking women, diagnosed with TNM Stage I, II, or III (nonmetastatic) breast cancer, with no major underlying medical problems (e.g., cardiac or renal disease) or previous history of cancer, with the exception of non-melanoma skin cancer, who enter the study 2–3 weeks following surgery. English-speaking subjects are necessary to allow participation in the study and to ensure that directions related to the research instruments are understood. Women having surgery within the past 2–3 weeks are actively involved in treatment regimens (recent surgery, radiation, chemotherapy). For the purposes of this project, surgery refers to the date of last surgery for mastectomy/lumpectomy and/or lymph node dissection. Limiting the sample to subjects with Stage I, II, or III (nonmetastatic) breast cancer with no major underlying medical problems will decrease attrition resulting from inability to participate due to other health problems or the severe symptoms associated with metastasis.

Recruitment. A sample of 174 subjects will be recruited. Allowing for a 10% attrition rate based on our recently completed study [Samarel, Fawcett, and Tulman, 1997], this yields a final sample size of 156 subjects, or 52 subjects per treatment group. This final sample size provides a power of .80 given an alpha of .05 and an estimated medium effect size of $f = .25$ (Cohen, 1988) for tests of main effects of variance. Our previous study had an effect size of $f = .16$, which is a small-to-medium effect size for the intervention. However, this study proposes a more extensive intervention and therefore a medium effect size is estimated. Based on our past experience with recruitment of subjects with Stage I and II breast cancer, 174 subjects can be recruited in an 11-month period. Because we are including subjects with Stage III breast cancer in the proposed study, we anticipate no difficulty in recruiting the necessary 174 subjects in the required time frame.

Women from central and northern New Jersey (N.J.) under care of private physicians, attending clinics at several medical centers, and/or members of the American Cancer Society (ACS), N.J. Division, sample subset will be recruited for the study. Personnel at all sample recruitment sites have assured the investigators that sufficient numbers of patients will be available for the study, and the lack of difficulty in recruitment for our recently completed project and our ongoing pilot study confirms the availability of new subjects. Furthermore, the profile of the available subjects is consistent with the criteria required for study participation. That is, sufficient numbers of English-speaking patients are available who have been diagnosed with nonmetastatic breast cancer and are experiencing no major underlying medical problems. Letters documenting access to subjects are appended. All subjects will be female. In an effort to ensure a representative minority sample, a substantial number of subjects will be recruited from surgeons' offices and hospital-based practices in urban areas where a large proportion of ethnic minority women (African-American, Asian, and Hispanic) are treated. In addition, the ACS, N.J. Division, has approved the project for access to its sample subset in underserved counties in New Jersey. This includes all women in those counties diagnosed with breast cancer, thereby including minority representation.

The physicians, clinic directors, and ACS units will identify potential subjects for the study and invite them to contact the investigators. Explanations of the study will be provided, orally by telephone and in writing through the mail, to all women who contact us. Signed informed consent will be obtained by mail. Each subject will be informed on entry into the study that she will be assigned to one of three study treatment groups. All subjects completing the study will be remunerated in appreciation for their time in completing the data-collection instruments.

Randomization. An alternative to simple randomization is necessary to ensure no unbalanced subject assignments to any one study treatment group, which could result from long, unbroken runs of assignment to one group. For example, simple randomization may result in consecutive assignment of six or seven subjects to control treatment groups 1 and 2 (no group social support), followed by randomization of one or two subjects to the experimental treatment group (group social support), followed by randomization of the next six or eight subjects to control treatment groups 1 and 2. Because of a brief time window (2–3 weeks) postsurgery for beginning a cohort, it would not be possible to delay the start of the intervention for these subjects, resulting in the need to have one experimental treatment cohort of only one or two subjects. It is not possible to adequately provide group social support in a group of one or two individuals, nor is it fiscally responsible to assign two research assistants to a cohort consisting of two subjects. Therefore, using a permuted block design for randomization (Rudy, Vaska, Daly, Happ, and Shiao, 1993), subjects will be assigned to study treatment groups In blocks or cohorts, rather than on an individual basis. Such a plan for randomization is effective in preventing grossly unbalanced subject assignments.

Each cohort will consist of four to eight subjects. Once four to eight subjects have been recruited, the entire cohort will be randomly assigned to one of the three study treatment groups using the sealed opaque envelope technique. When the next four to eight subjects have been recruited, that cohort will be assigned, using the two remaining sealed opaque envelopes, to one of the two remaining study treatment groups. The next cohort of four to eight subjects will be assigned to the remaining study treatment group. After the first three groups have been filled, the process will start again. We anticipate, based on our initial N of 174, that 24 to 27 cohorts will receive study treatments. Selection bias will be avoided by using a separate research assistant to assign cohorts to treatment groups following the return of baseline data, thereby blinding the recruiter to group assignment. Subjects will not be informed of their group assignment until they have agreed to participate in the project, their cohort is filled, and their signed informed-consent forms and baseline data are returned. Subject recruitment will continue, with assignment to study treatment groups taking place after each four to eight subjects are recruited, until all 174 subjects have been recruited and assigned to study treatment groups. On the basis of our on-going study, we anticipate that 12 to 16 subjects can be accrued within one month. (Samarel et al., 1995–1997)

The next example, taken from a research report published in a journal, illustrates the description of the sample in narrative form and includes the power analysis calculation for sample size. The correlational research was designed to test an explanatory theory of correlates of grief responses. The theory was derived from Roy's Adaptation Model (Roy and Andrews, 1991).

■ Example: **NARRATIVE DESCRIPTION OF THE SAMPLE, WITH A POWER ANALYSIS, IN A JOURNAL ARTICLE**

The convenience sample consisted of 65 women between the ages of 45 and 84 with a mean of 64.8 years ($SD = 10.7$). Formal education ranged from 7 to 16 years ($M = 11.6$ years, $SD = 2.3$). The range of years married was 1–65 years with a mean of 38.8 years ($SD = 14.9$). Of the sample, 8% were Afro-American and 92% were Euro-American; 9% were Catholic and 91% were Protestant. The range of annual income of the sample was 29% below $10,000; 38% between $10,000 to $20,000; and 32% above $20,000. The range of months since the spouse's death was 13 to 24 months with a mean of 18.74 ($SD = 3.7$). Sixty-two percent of the sample had husbands who died from cancer, 15% from heart disease, 9% from respiratory disease, and 13% from other causes. The sample size ($N = 65$) exceeded the requirement of 57 subjects as determined by a power analysis for multiple regression with 6 variables, estimating a medium-size effect with alpha set at .05 and power of .80 (Cohen and Cohen, 1983). (Robinson, 1995, p. 160)

The following example, also taken from a research report published in a journal, illustrates the description of the sample in narrative form with important sample characteristics for each of two study groups summarized in a table. In addition, the informed-consent procedure is explained. The excerpt is from correlational research designed to test an explanatory theory of pain experienced by Mexican-American and Anglo-American women undergoing elective surgery. The theory was based on Roy's Adaptation Model (Roy and Andrews, 1991).

■ Example: **DESCRIPTION OF THE SAMPLE IN NARRATIVE AND TABLE FORMS, WITH THE INFORMED-CONSENT PROCEDURE, IN A JOURNAL ARTICLE**

Thirty-eight Anglo-American (white non-Hispanic) female patients and 22 Mexican-American female patients were included in the study. The method

Table 5–3 ■ SAMPLE CHARACTERISICS PRESENTED IN A TABLE

Characteristics	Mexican-American (n = 22)		Anglo-American (n = 38)	
Place of birth	Mexico	73%	U.S.	100%
Age (x)	35 years		37 years	
Marital status	married	73%	married	50%
Children (x)	2		2	
Education	≤ 8th grade	41%	high school	50%
Occupation	housewife	64%	housewife	42%
Family income	<$20,000	77%	<$20,000	62%
Religion	Catholic	77%	Protestant	66%
Previous hospitalizations	82%		68%	
Previous surgeries	41%		28%	

Source: From Calvillo and Flaskerud, 1993, p. 122, with permission.

of sampling was purposive, based on the principle of selecting individuals for the sample according to control criteria. The patient participants were selected for an interview and chosen on the basis of the following criteria: (a) women identified as either Mexican-American or Anglo-American and (b) scheduled for an elective cholecystectomy. Any patient whose recovery was complicated was excluded as the study progressed. Complications included infection, hemorrhage, obstruction of the T-tube, respiratory complications, circulatory complications, or cancer. Patients having an emergency cholecystectomy were not considered. Patients having incidental appendectomies were included, but all other surgery combinations were excluded.

Sociodemographic variables for the purposes of description, correlation, and theory testing were recorded. These variables included place of birth, age, marital status, spouse's occupation, husband's place of birth, number of children, education, occupation, family income, religion, number of hospitalizations, number of previous surgeries, and admission weight. Table [5–3] displays [some of the] sample characteristics.

Permission to conduct the study was obtained from the institutional review boards of each of the facilities where data were collected. Each subject was given a full explanation of the study and signed a consent form. (Calvillo and Flaskerud, 1993, p. 122)

The final example of the sample subsection illustrates presentation in a research report of a power analysis prior to the study to calculate sample size, and determination of the obtained power based on the study results. The report is of experimental research designed to test a predictive theory of the effects of walking exercise on physical functioning, exercise level, emotional distress, and symptom experience of women with breast cancer who were receiving radiation therapy. The theory was based on Roy's Adaptation Model (Roy and Andrews, 1991) and on findings from previous research. The sample included 46 women who had breast cancer. Following random assignment of the first subject, subsequent subjects were alternatively assigned to an experimental moderate-exercise treatment group ($n = 22$) or a control usual-care treatment group ($n = 24$).

■ Example: **DESCRIPTION OF POWER ANALYSIS IN A JOURNAL ARTICLE**

A priori power analysis, based on pilot work with the exercise intervention, determined that 50 subjects, randomly assigned to two groups, would provide a power of 0.80 to detect a large effect size at an alpha level of 0.05. This power analysis was calculated for a multivariate analysis of covariance (MANCOVA) procedure with five dependent variables (Stevens, 1980). Post hoc power analysis revealed an actual power of 1.00 on the MANCOVA test with the 46 subjects who completed the study. (Mock et al., 1997, p. 993)

Instruments

The instruments subsection includes the name and psychometric properties of each instrument. A statement is included that links the instrument with the concept it measures. Evidence of validity and reliability also is included. Reports of completed research present reliability coefficients for the study sample. A brief description of the items for each questionnaire and the scale used to rate the items should be given. The range of possible scores is noted, and the interpretation of the scores is explained. The same information should be given in both research proposals and journal articles reporting the results of the completed research.

The example features a description of an instrument presented in a journal article reporting the results of correlational research designed to test an explanatory theory of the relationship of human field motion, human field rhythms, creativity, and sentience to adolescents' perceived health status. The theory was derived from Rogers' Science of Unitary Human Beings (Barrett, 1990).

■ Example: **DESCRIPTION OF AN INSTRUMENT**

Creativity is the personal assessment of attributes, such as imaginative and complicated, which are characteristic of creativity, and is measured by the Creativity Scale of the Adjective Checklist (CrScaleACL). The CrScaleACL was used as a measure of creativity (Cough and Heilburn, 1983). The CrScale measures the extent to which individuals describe themselves as possessing characteristics indicative of creativity, such as being complicated and imaginative. Based on items that discriminated between creative and noncreative groups in earlier studies of high school and college students, Yonge (1975) extracted a 19-item scale for creativity from the ACL. Yarcheski and Mahon (1991) had deleted two of the items from the 19-item scale based on a review for content validity by three seventh- and eighth-grade school teachers, all of whom agreed that seventh and eighth graders (early adolescents) would not comprehend the meaning of cynical and unconventional. For purposes of consistency, these two adjectives were deleted from the present analysis for all three samples. The possible range of scores for the CrScale is 1 to 17; higher scores indicate higher levels of creativity. Yonge (1975) reported evidence of construct validity for the CrScale from appreciable correlations found between the scale and subscales of the Temporal Experiences Inventory and the Personal Orientation Inventory. He reported a KR-21 reliability of .83 among 80 college students, whereas Cowling (1986) reported a reliability of .85 among 160 undergraduates. Yarcheski and Mahon (1991) reported KR-20 reliabilities of .70, .78, and .80 for early, middle, and late adolescents, respectively. In the present study, the KR-20s were .69, .77, and .80 among early, middle, and late adolescents, respectively. (Yarcheski and Mahon, 1995, pp. 387, 389–390)

Procedure

The procedure subsection provides a concise but detailed description of the data-collection procedures. The procedure used to recruit participants is explained if it has not been noted in the sample subsection. Data collectors are identified and any special training required for data collection is explained. The setting for data collection is identified and, if more than one instrument is used, the order of administration may be noted. The time required for data collection also is noted, as is any financial compensation given to participants. Furthermore, the procedure for obtaining informed consent is explained in this subsection if it has not been explained previously in the sample subsection. In experimental studies, the procedure subsection may present a description of the experimental and control conditions. Alternatively, the experimental and control conditions can be included as part of the instruments subsection.

This subsection usually is shorter in a journal article than it is in a research proposal or unpublished report, such as a dissertation. Regardless of space limitations, however, the essential information about the procedure used to collect the data is required.

The first example is the procedure subsection from a funded research proposal for an experimental study designed to test a predictive theory of the effects of different types of social support and education on emotional and interpersonal adaptation to breast cancer. The theory was based on Roy's Adaptation Model (Roy and Andrews, 1991).

■ Example: **DESCRIPTION OF PROCEDURE, INCLUDING EXPERIMENTAL AND CONTROL CONDITIONS, IN A RESEARCH PROPOSAL**

Experimental Treatment Group (extended-duration combined individual telephone and group social support and education; $n = 58$)

Each offering of the experimental treatment group will include a minimum of four and a maximum of eight subjects. The group size is based on our experience with support groups (Samarel, Fawcett, and Tulman, 1993). Study treatment-group size of four to eight subjects will permit the continuation of treatment during times of low subject recruitment.

The experimental treatment was selected based on a review of the literature and of the data obtained from interviews of subjects in our recently completed study. The combination of individual and group social support and education will maximize attention to both individual and collective experiences of women with breast cancer. The experimental treatment was specifically designed to provide more intense support during times identified by subjects in our recently completed study as times of peak need. More specifically, the experimental treatment provides an intense period of weekly social support and education via telephone to each individual subject in the early months following surgery; increases in intensity through weekly group social support and education for 8 weeks during the period of adjuvant therapy; decreases in intensity to twice-monthly individual social support and education via telephone as treatment continues; and further decreases to once-monthly individual social support and education via telephone after adjuvant treatment has been completed. The social support and education offered in this study emphasize reducing and/or managing unpleasant emotional symptoms related to treatment; stress management; dealing with fear of recurrence; issues of self-image and sexuality; and enhancing communication and problem-solving techniques designed to improve interpersonal communication. Subjects assigned to the experimental treatment group will receive a 13-month (extended duration) intervention consisting of four phases:

Phase I, beginning 2 to 3 weeks following surgery, will consist of weekly individual social support and education via telephone from an oncology nurse or oncology social worker for 9 to 10 weeks, until the start of the group social support and education phase. Interviews of subjects in our recently completed study revealed that women need assistance with adaptation within the first few months following surgery but that group support at this time may not be practical because women may not feel comfortable traveling to evening sessions due to fatigue and/or discomfort from surgery and anesthesia; may have time conflicts with the required commitment to a group due to numerous scheduled consultative visits with radiologists, oncologists, and follow-up visits with their surgeons; and may not yet be ready emotionally to accept and confront their breast cancer in a group setting.

Individual social support and education (telephone support) in phase I will focus on the subjects' experiences and immediate concerns regarding breast cancer diagnosis, surgery, and treatment decisions. The calls will be initiated weekly by either the oncology nurse or oncology social worker (research assistants, or RAs) and will be designed to assist subjects to adapt in the self-concept and interdependence response modes of Roy's Adaptation Model; that is, emotionally and interpersonally. Each RA will be assigned to two to four subjects (one-half of a cohort of four to eight subjects), providing a consistent primary telephone contact for each subject. In addition to the RA-initiated telephone support, each subject will be encouraged to initiate telephone contact with her RA should she have a question or require additional assistance with adaptation between RA-initiated telephone calls.

The telephone support providers (RAs) are the expert oncology nurse clinicians and social workers who inform and support the subjects, enabling them to make and/or participate in decisions affecting their emotional and interpersonal adaptation. The RAs will assist subjects in dealing with specific problems that may confront them. They will not, however, give advice regarding specific treatment decisions.

To ensure consistency and standardization among all cohorts, RAs will use objectives and guides that have been developed by the investigators specifically for telephone support. The objectives for each phase of the telephone support and the corresponding Roy's Adaptation Model response modes they address are in the Appendix (Telephone Support Objectives). Each RA will maintain a log of all telephone contacts with each subject to record the date, time, and duration of each contact; who initiated the contact; problems or topics discussed; outcomes; and continuing problems. Telephone Support Guides and Telephone Log Sheets are in the Appendix.

Phase II will consist of group social support and education (group support), which will be co-facilitated by the same RAs providing the telephone support in phase I. Groups will begin approximately 3 months after surgery, following 9 to 10 weeks of telephone support. Most women in our recently completed study began group support between 2.5 and 3.5 months after surgery and indicated this was the most advantageous time for such an intervention. The group support will consist of eight weekly 2-hour-long meetings, which is consistent with our recently completed project and was selected to provide adequate time to present information and promote subjects' sharing of their experiences, but to minimize attrition from the group component due to difficulties with transportation and scheduling. Phase II will contain a particularly strong educational component that will include information manuals for each subject in addition to the social support.

Group-support objectives and content for phase II were designed by the investigators to assist women with breast cancer to adapt in the self-concept and interdependence response modes of Roy's Adaptation Model. The objectives and content of the group support are based on our recently completed research and specific responses of women with breast cancer noted in the literature. Content validity and appropriateness of the order of presentation of content were initially determined by a review of six experts in cancer, cancer education, or support groups. Subjects in our ongoing pilot continue to validate the appropriateness of content. Content of the group support includes: management of emotional symptoms resulting from treatment–related problems; stress management techniques; communication and problem solving; dealing with fear; and issues of self-image and sexuality. Learning will be enhanced through the use of audiotapes, videotapes, and group participation. The behavioral objectives of the group support, the corresponding Roy's Adaptation Model response modes they address (self-concept and interdependence), and the schedule to accomplish the objectives are in the Appendix.

The *Breast Cancer Informational Manual*, developed by the investigators for the education component of the intervention, includes an introduction to and overview of the manual, and informational content arranged into eight chapters. These manuals, along with audiovisuals to enhance learning, will be used in the conduct of the group support to facilitate clarification and understanding of content with a minimum of note-taking required of the subjects. To ensure consistency and standardization of all experimental treatment groups, the investigators developed an additional manual for group facilitators (RAs). The *Breast Cancer Group Support Manual for Facilitators* is to be used as a supplement to the subjects' manual and is designed as a guide for the RAs following their initial orientation. This manual includes an introduction, general comments and remarks about facilitating the groups, and session-by-session information and hints for the RAs. Items discussed in the "General Comments" section include specific information about the session format, time frame, and subject participation. The session-by-session section provides suggested reading, lists of materials needed, and additional helpful comments. The content of both manuals reflects the self-concept and interdependence response modes of Roy's Adaptation Model. Sample chapters from both manuals are in the Appendix.

The role of the group facilitators (RAs) is identical to the role of the telephone support providers. In addition, the RAs act as group facilitators, change agents, and consumer advocates. As group facilitators and change agents, the RAs provide information to women with breast cancer and teach strategies that facilitate adaptation to breast cancer. As consumer advocates, the RAs inform and support the subjects, enabling them to make and/or participate in decisions affecting their health and adaptation.

During phase II, subjects will be encouraged to contact the RAs by telephone to discuss any questions, problems, or concerns that may arise between group support sessions. As in phase I, each RA will continue to maintain a log of all telephone contacts with each subject.

Phase III will begin approximately 5 months after surgery, immediately following the termination of the group support, and continue for 3 months. Phase III will consist of individual telephone support initiated by the RAs who provided the phase I telephone support and phase II group support. Telephone calls will be initiated twice each month. Women in our recently completed research reported that they felt "lost" at the termination of 8-week group support and still needed assistance with adaptation, but indicated that weekly group support was no longer needed. They proposed a less intense type of support, such as telephone contact. The twice-monthly telephone support will extend through the entire time span of adjuvant chemotherapy for women receiving it. In addition to the RA-initiated telephone support, each subject will be encouraged to initiate telephone contact with either of the RAs who co-facilitated the group support should she have a question or require additional assistance with adaptation between RA-initiated telephone calls. In this way, each subject will continue to have the benefit of both nursing and social work experience and expertise, being able to receive information related to the emotional and interpersonal sequelae of breast cancer. Moreover, having sources for additional telephone contact ensures continuity in the event of RA attrition from the study. Telephone support in phase III will focus on the subject's evolving emotional and interpersonal experiences and needs. For example, a common concern expressed by subjects at this time is the fear that termination of chemotherapy may result in recurrence. In addition to provision of social support, educational information will be provided in response to any questions raised by the subjects. Telephone logs will be continued to be maintained by RAs.

Phase IV will begin approximately 8 months after surgery, immediately following phase III, and consist of individual telephone support, by the same RAs, once a month for 5 months. Phase IV is designed to provide assistance with emotional and interpersonal adaptation past the anniversary of initial diagnosis and surgery. Women in our recently completed study reported that the 1-year anniversary was a "difficult" time for them. Monthly telephone support in phase IV will begin the termination phase of the RA-subject relationship and provide reassurance and encouragement in the form of social support and education for long-term emotional and interpersonal adaptation to breast cancer. (See Telephone Support Objectives and Guides in the Appendix). To ensure consistency, telephone logs will be maintained by RAs.

Control Treatment Group 1 (extended-duration individual telephone social support and education only, *n* = 58)

Subjects assigned to control treatment group 1 will receive 13 months (extended duration) of telephone support consisting of four phases. They will not receive the group social support and education component of the experimental treatment.

Phase I, identical to the phase I of the experimental treatment group, will begin 2 to 3 weeks following surgery and consist of weekly individual social support and education via telephone for 9 to 10 weeks.

Phase II will consist of continued individual telephone support, by the same RAs providing the phase I telephone support, once a week for 8 weeks, beginning approximately 3 months following surgery. At the start of this phase, the second RA for the cohort will telephone the subject to introduce herself and inform her that both RAs will be available for telephone support. As with subjects in the experimental treatment group, subjects in control group 1 will have the benefit of both nursing and social work experience and expertise. At the beginning of this phase, the *Breast Cancer Informational Manual*, identical to the manual used for the experimental treatment group, will be mailed to each subject along with the same audiovisual materials used to enhance learning for the experimental treatment group. In the event that any subjects do not own audiotape or videotape players, they will be encouraged to listen to or view the tapes with friends or relatives, if possible. The focus of this phase of the telephone support will be on the manual content, following the same schedule of content provided for subjects receiving group support.

Phases III and IV will consist of individual telephone support identical to the telephone support provided for the experimental treatment group.

Telephone support in phases I, III, and IV will be conducted in a manner identical to the telephone support for each corresponding phase in the experimental treatment group and meet the same objectives. RAs for control group 1 will use telephone support objectives and guides that are identical to the telephone support objectives and guides used in the experimental treatment group for phases I, III, and IV. The behavioral objectives for phase II of the telephone support for control group I are similar to the objectives for phase II of the group support for the experimental treatment group. The telephone support guide for phase II will provide more structured guidance for RAs to use when following the content of the *Breast Cancer Informational Manual*, which will be identical to the manuals used for the experimental treatment group. Identical telephone log sheets will be maintained for control group I subjects and experimental treatment group subjects. Roles of the RAs in control group I are identical to the roles of the RAs in the experimental treatment group.

Control Treatment Group 2 (education only, n = 58)

Subjects assigned to control treatment group 2 will receive education via mailed manuals. The same *Breast Cancer Informational Manual* used for the experimental treatment and control treatment I groups will be mailed to each subject, along with the audiovisual materials to enhance learning, approximately 3 months following surgery. Subjects will be informed that they may contact the project office to speak with an oncology nurse or oncology social worker if they have any questions related to manual content. Logs will be maintained for all telephone calls, which will be limited to educational information related to the content of the manual.

RESEARCH ASSISTANTS. Each cohort in the experimental treatment group and control treatment group I will be led by two RAs, one oncology clinical nurse specialist, and one oncology social worker, who have experience and expertise in facilitating cancer support groups and/or working with women with breast cancer. The nurse will bring nursing and medical expertise and be able to provide information and answer questions related to the physical and psychosocial sequelae of breast cancer. The social worker will focus on the psychosocial sequelae of breast cancer. There are distinct advantages to having two facilitators for each cohort. In addition to broadening the areas of expertise, the possibility of subject attrition due to inability to relate to one facilitator is significantly reduced. Our experience with our recently completed study of short-term group support has clearly demonstrated the value of nurse and social worker dyads for group facilitation. All RAs will be blinded to the study design and hypotheses. To ensure continuity in each cohort, the same two facilitators will be assigned for the duration of subject study participation. To control for potential bias and contamination, different pairs of RAs will be used for the experimental treatment groups and for control treatment groups I. Both treatment groups will, however, adhere to the same schedule and format of telephone support in phases I, III, and IV. The experimental treatment group and control treatment group I will adhere to the same schedule for phase II, although experimental treatment group RAs will conduct phase II through group support, whereas control treatment group I RAs will conduct phase II via telephone support. All RAs will be rigorously trained by the investigators. Other RAs, who are blinded to the study design and hypotheses, will interview subjects at the end of their study participation.

DATA COLLECTION. Data collection for all subjects will be by mail, with the exception of the interviews, which will be conducted via telephone. Prior to randomization to study treatment groups and to initial telephone support for experimental treatment group and control treatment group 1 subjects, baseline data will be collected from all subjects. Data will be collected at four points over a 13-month period for all subjects: at entry into the study (baseline) and at the termination of phases I, II, and IV to determine the effectiveness of each phase of the experimental and control interventions. Data will be collected from subjects in control treatment group 2 (education only) at the same collection times. If the preliminary data from the proposed study look promising, additional funding will be obtained for follow-up data which will be collected at two additional data points, at 18 months and 24 months following entry into the study. This follow-up will be used as preliminary data to determine the long-term effects of individual and group social support and education. Data collection points are shown in Table [5–4].

Prior to mailing each set of questionnaires at data collection points two through seven, an RA who is not a nurse or social worker and who is blinded to the study design will contact each subject by telephone to alert the woman to the forthcoming packet of questionnaires and request her continued participation in the study. No social support or educational information will be provided during this telephone contact. An additional measure to minimize attrition will be subject remuneration for each data collection point. (Samarel et al., 1995–1997)

Table 5–4 ■ DATA COLLECTION SCHEDULE

Data Points	1	2	3	4	5*	6*
Background Data Sheet	X					
Background Data Update		X	X	X	X	X
Profile of Mood States	X	X	X	X	X	X
Existential Well-Being Scale	X	X	X	X	X	X
Visual Analogue Scale-Worry	X	X	X	X	X	X
Relationship Change Scale	X	X	X	X	X	X
UCLA Loneliness Scale-Version 3	X	X	X	X	X	X
Subject Medication Record		X	X	X	X	X
Health Service Use Logs		X	X	X	X	X
RA Telephone Logs		X	X	X	X	X
Health Costs Interview	X	X	X	X	X	X
Open-Ended Interview				X		

Data Point
1 = Entry into study, 2–3 weeks postsurgery
2 = End of Phase I, 3 months postsurgery
3 = End of Phase II, 5 months postsurgery
4 = End of Phase IV, 13 months postsurgery
5 = 18 months postsurgery*
6 = 24 months postsurgery*
*pending continuing funding
Source: From Samarel et al., 1995–1997, with permission.

The next example was taken from a journal article reporting the results of completed research. The excerpt is from a study that used an ethnographic method to generate a descriptive naming theory of Mexican-American people's meanings and expressions of pain and associated self-care and dependent-care actions. The research was guided by Orem's (1991) Self-Care Framework.

■ Example: **DESCRIPTION OF PROCEDURE, INCLUDING INFORMED CONSENT, FOR THEORY-GENERATING RESEARCH IN A JOURNAL ARTICLE**

Informants were given an explanation of the nature and purpose of the study, how confidentiality would be ensured, and their rights in participating in the study. Those persons willing to participate in the study signed a written consent form and in the case of children, parental consent and verbal assent were obtained. The majority of key informants were interviewed in their homes, and all interviews were conducted by the investigator, who is both Mexican-American and bilingual, in the language preferred by informants. Interviews were conducted in English ($n = 10$), Spanish ($n = 5$), and also using a combination of both languages ($n = 5$). Key informants were interviewed at least twice. The time of each interview ranged from 45 min to 4 hrs; the cumulative observation and interview time with informants ranged from 4 to over 10 hr. In contrast, contact with general informants was generally a one-time occurrence, while the length of interviews ranged from 30 min to 2 hr. The length of interviews with key informants and the number of interviews with key and general informants over time served as a means to ensure the saturation of the data and to establish the credibility of findings. (Villarruel, 1995, p. 430)

The following example also was taken from a journal article. The excerpt is from a report of correlational research designed to test an explanatory theory of the relation of spirituality, perceived social support, and death anxiety to nurses' willingness to care for AIDS patients. The theory was derived from Rogers' (1992) Science of Unitary Human Beings.

■ Example: **DESCRIPTION OF PROCEDURE, INCLUDING INFORMED CONSENT, FOR THEORY-TESTING RESEARCH IN A JOURNAL ARTICLE**

Following the study's approval by the institution's review board, nurse managers were consulted to identify an appropriate time to provide staff with a verbal and written description of the study, including its purpose, the voluntary nature of participation, opportunity to withdraw from the study at any time, and agreement to the one-time completion of a questionnaire booklet requiring approximately 60 to 90 minutes. Anonymity was assured. Tacit consent was indicated by the mailed return of a completed questionnaire booklet. The survey design, which was based on the Dillman

Total Design Method (Dillman, 1978), motivates participants to respond and facilitates questionnaire completion. The questionnaire return rate was 82%. (Sherman, 1996, p. 208)

STUDY TIMETABLE. The procedure subsection of a research proposal also may include a timetable for the study. The timetable indicates how long each phase of the study is expected to take, including training of research assistants, participant recruitment, data collection, data analysis, and preparation of the research report. An example of a timetable was taken from a funded research proposal for an experimental study designed to test a predictive theory of the effects of different types of social support and education on emotional and interpersonal adaptation to breast cancer. The theory was based on Roy's Adaptation Model (Roy and Andrews, 1991).

■ Example: **STUDY TIMETABLE IN A RESEARCH PROPOSAL**

The proposed study will take 24 months to complete. It is expected that there will be time periods when there will be a pause in recruitment, during the holidays of Thanksgiving and Christmas when many subjects will be otherwise involved. Planning of group support during such times would lead to low attendance and high attrition. It may be possible, too, that there will be an occasional short hiatus (1 or 2 weeks) between groups to recruit the necessary subjects for the next cohort. The tentative timetable is presented in Table [5–5] (Samarel et al., 1995–1997).

Table 5–5 ■ **TIMETABLE FOR STUDY OF EFFECTS OF DIFFERENT TYPES OF SOCIAL SUPPORT AND EDUCATION ON EMOTIONAL AND INTERPERSONAL ADAPTATION TO BREAST CANCER**

Prefunding	Recruit and train research assistants
	Complete pilot ($n = 30$)
Months 1–3	Begin subject recruitment
	Begin data collection and study treatments
Months 4–10	Continue subject recruitment, study treatments, and data collection
	Begin quantitative data entry on computer
Month 11	Complete subject recruitment
Months 12–13	Continue study treatments, data collection, and data entry
	Begin transcription of qualitative data
Months 14–22	Begin preliminary data analysis
	Continue study treatments, data collection, and data entry
	Continue transcription of qualitative data
Months 23	Complete study treatments
	Continue data analysis and transcription of qualitative data
Month 24	Complete data collection and entry on computer
Post-funding Phase	Complete final statistical data analysis
	Complete content analysis of qualitative data
	Prepare research reports
	Prepare manuscripts for publication

Source: From Samarel et al., 1995–1997, with permission.

HUMAN SUBJECTS PROTOCOL. Research proposals frequently include a detailed discussion of the protocol for obtaining informed consent and protection of human subjects. When a study involves animals rather than or in addition to human beings as participants, procedures are included for the care of the animals. The following example was taken from a funded research proposal for a correlational study designed to test an explanatory theory of correlates of functional status that used a sample of pregnant and postpartal women. The theory was based on Roy's Adaptation Model (Andrews and Roy, 1986).

■ Example: **HUMAN SUBJECTS PROTOCOL**
IN A RESEARCH PROPOSAL

1. CHARACTERISTICS OF THE SUBJECT POPULATION
Subjects recruited will be married English-speaking women over 18 years of age who are in the first trimester of pregnancy and who have no underlying medical problems (e.g., diabetes, chronic renal or cardiac disease). Each subject will be followed from the end of the first trimester of pregnancy through 6 months postpartum. Pregnant women are necessary subjects because the study is an investigation of functional status during pregnancy and after childbirth.

2. SOURCES OF RESEARCH MATERIAL
Subjects will be identified only by code numbers. No reference to individuals will be made in any published reports of the proposed study. Data will be obtained only for research purposes.

3. RECRUITMENT OF SUBJECTS AND CONSENT PROCEDURES
Potential subjects will be approached while having a prenatal visit with their obstetrician or nurse-midwife. The proposed study will be explained to potential subjects by a trained research assistant. Potential subjects will be asked to review the consent form with the research assistant and sign the consent form if they wish to participate in the study. Potential subjects will be told that willingness to participate or not participate in the study will in no way affect their medical or nursing care. Subjects will be compensated a modest sum ($85) for their time spent during the seven 1-hour data collection sessions. Letters confirming access to the subject recruitment sites are in the Appendix. A copy of the consent form is in the Appendix.

4. POTENTIAL RISK
There is minimal risk involved.

5. PROTECTION OF SUBJECTS
Confidentiality will be safeguarded through a system of coding on all research instruments. Subjects will be identified only by code numbers on research instruments. A master list will contain the names, addresses, and telephone numbers of subjects and their corresponding code numbers. This list will be kept in a locked file and be made available only to the investigators and research assistants. The master list will be destroyed at the earliest possible time after all data are collected and a summary of the study

results is mailed to subjects who have requested them. No reference to individuals will be made in any published reports of the proposed study. Data
will be obtained and used only for research purposes.
6. RISK/BENEFIT RATIO
    There are no specific direct benefits, other than a modest sum of money
for study participation, to be gained by individual subjects. Societal benefits
would include objective data upon which to base maternity leave/compen-
sation policies and legislation and interventions to facilitate improved functional status during pregnancy and after delivery. The potential benefits of
the proposed study to society far outweigh the potential of minimal risk
for individual subjects. (Tulman and Fawcett, 1990–1993)

Data-Analysis Plan

The subsection for the data-analysis plan includes an explanation of how the
data will be or were processed. When qualitative data are collected, the data-analysis plan specifies the specific content analysis techniques used. When the data are
quantitative, the plan may include measures of central tendency and variability, a
correlation matrix of all major research variables, and the inferential statistical test
for each relation being examined.

Research proposals typically include a subsection for the data-analysis plan.
Journal articles that report the results of completed research do not necessarily include a separate subsection for the data-analysis plan, especially if the data-analysis techniques are well-known. If the techniques used are well-known, they simply
can be named in the results section of the report. If more detail is required, the techniques can be explained in the procedure subsection or can be presented in a separate subsection for the full data-analysis plan. Regardless of the level of detail given
and the location of the data-analysis plan in the research document, the a priori alpha level selected for inferential statistical tests should be stated (American
Psychological Association, 1994).

The following example of a data-analysis plan is from a funded research proposal
for an experimental study designed to test a predictive theory of the effects of different
types of social support and education on emotional and interpersonal adaptation to breast
cancer. The theory was based on Roy's Adaptation Model (Roy and Andrews, 1991).
The excerpt includes the plan for analysis of both quantitative and qualitative data.

■ Example: **DATA-ANALYSIS PLAN FOR THEORY-TESTING
RESEARCH IN A RESEARCH PROPOSAL**

Quantitative data will be coded and entered into a personal computer
using the latest version of Statistical Package for the Social Sciences
(SPSS/PC+). Frequency distributions and measures of central tendency and

variability will be calculated for all variables. Normality and equality of variances will be assessed in the relevant continuous variables and normalizing transformations will be considered where appropriate. Correlation matrices will be constructed for all variables, including demographic variables, attendance and attrition rates, amount of telephone support, and use of medication and health services. Comparison of the three groups for differences in demographic and baseline outcome measures will be done to determine whether there was selective experimental mortality or group assignment bias. Internal consistency reliabilities will be calculated for the Profile of Mood States, Existential Well-Being Scale, Relationship Change Scale, and UCLA Loneliness Scale-Version 3 for the study subjects. Interrater reliability will be established for the Visual Analogue Scale-Worry and for the content analysis of transcripts of the open-ended interviews. If the treatment groups are different with regard to age, education, socioeconomic status, health variables, or baseline measures of the outcome variables, and these are found to be statistically significantly associated with the dependent variables, analysis of covariance procedures, rather than analysis of variance procedures, will be used to statistically control for the differences.

Data related to Hypotheses 1 and 2 will be tested by MANOVA with repeated measures (group $\times$ time) for those outcome variables found to be significantly correlated. Separate ANOVAs will be conducted for each dependent variable if the overall F-ratio for the MANOVA is significant at the .05 level. ANOVA will be done for those dependent variables found to be uncorrelated with other outcome variables. A Bonferroni adjustment (alpha $\div$ number of tests) will be used to correct for an inflated p value if multiple ANOVAs are performed.

To answer the question pertaining to breast cancer–related economic costs, the following will be calculated: 1) intervention costs, including personnel costs, materials and supplies, and expenses such as telephone charges and support services for group support meetings, will be allocated to participants in each group based on the proportion of use by each participant. RA telephone logs and group support attendance records will be used to assign costs to each participant based on time; 2) breast cancer–related health care costs, including health care provider services and medications, will be estimated for the study period, whether paid for by the subject or by a third-party payer; and 3) indirect economic costs associated with productivity loss will be assessed using data from the health costs interviews.

Intervention costs, breast cancer-related health care costs, and indirect economic costs will be summed for each subject. Costs will be based on estimated cost of services provided using relative value-based Medicare fee schedules available from the Health Care Financing Agency (HCFA). Cost of health provider encounter will be obtained from the Medicare fee schedule for the provider visit category. Costs of medications will be estimated using wholesale prices of the generic brand of the drug. If any participants are hospitalized, the average reimbursement of the DRG (diagnostic-related group) in New Jersey will be used. The mean cost for subjects in each of the three study treatment groups will be determined. Descriptive statistics will be provided for each of the three study treatment groups for intervention cost and for cost of breast cancer–related health care costs. In addition, descriptive statistics will be provided for breast cancer–related costs (the sum of the intervention and breast cancer–related health care costs). ANOVA will be used to test for significant differences in the direct and indirect breast cancer–related costs of health care.

Analysis of follow-up data (pending additional funding) will continue to examine the study outcomes and cost analysis with regard to long-term effects of the experimental and control interventions.

Additional Analyses. To determine the subjects' perceptions of their adaptation to breast cancer and their experiences in the research project, qualitative data from the open-ended interviews will be transcribed from the audiotapes and systematically analyzed by means of content analysis. The initial content analysis will be guided by the interview questions with the self-concept and interdependence response modes of Roy's Adaptation Model used as the a priori category scheme. The units of analysis will be words, phrases, or sentences that reflect adaptive or ineffective responses within these modes. Adaptive responses are those that promote the integrity of the human adaptive system by meeting the goals for survival, growth, reproduction, and mastery; ineffective responses do not meet these goals (Roy and Andrews, 1991). The data also will be examined for responses that lie outside Roy's model categories and additional categories will be developed, if necessary. Frequency of responses will be examined to determine whether there are any significant differences among the treatment groups. This method of data analysis permits systematic and objective treatment of the qualitative responses to the interview questions (Kerlinger, 1986). It should be noted that all three investigators for the proposed study have used content analysis in other studies (Fawcett, 1981; Samarel, 1991; Tulman and Fawcett, 1991).

Additional data analysis also will consist of content analysis of the telephone logs to identify categories representing general themes and specific needs and problems of women with breast cancer, as well as strategies suggested by the RAs and strategies used by the subjects (Krippendorff, 1980; Weber, 1990). Frequencies will be calculated for the coded categories. Those data will be useful in the planning of future interventions for breast cancer survivors. (Samarel et al., 1995–1997)

The next example was taken from a journal article reporting the results of completed research. The excerpt exemplifies the data-analysis plan for theory-generating research using an ethnographic method. The study, which was guided by Orem's (1991) Self-Care Framework, was designed to generate a descriptive naming theory of Mexican-American people's meanings and expressions of pain and associated self-care and dependent-care actions. A special feature of this example is the investigator's discussion of efforts to limit bias in the data-analysis phase of the study.

■ Example: **DATA-ANALYSIS PLAN FOR THEORY-GENERATING RESEARCH IN A JOURNAL ARTICLE**

Leininger's phases of analysis for qualitative data (1990, 1991a) were used to guide the analysis and conduct of the study. In addition, evaluative criteria for qualitative studies, including credibility, confirmability, saturation, meaning-in-context, transferability, and recurrent patterning were used throughout the phases of analysis to substantiate findings (Leininger, 1992; Lincoln and Guba, 1985). In the first phase, raw data, condensed field notes from observations, and interviews of general and key informants were recorded, expanded, and entered into the computer, using the software program HyperQual (Padilla, 1988). Reflections of the investigator, and beginning coding and interpretations of the data also were recorded.

In the second phase, data were coded further according to pain meanings, pain expressions, care of self, care of others, and care received from others. Descriptors that reflected the perspective of informants (emic perspective) and interpretations by the researcher (etic perspective) were identified and examined for similarities, differences, and meanings-in-context. In the third phase of analysis, data were examined further to discover saturation of ideas, recurrent patterning, and consistencies in meaning across contexts. In the fourth phase, major themes were abstracted from previous phases of analysis. This required an intense reexamination and synthesis of the data to ensure the credibility and meaning-in-context of the results. Once major themes were formulated, further examination of themes, patterns, descriptors, and raw data was undertaken to identify differences and similarities according to gender and extent of acculturation. Throughout all phases of analysis, the reflections, impressions, and questions that emerged were confirmed with general and key informants. (Villarruel, 1995, p. 430)

The following example of a brief data-analysis plan was taken from a journal article reporting the results of theory-testing research. The excerpt is from a report of correlational research designed to test an explanatory theory of the relation of spirituality, perceived social support, and death anxiety to nurses' willingness to care for AIDS patients. The theory was derived from Rogers' (1992) Science of Unitary Human Beings. The data-analysis plan was given at the end of the procedure subsection.

■ Example: **BRIEF DATA-ANALYSIS PLAN FOR THEORY-TESTING RESEARCH, WITH SPECIFICATION OF LEVEL OF STATISTICAL SIGNIFICANCE, IN A JOURNAL ARTICLE**

Using SPSS/PC, all data were entered twice for verification. Statistical analyses were conduced using the Statistical Package for the Social Sciences (SPSS/PC+, Version 4.0), with the level of statistical significance set at .05. (Sherman, 1996, p. 208)

The next example presents a data-analysis plan in more detail, which facilitates the reader's understanding of a complex statistical technique. The excerpt was taken from a journal article reporting the results of a completed correlational study designed to test an explanatory theory of the relation of severity of illness, hardiness, perceived control over visitation, and state anxiety to length of stay in an ICU. The theory was derived from Roy's Adaptation Model (Roy and Andrews, 1991).

■ Example: **DETAILED DATA-ANALYSIS PLAN FOR THEORY-TESTING RESEARCH IN A JOURNAL ARTICLE**

Path analysis was used in testing the [theory] [Figure 5–2, p. 160]. Before path analysis, a correlational matrix was generated and examined for multicollinearity of the independent variables. Gorden's (1968) criteri[on] of $r < .65$ for correlation of variables entered in the same equation was used. Residuals were checked against assumptions of the multiple regression statistic (Gorden, 1968). The sample size of 60 allowed for about 15 subjects per independent variable and was adequate for preliminary examination (Cohen and Cohen, 1983). A criterion level of $p < .10$ was used for both the standardized multiple regression coefficients and the R^2 for retaining variables in the [theory]. The primary interest in the first testing of this [theory] was to examine the relationships within the [theory], thus the lower significance level. (Hamner, 1996, p. 217)

RESULTS

The results section is structured according to the specific aims or hypotheses of the research. The results section of theory-generating research reports presents the concepts and propositions that emerged from the data analysis. In theory-testing research, this section starts with descriptive statistics for the major concepts of the theory, including measures of central tendency and variability. Statistical procedures used to test each hypothesis or analyze the data related to each specific aim are identified if a separate data-analysis plan is not included in the report. The findings for each statistical test are presented, and a definitive conclusion is drawn with regard to the support or lack of support for each hypothesis that was tested.

Tables and figures can be used to supplement the narrative research results (Table 5–2, Guidelines for Constructing Tables and Figures). Regardless of the format(s) used for presentation of the results, sufficient data should be presented to permit calculation of effect sizes for power analysis and integrative reviews.

Presentation of Theory-Generating Research Results

The following example illustrates the presentation of results from theory-generating research. The excerpt is from a journal article reporting theory-generating research using an ethnographic method. The study, which was guided by Orem's (1991) Self-Care Framework, was designed to generate a descriptive naming theory of Mexican-American people's meanings and expressions of pain and associated self-care and dependent-care actions. The results section of this research report continued with a detailed discussion of the concepts of the theory (the four themes) and the dimensions of each concept (the patterns).

■ Example: **NARRATIVE PRESENTATION OF THEORY-GENERATING RESEARCH RESULTS**

From the analysis of data, four themes concerned with pain meanings, expressions, care of self, care of others, and care by others were identified. Within this study, intracultural variation by gender and extent of acculturation were examined. Major gender differences in the expression of pain, care of self, and care for others were identified. Conversely, there was no variation by extent of acculturation in themes or patterns and only subtle variations in descriptors related to pain meaning and care. The four themes identified from the analysis of data are presented in detail and, within this context, variations by gender and extent of acculturation are identified. For each theme, the major patterns identified in phase three [of data analysis], descriptors and components identified in phase two [of data analysis], and raw data are included. The presentation of study results in this manner facilitated decisions about the transferability of findings to a similar context or situation. (Villarruel, 1995, p. 430)

The next example demonstrates how the narrative presentation of theory-generating research results can be supplemented by a table. The excerpt was taken from a journal article reporting theory-generating research using a hermeneutic method. The study was designed to generate a descriptive classification theory of the personal power experienced by people with schizophrenia. The research was based on Barrett's (1983) concept of power, which was derived from Rogers' (1982, 1983) Science of Unitary Human Beings. Data were collected via interviews, which were guided by a semi-structured, topic-based protocol, and administration of the Power as Knowing Participation in Change Test. In the journal article, two tables were used to present the major concepts of the theory (the themes across the topics). A detailed narrative description of the concepts accompanied the tables.

■ Example: **PRESENTATION OF THEORY-GENERATING RESEARCH RESULTS IN NARRATIVE AND TABLE FORMS**

Hermeneutic analysis yielded thematic responses to the protocol topics and hierarchical clusters that transcended individual topics to describe the essential structure of participants' power. Some participants were relatively powerful, participating knowingly in change. Others seemed relatively less powerful; that is, as waiting for, rather than as initiating change, and demonstrating little knowing involvement in directing their lives.

Themes that emerged in response to each power topic in the protocol are listed in [Table 5–6]. . . . Three themes —integrality or directedness toward the world, awareness of integrality, and mundaneness—characterized responses to the protocol items. These themes and examples from the interviews are summarized in [Table 5–7]. (Dzurec, 1994, pp. 156, 158)

Table 5–6 ■ SUMMARY OF PROTOCOL TOPICS AND THEMES

1. What kinds of choices do you make on a day-to-day basis?
   a. Choices about daily activities
   b. Choices about interacting:
      1. From a giving perspective
      2. Because I am forced to interact
2. Do the choices you make, make a difference in what happens to you?
   a. Yes, in context
   b. I don't know
3. Do you feel free to make the choices you want to make?
   a. Completely free
   b. Restricted by:
      1. Family
      2. Discrimination
      3. Physical pain
   c. No freedom
4. Have you felt able to change things in your life?
   a. Yes, with direction
   b. No
5. What is your view of your life?*
   a. Process—something in which I engage
   b. Product—something that I can describe, not change
6. What is a good day like for you?*
   a. Process
      1. Engaging in activities
      2. Being with people
   b. Product
      1. Physical characteristics of the day
      2. A function of state-of-mind
7. What is important in your life?
   a. Connectedness (integrality) through:
      1. Reading
      2. God
      3. People
      4. Decreasing stress
8. What do you think your future will be like?
   a. Uncertain
   b. Better
9. What are you thinking about as we talk about these things?
   a. Only the interview

---

*The notions of process and product as they are presented in Topics 5 and 6 represent the investigator's imposition of labels on the themes expressed by participants. Descriptions given for all other topics represent essentially verbatim responses of participants.

Source: From Dzurec, 1994, p. 157, with permission.

Table 5–7 ■ SUMMARY OF THEMES
ACROSS TOPICS: THE
STRUCTURE OF
PARTICIPANTS' POWER

Integrality
Relationships with God
Relationships with people
Reading and studying
Living in the world
   As limiting
   As enriching
Quality of integrality reflected in:
   Belongingness
   Loneliness
   Uncertainty
Awareness
Certainty of integral role
Uncertainty of integral role
Mundaneness
Relatively little leverage in influencing others

Source: From Dzurec, 1994, p. 158, with permission.

Presentation of Theory-Testing Research Results

Theory-testing research reports present descriptive statistics for the theory concepts as well as the results of inferential statistical tests. Tables and figures (Table 5–2, Guidelines for Constructing Tables and Figures) frequently are used to summarize the results.

DESCRIPTIVE STATISTICS. The following two examples illustrate the presentation of descriptive statistics for concepts in theory-testing research. The examples were taken from a journal article reporting the results of research designed to test an explanatory theory of the relation of various concepts representing basic conditioning factors to the adjustment responses of children and their mothers to the children's cancer. The theory was directly derived from Orem's (1995) Self-Care Framework. The first example illustrates the presentation of measures of central tendency and variability; the second, a correlation matrix. In both examples, the narrative is limited to a reference to the relevant table.

■ Example: **PRESENTATION OF MEASURES OF CENTRAL TENDENCY AND VARIABILITY IN A TABLE**

Table [5–8] shows means, standard deviations, and ranges for the study's dependent variables. (Moore and Mosher, 1997, p. 521)

Table 5–8 ■ MEANS, STANDARD DEVIATIONS, AND RANGES FOR ADJUSTMENT RESPONSES OF CHILDREN AND MOTHERS

Dependent Variable	$\bar{x}$	SD	Observed Ranges
Children			
Self-care practices	207.77	16.77	161–243
State anxiety	29.33	5.75	20–44
Trait anxiety	33.22	7.25	20–50
Mothers			
Dependent-care practices	242.75	18.99	195–274
State anxiety	36.45	11.59	20–74
Trait anxiety	36.73	8.91	20–64

n = 74

Source: From Moore and Mosher, 1997, p. 521, with permission.

■ Example: **PRESENTATION OF CORRELATIONS IN A TABLE**

Table [5–9] shows correlations. (Moore and Mosher, 1997, p. 521)

Table 5–9 ■ PEARSON CORRELATIONS BETWEEN VARIABLES

	Age	SES	SCP	CSA	CTA	DCA	MSA	MHA
Child's age	1.00							
Socioeconomic status (SES)	0.16	1.00						
Self-care practices (SCP)	−0.37**	−0.07	1.00					
Child state anxiety (CSA)	0.38**	0.04	−0.12	1.00				
Child trait anxiety (CTA)	0.05	−0.10	−0.28*	0.15	1.00			
Dependent-care agent practices (DCA)	−0.07	0.05	0.04	−0.09	−0.37**	1.00		
Mother state anxiety (MSA)	0.09	−0.09	0.20	0.12	−0.07	0.13	1.00	
Mother trait anxiety (MTA)	0.02	−0.08	0.05	0.05	0.21	−0.07	0.73**	1.00

n = 74 (children and mothers); * p < 0.01; ** p < 0.001.

Source: From Moore and Mosher, 1997, p. 521, with permission.

RESULTS OF STATISTICAL TESTS. Three examples are given to illustrate various ways to present the results of inferential statistical tests for theory-testing correlational and experimental research. The first example illustrates how results can be presented in a narrative that is supplemented with a table. The excerpt is from a journal article reporting the results of correlational research designed to test an explanatory theory of the relation of human field motion, human field rhythms, creativity, and sentience to adolescents' perceived health status. The sample was divided into the three phases of the adolescent years: 12 to 14 represented early adolescent years; 15 to 17, middle adolescent years; and 18 to 21, late adolescent years. The theory was derived from Rogers' Science of Unitary Human Beings (Barrett, 1990). The narrative includes an explanation of how the data were analyzed, and the results are organized according to the specific aims of the study, which were stated in the form of research questions.

The second example illustrates how results can be presented in a narrative that is supplemented with a table and a figure. The excerpt was taken from a journal article reporting the results of correlational research designed to test an explanatory

---

■ Example: **PRESENTATION OF RESULTS OF STATISTICAL TESTS IN NARRATIVE AND TABLE FORMS FOR THEORY-TESTING CORRELATIONAL RESEARCH**

Data were analyzed using Pearson correlations, with a two-tailed test of significance. The results are presented in Table [5–10]. With respect to the first research question, perceived field motion was statistically significantly and positively related to perceived health status in early, middle, and late adolescents. The Z test for the difference between two independent correlations (Shelley, 1984) was calculated between early and middle adolescents, early and late adolescents, and middle and late adolescents. None was statistically significant. With respect to the second research question, human field rhythms were statistically significantly and positively related to perceived health status in late adolescents only. In addition, none of the Z tests were statistically significant. With respect to the third research question, creativity was statistically significantly and positively related to perceived health status in late adolescents only. None of the Z tests were statistically significant. With respect to the fourth research question, the inverse relationship found between sentience and perceived health status was not statistically significant in early, middle, or late adolescents. (Yarcheski and Mahon, 1995, pp. 390–391)

Table 5–10 ■ **CORRELATIONS COEFFICIENTS BETWEEN ROGERS' FIELD MANIFESTATIONS AND PERCEIVED HEALTH STATUS IN EARLY ($N = 106$), MIDDLE ($N = 111$), AND LATE ($N = 113$) ADOLESCENTS**

	Perceived Health Status Adolescents		
Variables	**Early**	**Middle**	**Late**
Perceived Field Motion	.24*	.26**	.44**
Human Field Rhythms	.06	.10	.23*
Creativity	.01	.01	.20*
Sentience	−.06	−.16	−.03

*$p < .05$. **$p < .01$.

Source: From Yarcheski and Mahon, 1995, p. 391, with permission.

theory of the relation of severity of illness, hardiness, perceived control over visitation (PCV), and state anxiety to length of stay in an intensive care unit. The theory was derived from Roy's Adaptation Model (Roy and Andrews, 1991). The narrative includes a detailed explanation of how the data were analyzed.

■ Example: **PRESENTATION OF RESULTS OF STATISTICAL TESTS IN NARRATIVE, TABLE, AND FIGURE FORMS FOR THEORY-TESTING CORRELATIONAL RESEARCH**

Testing of the [theory] [Figure 5–3] began with a series of regression analyses with blocks of independent variables. The focal stimulus (severity of illness) was entered into the equation first, the contextual stimuli (PCV and state anxiety) were entered second, and the residual stimulus (hardiness) was entered third. Results are summarized in Table [5–11].

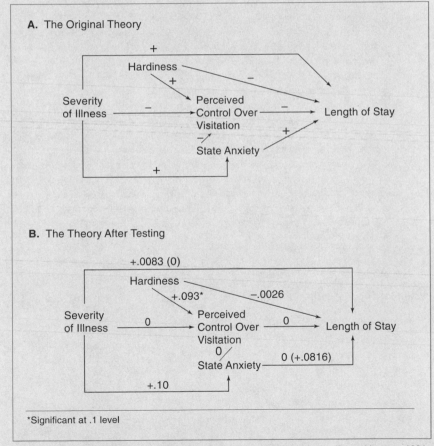

Figure 5–3 ■ Diagrams of the proposed (A) and tested theory (B). (From Hamner, 1996, pp. 216, 218, with permission.)

Table 5–11 ■ BLOCKED REGRESSION ANALYSIS OF SEVERITY OF
ILLNESS, PERCEIVED CONTROL OVER VISITATION (PCV),
STATE ANXIETY, AND HARDINESS ON LENGTH OF STAY

	R^2	Signif. F	B	Signif. T
Block 1				
Severity of illness	.02	.24	.0085	.237
Block 2				
State Anxiety	.13	.05	.0083	.01
PCV	(both variables)		.0013	.76
Block 3				
Apache	.18	.03	.0094	.177
State Anxiety	(all variables)		.0126	.002
PCV			−.0009	.985
Hardiness			.0032	.073

Source: From Hamner, 1996, p. 217, with permission.

Next, a series of multiple regression analyses were done in order to estimate certain coefficients in the [theory]. Table [5–12] describes these
analyses. The first step was to regress the dependent variable on the exogenous variables, that is, the variables whose variability is assumed to be
determined by causes outside the [theory]. In this case, neither severity of
illness nor hardiness proved significant in predicting LOS [length of stay].

The second step was to ascertain which variables in the [theory] contributed
to the explanation of the endogenous variables, or the variables explained by
the [theory]. In addition to LOS, state anxiety and PCV are endogenous.
Hardiness and severity of illness were exogenous variables with paths to PCV;
therefore, PCV was regressed on these two variables and it was found that 10%
of the variance was explained at a significant level. The second part of this step
was to examine the endogenous variable of state anxiety. The only path leading to state anxiety in the model was severity of illness, therefore state anxiety
was regressed on severity of illness, again with no significant variance explained.
[Figure 5–3 also depicts the theory after testing.] (Hamner, 1996, p. 217)

Table 5–12 ■ MULTIPLE REGRESSION SERIES FOR PATH ANALYSIS

Independent Variables	Dependent Variables	R^2	Signif. F	B	Signif. T
Hardiness		.03	.49	−.00026	.858
Severity of illness	Length of Stay	(both variables)	(both variables)	.00834	.255
Severity of Illness	Perceived Control over	.10	.05	.238	.24
Hardiness	Visitation	(both variables)	(both variables)	.093	.02
Severity of Illness	State Anxiety	.002	.72	.102	.7225
Hardiness	Perceived	.108	.09	.067	.195
Severity of Illness	Control over	(3 variables)	(3 variables)	.229	.262
State Anxiety	Visitation			−.094	.425

Source: From Hamner, 1996, p. 217, with permission.

The third example illustrates presentation of the results for the test of the main hypothesis from experimental research that tested a predictive theory of the effects of walking exercise on physical functioning, exercise level, emotional distress, and symptom experience of women with breast cancer who were receiving radiation therapy. The theory was based on Roy's Adaptation Model (Roy and Andrews, 1991) and findings from previous research. The investigators hypothesized that "women who participated in a moderate walking exercise program during radiation therapy treatment would have a higher level of physical functioning [and exercise level] and lower levels of distressful symptoms [emotional distress and symptom experience] than a control group receiving usual care" (Mock et al., 1997, p. 992). Physical functioning was measured by the 12-Minute Walk Test; exercise level, by the Exercise Rating Scale; emotional distress, by the Symptom Assessment Scale (SAS); and symptom experience, by the SAS and the Piper Fatigue Scale. The narrative includes a brief explanation of how the data were analyzed; a detailed explanation had already been presented in the method section.

■ Example: **PRESENTATION OF RESULTS OF STATISTICAL TESTS FOR THEORY-TESTING EXPERIMENTAL RESEARCH**

Testing of the basic hypothesis by means of MANCOVA revealed highly significant differences between the two groups on physical functioning and symptom intensity outcomes, $F(1,39) = 9.67$, $p < 0.001$. Univariate analyses of covariance, with the baseline pretest measurement as the covariate, indicated significant differences in the pre- to post-test values between the groups on both physical functioning outcomes and the most frequent symptoms—fatigue, anxiety, and difficulty sleeping. Only depression failed to show a significant difference between groups (Table [5–13]). (Mock et al. 1997, p. 995)

Table 5–13 ■ **ANALYSIS OF COVARIANCE ADJUSTED FOR BASELINE VALUES ON 12-MINUTE WALK TEST, EXERCISE LEVEL, AND FREQUENT SYMPTOMS**

Variable	Exercise $\overline{X}$	Usual Care $\overline{X}$	F	p
12-Minute Walk Test (feet)	33.71	30.89	9.69	0.003
Exercise level	4.51	0.92	48.32	<0.001
Fatigue	24.72	45.49	6.10	0.018
Difficulty sleeping	12.38	32.58	5.39	0.027
Anxiety	10.44	26.93	5.11	0.029
Depression	9.51	21.05	2.77	0.104

Source: From Mock et al., 1997, p. 995, with permission.

DISCUSSION

The discussion section also is structured according to specific aims or hypotheses. Results are not repeated in the discussion section, although they may be summarized for clarity.

This section of a research report frequently includes a comparison of the study findings with results from related research. In theory-generating research, a comparison of the theory that was generated with extant theories may be included. In theory-testing research, the results may be compared with those of previous research.

The discussion section should include a definitive conclusion regarding the empirical adequacy of the middle-range theory and the credibility of the conceptual model. This section also may include alternative methodological and/or substantive explanations for the study findings.

The discussion section frequently ends with the investigator's recommendations for future research designed to test the empirical adequacy of the theory, as well as to extend the theory. In addition, the final part of the discussion section may include conclusions about the pragmatic adequacy of the theory that was tested. More specifically, a recommendation may be offered regarding the implications of the study findings for clinical practice, such as formulation of practice guidelines or health policies.

Discussion of Theory-Generating Research Results

The following example illustrates the discussion section for theory-generating research. The excerpt was taken from a journal article reporting theory-generating research using a hermeneutic method. The study was designed to generate a descriptive classification theory of the personal power experienced by people with schizophrenia. The research was based on Barrett's (1983) concept of power, which was derived from Rogers' (1982, 1983) Science of Unitary Human Beings. The investigator used the discussion section to summarize and interpret the theory that was generated, compare the theory to the works of other scholars, and relate the theory to Rogers' Science of Unitary Human Beings. In addition, the investigator offered suggestions for future research to test the empirical adequacy of the theory that was generated, to progress to development of an explanatory theory. Finally, the investigator addressed the potential use of the theory in clinical practice.

■ Example: **DISCUSSION OF THEORY-GENERATING RESEARCH RESULTS**

Power characterizes and directs life experience. For people with schizophrenia, life experience is characterized by relative powerlessness—dependence, uncertainty, domination. Little attention has been paid to the characteristic of power for people with schizophrenia. This study represents a first step in such an effort.

For participants in the study, integrality, or directedness toward the world, was the essence of power; awareness of one's integrality gauged relative degree of power; and mundaneness characterized participants' range of power. Participants' power, variable yet limited, is probably similar to all people's power, but it is different from others' power in that it is restricted to mundane considerations. Although this single and basic study does not fully disclose the nature of the power for people with schizophrenia, it does offer a workable and testable view of power for people with schizophrenia. The characterization of power, especially its mundaneness, is important to understanding the tenacity of schizophrenia. As Strauss (1989) noted, one's feeling about a disorder and its course affect its evolution. People with schizophrenia, pathophysiology notwithstanding, might behave in ways that perpetuate their relative powerlessnss, because they perceive themselves as powerless. This finding is consistent with others' views. (Foucault, 1965, 1977, 1989; Ingleby, 1980; Rogers, 1982, 1983)

Future research might build on this basic work to extend or refute this characterization of power and to examine the relation between power and other phenomena for people with schizophrenia. For example, social and legal mandates have severely restricted opportunities for people with schizophrenia to reside in hospitals. Living in communities outside hospitals, people with schizophrenia are required to use power skills to negotiate for jobs and housing, and to manage interpersonal situations. The successes of mentally ill people to negotiate community life are limited, at best. Some researchers (Champney and Dzurec, 1992; Ciompi, 1980; Harding, Brooks, Ashikaga, Strauss, and Brier, 1987) have suggested that community adjustment for people with severe mental disabilities such as schizophrenia depends on appropriate social supports. One could argue that the most appropriate social supports involve assessing clients' relative power, teaching them about the pervasiveness of power, and assisting them to use their power most effectively. (Dzurec, 1994, p. 159)

Discussion of Theory-Testing Research Results

The following excerpt exemplifies discussion of the empirical adequacy of an explanatory theory of the relation of severity of illness, hardiness, perceived control over visitation (PCV), and state anxiety to length of stay in an intensive care unit. The statistical technique of path analysis was used to test the theory. The excerpt also exemplifies discussion of the credibility of Roy's Adaptation Model (Roy and Andrews, 1991), the conceptual model from which the theory was derived.

■ Example: **DISCUSSION OF THEORY-TESTING RESEARCH RESULTS, WITH CONCLUSIONS ABOUT THE EMPIRICAL ADEQUACY OF A THEORY AND THE CREDIBILITY OF A CONCEPTUAL MODEL**

The proposed [theory] demonstrated inadequate support. Only one path (the path between hardiness and PCV) could be supported at the significance level of .1.

The study was based on the proposition: Freedom of communication patterns will positively influence the adequacy of seeking and receiving affection. However, PCV did not perform in the regression analysis or [theory] testing as hypothesized. Thus, the proposition from the Roy Adaptation Model cannot be supported. (Hamner, 1996, p. 219)

The next example illustrates an alternative substantive explanation. The excerpt was taken from a journal article reporting the results of a test of an explanatory theory of the relation of various concepts representing basic conditioning factors to the adjustment responses of children and their mothers to the children's cancer. The theory was directly derived from Orem's (1995) Self-Care Framework. At the time of the study, 42% of the children were receiving cancer–related therapy; the remainder had completed cancer therapy and were considered off therapy.

■ Example: **DISCUSSION OF THEORY-TESTING RESEARCH RESULTS, WITH AN ALTERNATIVE SUBSTANTIVE EXPLANATION AND RECOMMENDATIONS FOR FUTURE RESEARCH**

Children who have completed treatment for cancer have better adjustment responses than those currently receiving treatment. A comparison of children on therapy and off therapy had not been documented in previous research. As expected from clinical observation, children's state anxiety was significantly higher in the on-therapy group. Because state anxiety reflects how an individual is feeling at the moment, it seems reasonable that having cancer, as well as being scheduled for chemotherapy or another treatment procedure at the time of testing, would create more anxiety for the child. No significant differences existed between the self-care practices and the trait anxiety levels in the on- and off-therapy groups. Perhaps children think that self-care practices and health promotion are as important while receiving therapy as when they have completed treatment. Trait anxiety is more of a personality characteristic and, therefore, is more constant and less influenced by particular situations or diagnoses. Further study is needed to investigate the self-care practices of children with cancer, possibly in a qualitative study, as well as to compare the self-care practices and trait anxiety of children with cancer to a normative sample of children. Such research would help clinicians understand whether children with cancer differ from children without cancer. (Moore and Mosher, 1997, p. 523)

Methodological explanations for study findings are exemplified by the following two excerpts. The first excerpt, which illustrates discussion of the sample, was taken from a journal article reporting the results of correlational research designed to test an explanatory theory of the relation of the basic conditioning factors of maternal age, socioeconomic status, marital status, maternal employment hours, ethnic group, only child, child age, child gender, birth order, number of children, child health problems, and child status (biologic, adopted, stepchild) to the dependent-care agency of mothers' performance of health promotion and child self-care activities. The theory was directly derived from Orem's (1995) Self-Care Framework. The sample included 380 mothers, 3.2% of whom were Asian; 15.5%, African-American; 5%, Hispanic; 75.3%, white; and 1%, other.

■ Example: **DISCUSSION OF THEORY-TESTING RESEARCH RESULTS, WITH A METHODOLOGICAL EXPLANATION RELATED TO THE SAMPLE AND RECOMMENDATIONS FOR FUTURE RESEARCH**

A second recommendation for future research is more precise measurement of specific variables, for example, more precise identification of a subject's cultural background. In the present study, for example, mothers who selected the ethnic option of "white" included women from many nations, such as the United States, Egypt, and Afghanistan. On an issue as culture-bound as a mother's care for her child, further delineation would help identify differences and, thus, provide a more sound empirical base for clinical decision-making in cross-cultural practice settings. Incorporating these measurement revisions into subsequent investigations of dependent care agent performance may account for an additional percentage of the variance, therefore providing more support for the theory.

A third recommendation relates to sample selection. In the present study, individual basic conditioning factors that significantly influenced a mother's dependent care agent performance were child age and ethnic group. As anticipated, increasing child age was significantly associated with decreased levels of maternal dependent care agency performance. This finding might be explained by the fact that mothers of adolescents generally spend less time with them than mothers of younger children spend with theirs. An expanded explanation is that older children may be viewed by their mothers as having greater self-care skills, therefore requiring dependent care agent performance that is either less than, or different in character than, that required during early childhood years. Although ethnic group was shown to be a significant influence, further study is needed with samples that include a greater representation of individuals from a wider range of more specifically defined ethnic groups. Future studies of dependent care agent performance might use stratified random sampling by age and ethnic group. (Gaffney & Moore, 1996, pp. 163–164)

The next example illustrates an instrument-based explanation. The excerpt was taken from a journal article reporting the results of correlational research designed to test an explanatory theory of correlates of grief responses. The theory was derived from Roy's Adaptation Model (Roy and Andrews, 1991).

■ Example: **DISCUSSION OF THEORY-TESTING RESEARCH RESULTS, WITH A METHODOLOGICAL EXPLANATION RELATED TO THE INSTRUMENT**

> Spiritual beliefs were not found to be significantly related to the coping processes; this finding must be interpreted cautiously because of the reliability of the measure (.58). The instrument assessed current level of religious participation as one parameter of spiritual beliefs. This may not have been the best parameter to assess, given the changes that took place in the women's lives. The death of their spouse may have affected their religious participation; for example, lack of transportation may have led to less frequent attendance at services, in addition to their religious participation affecting their coping processes and grief response. (Robinson, 1995, p. 162)

Discussion of Pragmatic Adequacy

An example of a discussion of pragmatic adequacy is evident in the following excerpt from a journal article reporting the results of experimental research that tested a predictive theory of the effects of walking exercise on physical functioning, exercise level, emotional distress, and symptom experience of women with breast cancer who were receiving radiation therapy. The theory was based on Roy's Adaptation Model (Roy and Andrews, 1991) and findings from previous research.

■ Example: **DISCUSSION OF PRAGMATIC ADEQUACY**

> The low-risk, low-cost walking exercise program tested in this study can be quickly and easily taught and monitored by nurses or other health care professionals. The self-paced, home-based walking program provided an effective, convenient, and cost-efficient way for women in treatment for breast cancer to reduce their symptoms and exert a degree of personal control during a period that often is characterized by uncertainty (Ferrell, Grant, Funk et al., 1996). An intervention that maintains or improves functional status and decreases side effects of breast cancer treatment may improve QOL [quality of life] (Ferrell, Grant, Dean et al., 1996) and increase adherence to treatment protocols. (Mock et al., 1997, p. 999)

SUGGESTIONS FOR WRITING RESEARCH DOCUMENTS

Writing a research grant proposal, thesis or dissertation proposal, or a report of completed research can seem like an overwhelming task. The following suggestions, if followed, may facilitate the preparation of research documents and reduce the psychological and physical burden of the task.

First and foremost, the investigator must be very familiar with the research topic and the conceptual model that is to guide the study. Familiarity is achieved by immersing oneself in the literature about the conceptual model and the research topic. A comprehensive literature search should be done many months prior to a proposal deadline to provide adequate time for reading and thinking about the content of the conceptual model, the ways in which the conceptual model has been used to guide previous studies, and the particular research topic. In addition, the investigator should become familiar with the process of constructing conceptual-theoretical-empirical structures, which can be achieved by reading this book and analyzing and evaluating existing research documents.

Next, the investigator should assemble and have frequent communication with a research team consisting of co-investigators and consultants who are familiar with the conceptual model, the theoretical aspects of the research topic, and the methodology associated with the conceptual model and the research topic. If the research topic is clinical in nature, the research team also should include at least one clinical expert, so that the real world of the clinical situation can be addressed adequately and appropriately. In addition, a clinical expert may facilitate access to potential research subjects. All members of the research team should participate in the construction and refinement of the conceptual-theoretical-empirical (C-T-E) structure for the research.

Third, the investigator should become familiar with the format for the document. Virtually every university, funding agency or organization, and journal or book publisher requires submission of documents in a distinctive format that must be followed. The format encompasses the label for and the content of each section of the document, as well as the citation style within the narrative and in the list of references. Moreover, the investigator should select one or two existing research documents or the excerpts from existing documents given in this chapter to serve as a template for the new document.

Fourth, any preliminary research that is needed to support a research proposal should be carried out as soon as the research topic and empirical research methods are identified. Pilot studies are especially important and strengthen the proposal considerably. The specific purposes of a pilot study are to determine the adequacy of subject enrollment and retention strategies, check the feasibility of the design, check the validity and reliability of the instruments with the particular population to be sampled, and estimate the effect size for determining sample size for the larger study (Prescott and Soeken, 1989). The findings of a pilot study may strengthen the initial conceptualization of the study or require the research team to revise the original purpose of the research, the approach for subject recruitment and retention, the instruments to be used, or even the entire C-T-E structure.

In addition, a narrative or quantitative integrative review of existing relevant literature should be prepared, employing the strategies discussed in Chapter 4, and used as the literature review section of the document. If the purpose of the research document is to propose a new study or report the results of a completed study, the integrative review should be summarized in just a few concise paragraphs. If, on the other hand, the purpose of the research document is to propose an integrative review or report the results of such a review as a study itself, the entire process of an integrative review should be described (see Chapter 4).

The actual writing of the research document can be facilitated by preparing a diagram of the C-T-E structure and writing a sentence about each component. Each sentence then can be expanded into one or more paragraphs that will provide the required detail. Alternatively, an abstract can be written, and each sentence of the abstract then can be expanded into one or more paragraphs. The use of an abstract as the starting point is especially helpful if the investigator is progressing from brief notes and audiovisual aids used for a conference presentation, or from the great detail of a dissertation or thesis, to a journal article or book chapter.

Johnson (1996) suggested dictation as an especially efficient approach to writing a research document. She noted that a good dictaphone works better than a tape recorder, because tape recorders do not have sufficiently fine control for stopping and reversing the tape. The investigator, along with other members of the research team, can dictate the sentences and paragraphs that complete a diagram of the C-T-E structure or the paragraphs that expand the abstract. The investigator then can transcribe the dictated material or seek the services of a skilled secretary. If a secretary is employed, the investigator should take that person's other work responsibilities and commitments into account when negotiating a deadline. Once the dictated material is transcribed, the entire research team should read and participate in editing the document both for substance and writing style. Repeated readings of the document and many drafts may be required to achieve the necessary clarity. Each draft of the document should be systematically analyzed using the technique of C-T-E formalization described in Chapter 2 and then evaluated using the criteria for evaluation of C-T-E structures given in Chapter 3.

A dictaphone or small tape recorder also can be used to record ideas for revisions in the document as they occur to the investigator. Inasmuch as ideas about the document may occur when in the midst of other work or even during leisure time, it is prudent to always have the dictaphone or tape recorder close at hand.

In addition, the assistance of a colleague who is not part of the research team can be an invaluable contribution to the quality of a research document (Polit and Hungler, 1995). The colleague chosen, who should be an experienced and published researcher, should be asked to read and comment on the document from the perspective of a grant review committee, examination committee, or journal peer-reviewer.

Finally, writing a research document is greatly facilitated if the investigator keeps in mind that the document is not a great work that reflects exceptional creativity in writing. Rather, a research document is no more or no less than a clear and concise presentation of each component of a logically constructed C-T-E structure.

A NOTE ON THE LENGTH OF RESEARCH DOCUMENTS

The length of a research document frequently is dictated by the agency, organization, publisher, or university to which the document will be submitted. Investigators are cautioned to adhere to the required page limit, which can be achieved by writing clearly and concisely. Even if a page limit is not specified, clear and concise writing should be a goal.

Furthermore, the writers of theses and dissertations are encouraged to write concisely. Indeed, there is much to be gained, with regard to moving from the typical great detail of a thesis or dissertation to a publishable report, if the initial document is written as "a manuscript of appropriate form and length for publication" (Krathwohl, 1985, p. 155). For example, a thesis or dissertation could be written as one or more journal article(s), a book chapter, a monograph, or a full book. In making his suggestion for the publishable manuscript format of a thesis or dissertation, Krathwohl (1985) pointed out a comprehensive literature review, the raw data, and other similar documentation that might be requested by the examining committee or university could be placed in an appendix. The advantages of this suggestion are:

> ■ (1) learning journal format and how to reduce a complicated study to abbreviated length with the appropriate inclusion and exclusion of aspects of the argument and of detail, (2) doing so when not burdened with a new position and its unfamiliar demands, (3) having the guidance of experienced faculty members to facilitate learning, (4) having the dissertation "wrapped up" on getting the degree and the freedom to devote full energies to one's new tasks, . . . (5) possibly a publication on entering the first position, and (6) the reinforcement of successfully accomplishing these gains, which would make it more likely that future research will be seen as rewarding. (Krathwohl, 1985, p. 155)

CONCLUSION

The guidelines for writing research documents presented in this chapter continue the emphasis in this book on the relation of conceptual models to middle-range theories and empirical research methods. The guidelines were illustrated with examples drawn from both theory-generating and theory-testing research that was based on explicit conceptual models. The application of these guidelines should facilitate communication of what investigators plan to do and what they actually have done, always within the context of a conceptual-theoretical-empirical structure.

References

American Psychological Association. (1994). *Publication manual of the American Psychological Association* (4th ed.). Washington, D.C.: The Association.

Andrews, H.A., & Roy, C. (1986). *Essentials of the Roy adaptation model*. Norwalk, CT: Appleton-Century Crofts.

Barrett, E.A.M. (1983). *An empirical investiga-*

tion of Martha E. Rogers's principle of helicy: The relationship of human field motion and power. Unpublished doctoral dissertation, New York University.

Barrett, E.A.M. (Ed.) (1990). *Visions of Rogers' science-based nursing.* New York: National League for Nursing.

Breckenridge, D.M. (1997a). Decisions regarding dialysis treatment modality: A holistic perspective. *Holistic Nursing Practice, 12*(1), 54–61.

Breckenridge, D.M. (1997b). Patients' perceptions of why, how, and by whom dialysis treatment modality was chosen. *American Nephrology Nurses Association Journal, 24,* 313–319.

Brooks-Brunn, J.A. (1991). Tips on writing a research-based manuscript: The review of literature. *Nurse Author and Editor, 1*(2), 1–3.

Calvillo, E.R., & Flaskerud, J.H. (1993). The adequacy and scope of Roy's adaptation model to guide cross-cultural pain research. *Nursing Science Quarterly, 6,* 118–129.

Degner, L.F., & Beaton, J.I. (1987). *Life-death decisions in health care.* New York: Hemisphere.

Downs, F.S. (1994). Information processing [Editorial]. *Nursing Research, 43,* 323.

Dzurec, L.C. (1994). Schizophrenic clients' experiences of power: Using hermeneutic analysis. *Image: Journal of Nursing Scholarship, 26,* 155–159.

Gaffney, K.F., & Moore, J.B. (1996). Testing Orem's theory of self-care deficit: Dependent care agent performance for children. *Nursing Science Quarterly, 9,* 160–164.

Grant, G.E. (1997, June 30). *Memorandum to Directors of Offices of Sponsored Programs from the Director of the Office of Policy for Extramural Research Administration, Office of Extramural Research, National Institutes.* Bethesda, MD: National Institutes of Health.

Haller, K.B. (1992). Solving puzzles [Editorial]. *Journal of Obstetric, Gynecologic, and Neonatal Nursing, 21,* 444.

Hamner, J.B. (1996). Preliminary testing of a proposition from the Roy adaptation model. *Image: Journal of Nursing Scholarship, 28,* 215–220.

Hunter, S.M., Langemo, D.K., Olson, B., Hanson, D., Cathcart-Silberberg, T., Burd, C., & Sauvage, T.R. (1995). The effectiveness of skin care protocols for pressure ulcers. *Rehabilitation Nursing, 20,* 250–255.

Johnson, S.H. (1996). Dictation—The fastest way to write. *Nurse Author and Editor, 6*(1), 8.

Krathwohl, D. (1985). *Social and behavioral science research.* San Francisco: Jossey-Bass.

Langemo, D.K., Olson, B., Hunter, S., Hanson, D., Burd, C., & Cathcart-Silberberg, T. (1991). Incidence and prediction of pressure ulcers in five patient care settings. *Decubitus, 4*(3), 25–26, 28, 30, 32, 36.

Mock, V., Dow, K.H., Meares, C.J., Grimm, P.M., Dienemann, J.A., Haisfield-Wolfe, M.E., Quitasol, W., Mitchell, S., Chakravarthy, A., & Gage, I. (1997). Effects of exercise on fatigue, physical functioning, and emotional distress during radiation therapy for breast cancer. *Oncology Nursing Forum, 24,* 991–1000.

Moore, J.B., & Mosher, R.B. (1997). Adjustment responses of children and their mothers to cancer: Self-care and anxiety. *Oncology Nursing Forum, 24,* 519–525.

Neuman, B. (1995). *The Neuman systems model* (3rd ed.). Norwalk, CT: Appleton and Lange.

Orem, D.E. (1991). *Nursing: Concepts of practice* (4th ed.). St. Louis: Mosby YearBook.

Orem, D.E. (1995). *Nursing: Concepts of practice* (5th ed.). St. Louis: Mosby YearBook.

Polit, D.F., & Hungler, B.P. (1995). *Nursing research: Principles and methods* (5th ed.). Philadelphia: Lippincott.

Prescott, P.A., & Soeken, K.L. (1989). The potential uses of pilot work. *Nursing Research, 38,* 60–62.

Roberts, K.L., Brittin, M., Cook, M-A., & deClifford, J. (1994). Boomerang pillows and respiratory capacity. *Clinical Nursing Research, 3,* 157–165.

Robinson, J.H. (1995). Grief responses, coping processes, and social support of widows: Research with Roy's model. *Nursing Science Quarterly, 8,* 158–164.

Rogers, M.E. (1982). Beyond the horizon. In N. Chaska (Ed.), *The nursing profession: A time to speak* (pp. 795–801). New York: McGraw-Hill.

Rogers, M.E. (1983). *Nursing science: A science of unitary human beings. Glossary.* Unpublished paper, New York University.

Rogers, M.E. (1992). Nursing science and the space age. *Nursing Science Quarterly, 5,* 27–34.

Roy, C., & Andrews, H.A. (1991). *The Roy adaptation model. The definitive statement.* Norwalk, CT: Appleton and Lange.

Samarel, N., Fawcett, J., & Tulman, L. (1995–1997). *Effect of extended individual and group support for breast cancer.* Research grant proposal funded by the American Cancer Society, Grant No. PBR-64B.

Samarel, N., Fawcett, J., & Tulman, L. (1997). Effect of support groups with coaching on adaptation to early stage breast cancer. *Research in Nursing and Health, 20,* 15–26.

Schaefer, K.M., & Pond, J.B. (Eds.). (1991). *Levine's conservation model: A framework for nursing practice.* Philadelphia: F. A. Davis.

Sherman, D.W. (1996). Nurses' willingness to care for AIDS patients and spirituality, social support, and death anxiety. *Image: Journal of Nursing Scholarship, 28,* 205–213.

Tulman, L., & Fawcett, J. (1990–1993). *Functional status during pregnancy and the postpartum.* Research grant proposal funded by the National Institutes of Health, National Center for Nursing Research, Grant No. 1 R01-NR02340.

Tulman, L., & Fawcett, J. (1994). *Functional sta-tus during pregnancy and the postpartum.* Final report for Grant No. 1 R01-NR02340 submitted to the National Institutes of Health, National Center for Nursing Research.

Villarruel, A.M. (1995). Mexican-American cultural meanings, expressions, self-care and dependent-care actions associated with experiences of pain. *Research in Nursing and Health, 18,* 427–436.

Yarcheski, A., & Mahon, N.E. (1995). Rogers's pattern manifestations and health in adolescents. *Western Journal of Nursing Research, 17,* 383–397.

Additional Readings

Barnum, B.S. (1995). *Writing and getting published: A primer for nurses.* New York: Springer.

Blenner, J.L. (1990). Writing the qualitative grant proposal while meeting quantitative criteria: Walking on eggshells. *Florida Nursing Review, 4*(3), 5–9.

Creswell, J.W. (1994). *Research design: Qualitative and quantitative approaches.* Thousand Oaks, CA: Sage.

Fawcett, J. (1996). Putting the conceptual model into the research report. *Nurse Author and Editor, 6*(2), 1–4.

Fuller, E.O. (1983). Preparing an abstract of a nursing study. *Nursing Research, 32,* 316–317.

Haller, K.B. (1988). Writing effective research abstracts. *MCN, The American Journal of Maternal Child Nursing, 13,* 74.

Knafl, K.A., & Howard, M.J. (1984). Interpreting and reporting qualitative research. *Research in Nursing and Health, 7,* 17–24.

Reif-Lehrer, L. (1995). *The grant application writer's handbook.* Boston: Jones and Bartlett.

Sandelowski, M. (1998). Writing a good read: Strategies for representing qualitative data. *Research in Nursing and Health, 21,* 375–382.

Appendices

Introduction

Throughout the text, examples drawn from various research documents have been used to illustrate the steps of the analysis and evaluation of conceptual-theoretical-empirical structures for research. The appendix pulls together the text material by presenting complete analyses and evaluations of the conceptual, theoretical, and methodological elements of seven published research reports. Each report selected for inclusion in the appendix includes an explicit conceptual model that guides the middle-range theory-generating or theory-testing research.

Descriptive theory-generating research is exemplified by three reports that employ different descriptive research methods, including concept analysis, case study, and the interpretive method of naturalistic inquiry. They are: "The pediatric physiologic stress response: A concept analysis" (Rosenthal-Dichter, 1996); "Exploring music intervention with restrained patients" (Janelli, Kanski, Jones, and Kennedy, 1995); and "Patients' perceptions of why, how, and by whom dialysis treatment modality was chosen" (Breckenridge, 1997).

Descriptive theory-testing research is exemplified by two reports. One report, which employed psychometric analysis, is "The Inventory of Functional Status—Caregiver of a Child in a Body Cast" (Newman, 1997). The other report, which employed survey methodology, is "Stress experience of spouses of patients having coronary artery bypass during hospitalization and 6 weeks after discharge" (Artinian, 1991).

Explanatory theory-testing research is exemplified by a report that employed correlational methods, "Correlates of pain-related responses to venipunctures in school-age children" (Bournaki, 1997). Predictive theory-testing research is exemplified by a report employing an experimental method, "Boomerang pillows and respiratory capacity" (Roberts, Brittin, Cook, and deClifford, 1994).

A reprint of each research report is followed by an analysis of the conceptual-theoretical-empirical (C-T-E) structure for the research. The analysis employs the format for conceptual-theoretical-empirical formalization described in Chapter 2. Accordingly, each report was reviewed and the concepts of the conceptual model that guided the research, as well as the concepts of the middle-range theory that was generated or tested, were identified. Then the middle-range theory concepts were classified. Next, the propositions of the conceptual model and the middle-range theory were identified and classified. In addition, hierarchies of propositions were constructed and diagrams were drawn to illustrate the conceptual-theoretical-empirical structure. The criteria for evaluation of the conceptual-theoretical-empirical structure, which were discussed in Chapter 3, were then applied to determine specification adequacy, linkage adequacy, significance, internal consistency, parsimony, testability, operational adequacy, empirical adequacy, pragmatic adequacy, and conceptual model credibility.

An attempt has been made to share the line of reasoning with regard to decisions made at various points in the analysis and evaluation of each research report. The analysis and evaluation of the conceptual-theoretical-empirical structure for each research report facilitated understanding of the middle-range theory that was generated or tested, the role of one or more conceptual models in guiding the research, and the evidence provided by the research results with regard to the empirical adequacy and the pragmatic adequacy of the theory and the credibility of the conceptual model(s).

The terminology used in the research reports was repeated in the analysis and evaluation, including direct quotations where appropriate. Of note are the analyses that revealed that different researchers used different references and different terms

---

Table Appendix–1 ■ **SUMMARY OF STEPS IN THE ANALYSIS OF CONCEPTUAL-THEORETICAL-EMPIRICAL STRUCTURES FOR RESEARCH**

Component	Text Discussion
Step One: Identification of Concepts	Chapter 2, pp. 31–33
• Concept identification	pp. 31–32
• Pragmatics of concept identification	pp. 32–33
Step Two: Classification of Concepts	Chapter 2, pp. 33–39
• Classification by observability	pp. 34–35
• Classification by measurement characteristics	pp. 35–38
• Pragmatics of concept classification	pp. 38–39
Step Three: Identification and Classification of Propositions	Chapter 2, pp. 39–57
• Nonrelational propositions	pp. 40–45
• Relational propositions	pp. 45–53
• The hypothesis	pp. 53–55
• Pragmatics of proposition identification and classification	pp. 55–57
Step Four: Hierarchical Ordering of Propositions	Chapter 2, pp. 57–62
• Level of abstraction	p. 58
• Inductive reasoning	pp. 58–59
• Deductive reasoning	pp. 59–61
• Sign of a relationship	p. 61
• Pragmatics of hierarchical ordering of propositions	pp. 61–62
Step Five: Construction of Diagrams	Chapter 2, pp. 62–78
• Diagramming conventions	pp. 63–78
• Conceptual-theoretical-empirical structure	pp. 63–65
• Nonrelational and relational propositions	pp. 65–71
• Inventories of concepts and propositions	pp. 71–78
• Pragmatics of diagramming	pp. 75–78

to describe the content of the same conceptual model, in this case, Roy's Adaptation Model (see Janelli et al., Newman, Artinian, and Bournaki). The use of diverse terminology most likely reflects different interpretations of these abstract and general formulations.

Tables Appendix–1 and Appendix–2 summarize the steps of analysis and evaluation of C-T-E structures for research and cite the relevant chapters and pages for ready reference to the text material.

It is suggested that the reader first review each reprinted research report and carry out an analysis and evaluation of the C-T-E structure. The results then may be compared to those given here.

Table Appendix–2 ■ SUMMARY OF STEPS IN THE EVALUATION OF CONCEPUAL-THEORETICAL-EMPIRICAL STRUCTURES FOR RESEARCH

Criterion	Text Discussion
Step One: Evaluation of the Conceptual-Theoretical-Empirical Linkages	Chapter 3, pp. 86–88
• Specification Adequacy	pp. 86–87
1. The conceptual model should be identified explicitly.	
2. The conceptual model should be discussed in sufficient breadth and depth so that the relation of the model to the theory and empirical research methods is clear.	
• Linkage Adequacy	pp. 87–88
1. The linkages between the conceptual model, the theory, and the empirical research methods should be stated explicitly.	
2. The methodology should reflect the conceptual model.	
Step Two: Evaluation of the Theory	Chapter 3, pp. 88–90
• Significance	pp. 88–90
1. The theory should address a phenomenon of social and theoretical significance.	
• Internal Consistency	pp. 90–93
1. The theory concepts should be defined clearly, and the same concept names and definitions should be used throughout the theory.	
2. The theory should not contain redundant concepts.	
3. The propositions of the theory should be complete and free from redundancies, and they should follow the canons of inductive or deductive logic.	
• Parsimony	pp. 93–94
1. The theory should be stated clearly and concisely.	
• Testability	pp. 94–96
1. The concepts of the theory should be empirically observable.	
2. The propositions should be measurable.	
3. The hypotheses should be falsifiable.	
Step Three: Evaluation of the Research Design	Chapter 3, pp. 96–99
• Operational Adequacy	pp. 96–99
1. The sample should be representative of the population of interest.	
2. The empirical indicators should be valid and reliable.	
3. The research procedure should be appropriate.	
4. The data-analysis procedures should be appropriate.	

(continued on page 210)

Table Appendix–2 ■ SUMMARY OF STEPS IN THE EVALUATION OF CONCEPUAL-THEORETICAL-EMPIRICAL STRUCTURES FOR RESEARCH (Continued)	
Criterion	**Text Discussion**
Step Four: Evaluation of the Research Findings	Chapter 3, pp. 99–106 See also Chapter 4
• Empirical Adequacy	
1. Theoretical claims should be congruent with empirical evidence.	
2. Alternative methodological and substantive explanations should be considered.	
Step Five: Evaluation of the Utility of the Theory for Practice	Chapter 3, pp. 106–111 See also Chapter 4
• Pragmatic Adequacy	
1. Research findings should be related to the practical problem of interest.	
2. Implementation of innovative actions should be feasible.	
3. Innovative actions should be congruent with recipients' expectations.	
4. The practitioner should have the legal ability to implement and evaluate the innovation.	
5. The innovative actions should lead to favorable outcomes.	
6. The theory should serve as a catalyst for the development of clinical practice guidelines and public policies.	
Step Six: Evaluation of the Conceptual Model	Chapter 3, pp. 111–112 See also Chapter 4
• Credibility	
1. The discussion of research results should include conclusions regarding the credibility of the conceptual model.	

References

Artinian, N.T. (1991). Stress experience of spouses of patients having coronary artery bypass during hospitalization and 6 weeks after discharge. *Heart and Lung, 20,* 52–59.

Bournaki, M-C. (1997). Correlates of pain-related responses to venipunctures in school-age children. *Nursing Research, 46,* 147–154.

Breckenridge, D.M. (1997). Patients' perceptions of why, how, and by whom dialysis treatment modality was chosen. *American Nephrology Nurses Association Journal, 24,* 313–319.

Janelli, L.M., Kanski, G.W., Jones, H.M., & Kennedy, M.C. (1995). Exploring music intervention with restrained patients. *Nursing Forum, 30*(4), 12–18.

Newman, D.M.L. (1997). The Inventory of Functional Status-Caregiver of a Child in Body Cast. *Journal of Pediatric Nursing, 12,* 142–147.

Roberts, K.L., Brittin, M., Cook, M-A., & deClifford, J. (1994). Boomerang pillows and respiratory capacity. *Clinical Nursing Research, 3,* 157–165.

Rosenthal-Dichter, C.H. (1996). The pediatric physiologic stress response: A concept analysis. *Scholarly Inquiry for Nursing Practice, 10,* 211–234.

Analysis and Evaluation of a Descriptive Theory-Generating Study: The Method of Concept Analysis

The Pediatric Physiologic Stress Response: A Concept Analysis

Cathy H. Rosenthal-Dichter, R.N., M.N., C.C.R.N., F.C.C.M.

Pediatric nurses have had a long-standing interest in stress and its effect on infants and children. Recently, there has been increasing interest in the physiological stress response on the part of nurses. While in the pediatric critical care setting, nurses continually assess the physiologic stability of the critically ill child, as well as the child's responses to a variety of interpersonal interactions, clinical interventions, and treatments. This status is continually challenged by a multitude of stressors which induce subsequent responses by the child. Only through a better understanding of the age-appropriate physiologic stress response can nurses accurately confirm its presence and evaluate its potential consequences. A concept analysis of the pediatric physiological stress response was conducted, primarily using the strategy recommended by Walker and Avant (1988). Accordingly, this analysis included: (1) a literature review; (2) determination of possible uses of the concept; (3) selection of defining attributes; (4) identification of empirical referents; (5) identification of antecedents and consequences; (6) construction of model and alternative cases; and (7) review of implications for nursing research.

Pediatric nurses have had a long-standing interest in stress and its effect on infants and children. For over 25 years, research has been conducted on various aspects of the emotional responses of children to the stress of hospitalization and health care (Thompson, 1986). In recent decades, nursing research has

Reprinted from *Scholarly Inquiry for Nursing Practice*, *10*(3), 1996, 211–234, 1996, with permission.

expanded to include both the behavioral and the biologic responses to stress and illness (Fagin, 1987) in patients across the lifespan. This impetus to include a biologic or physiologic component in nursing research is expected to continue since the National Institute of Nursing Research has implemented a 10-year program to increase the use of biologic theory and measurements in nursing through a variety of funding mechanisms (Cowan, Heinrich, Lucas, Sigmon, & Hinshaw, 1993). The incorporation of biologic or physiologic components in nursing research is well suited to critical care settings, such as the pediatric or neonatal intensive care unit, given the nature and complexity of the environment and the availability of information derived from the use of invasive monitoring devices.

In the pediatric critical care setting, nurses continually assess the physiologic stability of the critically ill child as well as the child's responses to a variety of interpersonal interactions, clinical interventions, and treatments. Clinical parameters including, but not limited to, heart rate, respiratory rate, and blood pressure, are often used as barometers of physiologic status. This status is continually challenged by a multitude of stressors which induce subsequent responses by the child. Only through a better understanding of the age-appropriate physiologic stress response can nurses accurately confirm its presence and evaluate its potential consequences. In addition, many nursing interventions are evaluated for tolerance or effectiveness using the patient's physiologic stress response as a criterion. Without an understanding of the physiologic stress response of the neonate, infant, and child, one cannot adequately assess this response in the context of age and clinical condition.

PURPOSE OF THE CONCEPT ANALYSIS

The manifestations of stress include psychologic, behavioral, sociocultural, and physiologic responses (Lindsey, Carrieri-Kohlman, & Page, 1993). For the purpose of this analysis, only the pediatric physiological stress response, hereafter referred to as the stress response, is explored and any reference to the adult stress response is stated explicitly. This concept is selected due to its seemingly complex, ambiguous, and diverse nature noted in the literature and common references to the concept in the clinical arena. The analysis is conducted to clarify the meaning of the concept and its role in the author's program of research. It is intended that the stress response, its attributes, and measurement are illuminated during the analysis.

The process of selecting the method of concept analysis for this study included the following considerations: (1) the author's intent to use a method recommended by nurses and applied to concepts inherent to nursing; (2) the objective, versus subjective, nature of the physiologic concept which impedes the use of a method based on or incorporating qualitative approaches; and (3) congruence between the purposes of this study and the method of analysis to be selected.

This concept analysis begins with an orientation to the concept of stress and stress terminology presented without regard to age or development. After reviewing several methods, the strategy for concept analysis recommended by Walker and Avant (1988) was selected. Accordingly, this analysis will include: (1) a literature review; (2) determination of possible uses of the concept; (3) selection of defining attributes; (4) identification of empirical referents; (5) identification of antecedents and consequences; (6) construction of model and alternative cases; and (7) review of implications for nursing research.

LITERATURE REVIEW
An Orientation to Stress and Stress Terminology

Stress is a prevalent topic in today's society. Stress also is the subject of voluminous research and an ever increasing number of professional publications, conferences, and academic courses. Yet, despite numerous references to the word stress, there is little consensus regarding the meaning or definition of the term (Levine & Ursin, 1991). A commonly cited definition proposed by Selye (1993), generally regarded as the father of the concept (Harris, 1984), is that stress is "the nonspecific result of any demand upon the body" (p. 7). Selye's perspective of stress dictates a response-based definition, with the specific nature of the demand on the body being largely irrelevant (Weiner, 1992).

The multidimensional nature of stress has both facilitated and confounded the process of clarifying the concept of stress. Attempts to clarify a particular dimension of the term stress often result in the elucidation of that dimension's contribution to the concept of stress. The term stressor, in contrast to the word stress, is widely accepted and used to refer to the demand, challenge, or stimulus that elicits a stress response. A mediator or 'filter' is the process whereby an organism evaluates the stressor. Mediators have been the central theme in most contemporary writings on stress (Levine & Ursin, 1991). The stress response is the organism's reaction to the stressor. In sharp contrast to the other dimensions of stress, little is written on the definition of the end product, consequence, or outcome of stress. The challenge surrounding the concept of stress remains, since the dimensions interact with one another (Ursin & Olff, 1993) and the sum of the dimensions fail to adequately represent or clarify the concept of stress.

Illustrations of the dimensions of stress are offered by Levine and Ursin (1991) and by a model presented by the Institute of Medicine (IOM) on Research on Stress and Human Health (Elliot & Eisdorfer, 1982; IOM, 1981). Levine and Ursin (1991) describe stress as comprised of three dimensions: the input (stress stimuli); the processing systems, including the subjective experience of stress; and the output (stress response). The IOM model, as shown in Figure 1, depicts stress as comprised of a potential activator (stressor); mediators; and the reaction (the stress response). The IOM model differs from that proposed by Levine and Ursin (1991), as it also illustrates the consequences of the stress response. Whereas, the former (Levine & Ursin, 1991) depicts the stress response as the end product of stress, the latter, (IOM, 1981) depicts the consequences of stress as an end product, yielding a better representation of the continuum of stress. Consequences are defined as sequelae to the reactions, but of primary interest are changes in health (IOM, 1981). The IOM model diagrammatically represents the stress process as dynamic and sometimes circular, similar to the interactive process that occurs between the organism and the environment (Lowery, 1987). Although the descriptions of the dimensions of stress vary slightly in the literature, there is a congruent trend in the identification of most

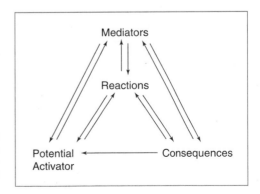

Figure I ■ Model Illustrating the Dimensions of Stress & Stress Terminology

(Reprinted with permission from *Research on Stress and Human Health*. Copyright 1981 by the National Academy of Sciences. Courtesy of the National Academy Press, Washington, DC.)

of the dimensions of stress, as well as in the temporal nature of these dimensions (see Table 1).

Selye and the General Adaptation Syndrome

Hans Selye began his pioneering studies of stress in the 1930s. Although during that time the primary impetus in medical science was identification of unique symptomatology, Selye noted the common elements in or reactions to various medical conditions. In a recent retrospective review, Selye (1993) stated "I was struck by how patients suffering from the most diverse diseases exhibited strikingly similar signs and symptoms . . ." (p. 9). He conceptualized stress as a nonspecific, uniform physiological pattern, consisting of hypertrophy of the adrenal cortex, atrophy of the thymus, spleen, lymph nodes and all other lymphatic structures, and gastric ulceration, occurring as a result of a variety of demands or challenges to an organism (Selye, 1946). These interdependent morphological changes were soon accepted as objective indices of stress. Subsequently, Selye described this nonspecific systemic reaction as one with three stages—alarm, resistance, and exhaustion—which he formally referred to as the General Adaptation Syndrome (GAS) (Selye, 1946, 1993).

The alarm reaction, the initial stage in the GAS, immediately calls into action the body's defensive forces to combat the imposed stressor to which the organism is not adapted. This stage is primarily the function of the sympathetic nervous system (SNS) activation. Cannon (1939) emphasized stimulation of the SNS during his investigations of homeostatic mechanisms and noted that activation of the SNS induces a bodily response which he termed a "fight or flight" response. As shown in Table 2, the effects of SNS activation are diverse. The effectors of the "fight or flight" response may be categorized as serving one of two primary functions: maintenance of cardiovascular and pulmonary function and energy or substrate mobilization (Lindsey et al., 1993). Epinephrine is also released from the adrenal medulla in response to SNS activation and serves to prolong and reinforce the "fight or flight" response.

The stage of resistance represents the body's attempts to reestablish stability or adaptation while still in the presence of the stressor. This stage of the stress response reflects the activation of the hypothalamic-pituitary-adrenal (HPA) axis and recruitment of numerous hormones including adrenocorticotrophic hormone (ACTH), glucocorticoids, mineralocorticoids, growth hormone, and antidiurectic hormone (see Table 2). The primary end product of the HPA axis is adrenal glucocorticoid release. The catabolic nature of glucocorticoids assists the organism by suppressing immunological responses while increasing the availability of energy substrates, including amino acids and glucose (Rhoades & Pflanzer, 1992). As detailed in Table 2, numerous hormones participate in the mobilization and distribution of energy and substrates during this stage of the stress response.

Table 1 ■ COMPARISON OF THE DIMENSIONS OF STRESS

Levine and Ursin (1991)	IOM Model (IOM, 1981)	Correlates to the Concept Analysis
Input: the stimuli	Potential activator	Antecedent
processing variables: input filters	Mediators	
Outcome variable: stress responses	The reaction	Concept of interest: the stress response
	Consequences	Consequences

Table 2 ■ **SELECTED EMPIRICAL REFERENTS FOR THE PHYSIOLOGIC STRESS RESPONSE**

Sympathetic Nervous System Activation "Fight or Flight Response"	Prepare for Continuation of Stress Response	Hypothalamus-Pituitary-Adrenal Axis Hormone Response
Maintain Cardiovascular Status:	Increase secretion of catecholamines from adrenal medulla*	Maintain Cardiovascular Status:
Increase HR		Increase HR via EPI
Increase myocardial force of contraction		Increase myocardial force of contraction via EPI
Increase BP		Increase BP via EPI
Dilation of coronary & skeletal muscle blood vessels		Dilation of skeletal muscle blood vessels via EPI
Constriction of cutaneous & visceral vasculature		Constriction of cutaneous & visceral vasculature via EPI
		Enhanced vascular responsiveness to catecholamines via GC
Maintain Respiratory Status		Maintain Respiratory Status:
Relaxation of smooth muscle		Relaxation of smooth muscle via EPI
Increase rate & depth of respiration		Provide Sources of Energy:
Provide Sources of Energy:		Glycogenolysis in liver & muscle via EPI
Glycogenolysis in liver & muscle		Gluconeogenesis via GH, GC
Lipolysis		Decrease tissue responsiveness to insulin via GH, GC
		Decrease glucose uptake in adipose & muscle via GH, GC
		Increase glycogen synthesis via EPI, GH
		Lipolysis via EPI, GH, GC
		Oxidation of fatty acids via GC
		Protein degradation via GC
Maintain Blood Volume:		Maintain Blood Volume:
Enhane blood coagulation		Increase Na retention via aldosterone
Contraction of spleen		Increase H2O reabsorption via ADH
Enhance CNS Alertness		Enhance CNS Alertness:
		Stimulate mental alertness via EPI

Key: NS—Sympathetic Nervous System; HR—heart rate; BP—blood pressure; GI—gastrointestinal; EPI—epinephrine; Na—sodium; H_2O—water; GH—growth hormone; GC—glucocorticoids (e.g., cortisol).
*Release of catecholamines from the adrenal medulla is a result of SNS activation, but is positioned in the table between the two columns to represent the role of catecholamines in reinforcing and prolonging the fight or flight response.

The last stage of the GAS, exhaustion, may occur when a stressor is extremely severe or persists for a sufficient amount of time to consume or deplete the body's reserves and defenses. The stage of exhaustion illustrates the finite nature of the body's ability to respond to a stressor. Selye (1993) stated "[b]ut just as any inanimate machine gradually wears out, so does the human machine sooner or later become the victim of constant wear and tear" (p. 10). Metaphorically, Selye (1993) equated the three stages of the GAS with three stages of the human life cycle: *childhood,* characterized by low resistance and an excessive response to any kind of stimulus (alarm stage); *adulthood,* characterized by an increased resistance and adaptation to the most commonly encountered agents; and *senility,* characterized by the loss of adaptation and eventual exhaustion (and death).

Possible Uses of the Concept

Although references to the adult physiologic stress response abound in the literature, references to pediatric physiologic stress response are more limited (Doswell, 1989). Most references to the concept of interest involve scant descriptions of the concept or a reiteration of what is known of the adult response with a brief discussion of the proposed differences that may exist between patients at different stages of development (Stidham & Bugnitz, 1992). A seminal review on the neonate's response to operative stress, conducted by Schmeling and Coran (1991), proved the most comprehensive. Although this review is comprehensive in one instance, it was limited in scope with regard to the type of stressor (surgical) and age (neonate).

Given the various disciplines concerned with the concept of interest, this author felt it was imperative to examine interdisciplinary applicable literature. This step in the analysis represents a departure from recommendations made by Walker and Avant (1988). There are differences among different disciplines, such as nursing, psychology, and medicine, with regard to conceptual framework, terminology of and references to the concept, intent of the research, and the type and frequency of empirical referents. These differences, which reflect the discipline's philosophy or worldview of stress and of the pediatric physiological stress response, are summarized in Table 3.

ATTRIBUTES, EMPIRICAL REFERENTS, ANTECEDENTS, AND CONSEQUENCES

Attributes

Attributes are defining characteristics or salient features that assist in identifying the occurrence of the concept. Attributes of the stress responses emerged as consistent themes upon review of the literature and in the examination of the model cases. The stress response is not an undesirable or atavistic response, but one that is an integral part of an adaptive biological system. It is considered protective, in fact, the stress response is categorized as a protective life process by Carrieri-Kohlman and colleagues (1993) in their textbook entitled *Pathophysiological Phenomena in Nursing*. It is categorized as such since the stress response assists in shielding the organism from stressors and altering the impact of stressors (Carrieri-Kohlman et al., 1993). The response, including the behavioral and physiological components, is necessary to the functioning and survival of the organism in a dynamic, complex environment (Ursin & Olff, 1993).

Activation of the stress response occurs when there is an imbalance in or challenge to the environment of the organism (Lindsey et al., 1993; Ursin & Olff, 1993). This activation serves as a warning system (or alarm), as well as the driving force that forces the organism to act to redirect energy and function during a time of need. The response is also graded, rather than an all or none response. Ursin and Olff (1993) state:

. . . when there is a discrepancy between the set value and the actual value for a particular variable, the alarm system or driving force will remain activated until there is an agreement between them, or until the brain gives a lower priority to the set value. (p. 9)

The composite of interrelated and interdependent neuroendocrine and metabolic events that comprise the stress response reflect the coordinating and integrating roles of the brain. The brain not only controls the autonomic nervous system, but also the central nervous system influences on stress response effectors, leading to endocrine, metabolic, and immunological responses (Ursin

---

Table 3 ■ **COMPARISON OF THE CONCEPT OF PEDIATRIC PHYSIOLOGIC STRESS RESPONSE IN NURSING, PSYCHOLOGY, AND MEDICAL LITERATURE**

Concept Characteristic	Nursing Literature	Psychology Literature	Medical Literature
Terminology Used for Concept	Physiologic arousal, Physiologic response, Psychophysiologic effects.	Adrenocorticoid response, cortisol response, physiologic responsivitiy, physiologic indicators of distress	Endocrine response, hormonal response, cortisol response, sympathoadrenal response, metabolic response
Conceptual Framework	Infrequent references to: Selye Cannon	Some references to: Selye	Some references to: Selye
Philosophy/World View	Organismic[1]	Organismic[1]	Mechanistic[1]
Purpose of Research	To describe a patient's actual or potential response to phenomena including: pain hospitalization parental presence/ anxiety preprocedural/ preoperative preparation	To describe the infant or child's response to: maternal separation hospitalization, preprocedural/ preoperative preparation	To describe the mechanism of the pediatric physiological stress response or components thereof. To contrast the response of the neonate and pediatric patient to the response of the adult patient. To explore methods of mitigating the response.
Type & Frequency of Empiric Referent	Varies from study to study. Predominantly noninvasive end organ effects or indicators such as heart rate, blood pressure, etc. Usually collected several times (3–5) in a repeated measures design.	Varies from study to study. Both hormone as well as end organ effects or indicators of response. Cortisol (serum and salivary) was common. Usually collected several times (2–3) in a repeated measures design.	Varies from study to study. A wide variety of specific hormones and metabolic substrates are collected. Usually collected many times (5–7) during the research protocol that may extend up to 72 hours.

[1]The organicism-mechanism dichotomy illustrates the divergent characteristics of two world views or philosophies to the study of the human-environment relationship. A few characteristics of organistic worldview include holism and expansionism and development that is quantitative and qualitative, whereas mechanistic worldview include elementarism and reductionism and development that is quantitative. *Source:* Fawcett, 1993.

& Olff, 1993). The magnitude and duration of the stress response, even to the same stressor, varies from individual to individual. Mediator processes are primarily responsible for this lack of linearity between the stressor and the stress response. This relationship between the stressor and the stress response is influenced by mediators, since the stressor is processed and evaluated before it gains access to the response (effector) system (Ursin & Olff, 1993). Mediators are generally categorized as those that evaluate the stressor and those that evaluate the resources to deal with the stressor (Ursin & Olff, 1993).

Consistent characteristics of the concept, derived through the review of the literature and the examination of the model cases, were assembled. Additionally, the "characteristics" of the [adult] stress response, as identified by Lindsey and colleagues (1993), assisted this author in refining attributes for this concept analysis. Attributes of the stress response, whether pediatric or adult, include the following:

The stress response begins as a normal, protective, and adaptive response to stressors.

The stress response is a graded, not an all or none, response.

The stress response consists of a composite of interrelated and interdependent neuroendocrine and metabolic events.

The magnitude and duration of the stress response, even to the same stressor, varies from individual to individual.

The magnitude and duration of the stress response can be influenced by multidisciplinary interventions.

Empirical Referents

Empirical references demonstrate how the concept exists in the real world and how the concept is measured (Rew, 1986; Walker & Avant, 1988). Empirical referents demonstrate the unquestionable existence of the concept through observable, measurable, and verifiable means. The classic signs and symptoms of the "fight or flight" response are empiric referents of the physiologic stress response since these may be observed, measured, and verified. Other examples of empirical referents abound in the literature and include all hormones and their precursors, metabolic substrates, and other endogenous mediators (i.e., opioids, prostaglandins, cytokines) involved in any aspect of the physiologic stress response. Empirical referents of the concept of interest vary greatly in the level of specificity (receptors versus hormones versus physiologic parameters such as heart rate) as well as origin (e.g., serum, urinary, or salivary). Examples of other empirical referents can be found in Tables 2 and 3, as well as in the model and borderline cases presented in this analysis.

Antecedents and Consequences

Antecedents are the incidents that occur prior to the concept of interest, whereas consequences are the result of the concept of interest. It is through the identification of the antecedents and consequences that the attributes of the concept become clearer, because attributes can be neither antecedents nor consequences (Walker & Avant, 1988). Antecedents of the stress response include all events, actual or perceived, that stimulate or induce such a response from the child. In other words, antecedents include any and all stressors. Antecedents are diverse in nature (physiologic and psychologic), duration, frequency, and intensity. Although it is beyond the scope of this concept analysis to list all possible stressors, common physiologic stressors for the pediatric critical care patient include sepsis, tissue injury (surgery or trauma), and respiratory infection (Yeh, 1992). Psychological stressors for the pediatric critical care patient include separation from parents, presence of unfamiliar personnel, and the complexity of critical care equipment and environment (Kidder, 1989; Wilson & Broome, 1989). Congruent with the notion that stress is more than a stimulus response, it is important to note that mediators (e.g., processes of cognitive appraisal and coping) may intensify a stress response if the stressor is evaluated as extraordinarily dangerous or if it is evaluated that there is an imbalance between the demand and the resources to attend to the demand.

Consequences include temporary and/or permanent conditions that occur as a result of the concept of interest (Walker & Avant, 1988). Given the lack of definition and clarity regarding the outcome dimension of stress, referred to earlier in this paper, it is no surprise that the identification of consequences to the stress response would be challenging. The stress response is considered an integral part of an adaptive biological system; consequently it is inherently considered a benign event with a salient purpose. Therefore, the consequence, in some instances, is optimal and results in the resolution of the stressor, the cessation of the stress response, and restoration of physiologic stability. There are also references in the literature to pathological consequences of the stress response. These consequences of the stress response have been noted for clinical states, such as the common cold, asthmatic attacks, anorexia nervosa, and obesity (Chrousos & Gold, 1992; Dorn & Chrousos, 1993; Lindsey et al., 1993). Pathophysiologic consequences appear to be associated with prolonged activation of the stress response (Ursin & Olff, 1993). The relationship between the stress response and these clinical states however, is one of association rather than causation (Lindsey et al., 1993).

Consequences of the stress response may be more detrimental in neonatal and pediatric patients due to their relative immaturity and their documented anatomical and physiological differences from older patients. Neonatal and pediatric patients are prone to metabolic instability due to (1) a greater body surface area necessitating greater heat production; (2) a larger brain-to-body-weight ratio, with increased obligatory glucose requirements, (3) a need to maintain somatic growth; and (4) relatively smaller reserves of protein, carbohydrate, and fat (Anand & Ward Platt, 1988). These developmental differences are greater in the neonate and decrease gradually with increasing age, yet they continue to exist to some degree throughout childhood.

MODEL AND ALTERNATIVE CASES
Model Cases
Model cases best represent the concept of interest and assist in the identification of the essential features of a concept (Avant, 1993). Although model cases may be fabricated patient situations or accumulations of information depicting ideal case studies (Goosen, 1989), the author strived to inductively select model cases relevant to the context of nursing and derived from the scientific literature. It is perceived that model cases with these characteristics would best fulfill the purpose in conducting this concept analysis. This step represents a modification of the process recommended by Walker and Avant (1988) in that cases are usually deductively constructed to illustrate the concept's attributes.

Examination of nursing studies or programs of research failed to identify a model case that exhibited the attributes of the concept of interest. Model cases presented in this concept analysis are extrapolated from research reports from medical programs of research conducted by Anand and colleagues (Anand & Hickey, 1992; Anand, Sippell, & Aynsley-Green, 1987) and other researchers exploring the stress responses of children to operative stressors (Wolf et al., 1993). Although the model cases were extrapolated from research addressing medical questions, the same methodology can be applied to answer nursing questions. For example, relevant studies would be the examination of the stress responses of children receiving two different nursing interventions or the effects of parental presence and separation on the stress responses of children in the pediatric intensive care unit.

Each of the model cases investigated the stress responses of children to operative stressors and is summarized in greater detail in Table 4. Three model cases are presented to illustrate the pediatric physiologic stress response across the continuum of development. These studies were randomized clinical trials that involved controlled, uniform surgical techniques and protocol-directed preoperative, perioperative, and postoperative care. A variety of serum hormones and metabolites, urinary metabolites, and indices of clinical course were collected throughout the protocols. Researchers then compared preoperative, perioperative and postoperative values of the selected empiric referents.

MODEL CASE #1. Anand and colleagues (1987) compared the operative stress responses of preterm neonates receiving different anesthetic regimens. Responses of the control group receiving a conventional anesthetic regimen, were compared to responses of a treatment group, receiving fentanyl in addition to the conventional anesthesia. Comparison of preoperative, perioperative and postoperative values revealed multiple hormonal responses to the operative stressor in both the control and treatment groups. In general, hormonal responses were significantly greater in the control group as compared to the treatment group. Although there were no significant differences between the two groups in cortisol responses, precursors to cortisol (corticosterone and 11-deoxycortisol) were significantly greater in the control group as compared to the treatment group. Significant differences in metabolic responses, specifically glucose, lactate, and pyruvate, were also noted between the groups. Although the differences in clinical course were not subjected to statistical analyses, the control group experienced more postoperative complications compared to the treatment group.

MODEL CASE #2. Anand and Hickey (1992) compared the operative stress responses of full-term term neonates receiving different anesthetic regimens. Responses of the control group, receiving a conventional anesthetic regimen, were compared to responses of a treatment group, receiving high dose suffentanil. Comparison of preoperative, perioperative and postoperative values revealed major hormonal responses to the operative stressor in both the control and treatment groups. In general, hormonal responses, including cortisol responses, were significantly greater in the control group as compared to the treatment group. Significant differences in metabolic responses, specifically glucose and lactate, were also noted between the groups. Statistically significant differences were noted in the clinical course and outcome between the groups, with the treatment group experiencing a lower incidence of complications and mortality.

MODEL CASE #3. Wolf and colleagues (1993) compared the stress responses of children ages 2 months to 4 years receiving extradural anesthesia to those of children receiving opioid anesthesia/analgesia while undergoing elective abdominal surgery. As reported in preterm (Anand et al., 1987) and term neonates (Anand & Hickey, 1992), the results of this study (Wolf et al., 1993) indicated that there were major hormonal responses in both groups to the operative stressor. All measured hormones, with the exception of norepinephrine (NE) increased significantly in both groups during surgery. In general, hormonal responses were significantly greater in the control group than the treatment group, as indicated by epinephrine, glucose, and ACTH. Although NE concentrations did not change significantly during or after surgery in either group, the treatment group had significantly lower NE levels than children in the control group. No group differences were found for cortisol, despite differences in ACTH responses.

DISCUSSION OF MODEL CASES. All attributes of the pediatric physiologic stress response are illustrated in these model cases, including the ability to mitigate

Table 4 ■ STUDIES COMPRISING THE MODEL CASES FOR THE PEDIATRIC PHYSIOLOGIC STRESS RESPONSE

Study/Conceptual Framework	Purpose/ Subjects	Methodology/ Stressor	Measures/ Definition	Findings
Wolf, Eyres, Laussen, Edwards, Stanley, Row, & Simon, 1993 Conceptual Framework: None specified	Purpose: To investigate the effects of extradural anesthesia/analgesia versus opioid anasthesia/analgesia on the child's stress response. Sample: N = 40, Children: ages 2 months to 4 years	Design: Experimental (randomized clinical trial) Randomized to receive general anasthesia supplemented during and after surgery with either: systemic opioids extradural bupivacaine Stressor Elective, major abdominal surgery	Measures: Measured the following serum hormone levels at baseline, 45 minutes after the start of surgery, l hour and 24 hours after the end of surgery: epinephrine (EPI) norepinephrine (NE) glucose adrenocorticotrophic hormone (ACTH) cortisol Bupivacaine levels in patients receiving bupivacaine were also measured at same intervals. Definitions: None specified for the study concepts	Baseline measures were within normal range. Patient characteristics were similar between groups. Perioperative increases in EPI, glucose and ACTH were significantly greater in the opioid group as compared to the extradural group. NE concentration did not change significantly during or after surgery in opioid group, but in extradural group they were significantly less than those in opioid group. The perioperative increase in cortisol was similar between the groups despite the difference noted in ACTH. ACTH increased in both groups during surgery, but was significantly greater in the opioid group.
Anand & Hickey, 1992 Conceptual Framework:	Purpose: To investigate the effects of deep opioid anesthesia on the	Design: Experimental (randomized clinical trial) Randomized to re-	Measures: Measured the following serum hormonal and metabolic sub-	No significant differences noted preoperatively. Suffentanil group had significantly, reduced re-

(continued on page 222)

Table 4 ■ STUDIES COMPRISING THE MODEL CASES FOR THE PEDIATRIC PHYSIOLOGIC STRESS RESPONSE (Continued)

Study/Conceptual Framework	Purpose/ Subjects	Methodology/ Stressor	Measures/ Definition	Findings
None specified	stress responses and clinical outcome of critically ill neonates. Subjects: N = 45, Neonates, term	ceive general anestheisa supplemented during and after surgery with either: halothane-morphine high dose suffentanil/fentanyl Stressor: Cardiac surgery including cardiopulmontary bypass and hypothermic cardiac arrest. Neonates experienced a variety of corrective or palliative repairs of congenital heart defects, such as transposition of the great vessels and Tetralogy of Fallot.	strate levels at six sampling points (at the end of the operation and at 6, 12, and 24 hours following the operation) after the preoperative baseline: EPI and NE, glucose, steroid hormones, insulin, glucagon, beta-endorphin, lactate and pyruvate, acetacetate, 3-hydroxybutyrate, alanine Outcome data was also recorded and included: postoperative mortality and morbidity, hypotension, atrial or ventricular arrhythmias, sepsis, DIC, and seizures Definitions: Operationally defined outcome criteria	sponses of beta-endorphin, NE, EPI, glucagon, aldosterone, cortisol, and other steroid hormones. Suffentanil group had greater insulin responses and greater insulin:glucagon ratios during the operation. Halothane-morphine group had more severe hyperglycemia and lactic acidemia during surgery and higher lactate and acetoacetate concentrations postoperatively. Suffentanil group had lower incidence of sepsis, metabolic acidosis, DIC, and postoperative deaths than the halothane-morphine group. 4 of the 15 in the halothane-morphine group died whereas none of the 30 in the suffentanil group died.
Anand, Sippell, & Aynsley-Green, 1987	Purpose: To compare the surgical stress	Design: Experimental (randomized clinical trial)	Measures: Measured the following serum hormonal	No significant differences between the groups preoperatively.

Conceptual Framework:
None specified

responses of preterm babies recieving two different anesthesia regimens.

Subjects:
N = 16
Neonates, preterm

Randomized to receive either:

anesthesia with nitrous oxide & curare alone
anesthesia with nitrous oxide & curare & fentanyl

Stressor:
Operative repair of the PDA

and metabolic substrate levels at six sampling points (at the end of the operation and at 6, 12, and 24 hours following the operation) after the preoperative baseline: EPI and NE, glucose, steroid hormones, insulin, glucagon, beta-endorphin, lactate and pyruvate, acetate, 3-hydroxybutyrate, alanine, triglycerides and glycerol

Concentrations of 3-methylhistadine and creatinine in the urine ($3MH/Cr$) were also measured.

Clinical course was also assessed to include: heart rate, respiratory support, incidence of bradycardia, peripheral circulation, oliguria, GI bleeding, metabolic acidosis, and paralytic ileus.

Definitions:
None specified for the study concepts

Hormonal responses to surgery were significantly greater in the non-fentanyl group than the fentanyl group as indicated by changes in EPI, NE, glucagon, aldosterone, insulin/glucagon ratio, blood glucose, lactate, and pyruvate levels.

There were no significant differences in cortisol between the two groups, however, corticosterone and 11-deoxycortisol responses were significantly greater in the no-fentanyl group than in the fentanyl group.

Compared to the fentanyl group, the no-fentanyl group had circulatory and metabolic complications noted postoperatively.

No-fentanyl group was more likely to require an increase in ventilatory support. Two neonates in the no-fentanyl group developed IVH.

Note. IVH = Intraventricular hemorrhage; PDA = Patent ductus arteriosus the physiologic stress response with interventions, specifically anesthetic regimens. The stress responses were induced as normal, adaptive, and protective responses to the operative stressor. Although summary measures are presented in the research reports, standard errors of the mean reflect the variance of individual responses in that measure and the graded response of each subject. The monitoring of the wide variety of hormones and metabolites used in these model cases facilitates the identification of a composite of hormonal and metabolic events.

These model cases illustrate not only that the response magnitude and duration vary from individual to individual, but also that they vary with the age or development of the patient, making these attributes applicable to individuals across the lifespan. Although it is beyond the scope of this concept analysis to comprehensively describe the quantitative and qualitative differences noted in the stress response across the continuum of development, a few differences are illustrated in the research that comprises the model cases. In general, hormonal responses of both the neonatal and older pediatric patients are greater in magnitude and shorter in duration than the responses of adults to similar procedures (Anand & Ward-Platt, 1988). Differences are also noted in the response of the preterm and term neonate. The most notable of these differences illustrated in the model cases is the cortisol response. In order to best evaluate the preterm infant's plasma steroid hormone response, steroid precursor hormones, including progesterone, 17-hydroxyprogesterone, 11-deoxy corticosterone, and 11-deoxycortisol, need to be taken into consideration. Term neonates respond with significantly greater cortisol during and after surgery, whereas preterm neonates respond with significantly greater precursor steroid hormones (Anand & Ward Platt, 1988). Preterm neonates exhibit a relative immaturity for steroid biosynthesis (Solomon, Bird, Ling, Iwamiya, & Young, 1967). Inasmuch as maturation of the hydroxylase enzymes occurs from the proximal to distal end of the steroid biosynthetic pathway (Solomon et al., 1967), the preterm neonate will display a diminished secretion of the final products of steroid biosynthesis (e.g., cortisol) and increased secretion of the precursor steroid hormones (Anand et al., 1987).

Borderline Cases
Borderline cases are those cases that cause difficulty in determining whether they are examples of the concept of interest. By understanding why these cases are difficult to classify, one can further clarify the concept of interest (Avant, 1939). The borderline cases presented in this concept analysis are extrapolated from nursing research and from a series of studies within a program of psychology research conducted by Gunnar and colleagues (Gunnar, Connors, Isensee, & Wall, 1988; Gunnar, Hertsgaard, Larson, & Rigatuso, 1992a). The two borderline cases are classified as such for different reasons.

BORDERLINE CASE #1. Acute pain is an example of a borderline case for the pediatric physiologic stress response. Nurse researchers have investigated several physiologic indicators of acute pain. According to Hester (1993), these studies were based upon the following axioms: (1) Stress arousal alters physiologic responses; (2) pain is a stress arousal; and (3) physiologic responses change with the presence of pain. The pediatric physiologic parameters examined in relationship to acute pain include changes in body temperature (Abu-Saad, 1984; Abu-Saad & Holzemer, 1981); heart rate or pulse (Abu-Saad, 1984; Abu-Saad & Holzemer, 1981; Dale, 1986; Froese-Fretz, 1986; Johnston & Strada, 1986; Mills, 1989); respiratory rate (Abu-Saad, 1984; Abu-Saad & Holzemer, 1981; Mills, 1989); blood pressure (Abu-Saad, 1984; Abu-Saad & Holzemer, 1981); transcutaneous oxygen (TcpO$_2$) (Froese-Fretz, 1986; Norris, Campbell &

Brenkert, 1982); skin color (Mills, 1989); and diaphoresis (Mills, 1989). These studies have yielded inconsistent results. The findings differ according to the type of pain (pain associated with tissue injury or surgery versus pain associated with medical procedures) and show a great degree of variability among individuals in the physiologic response to pain (Hester, 1993). Hester (1993) proposed that the changes in physiologic parameters may have occurred with other stress-arousing events (confounding variables) limiting these parameters as measures of pain. In addition, the relationship between physiologic responses, such as those measured by nurse researchers investigating pain, and neurohormonal and metabolic events has yet to be fully defined. Craig and Grunau (1993) point out that ". . . physiologic events are multidetermined. They can vary with a multitude of physiological and psychological events" (p. 82).

One could argue that acute pain illustrates most of the defining attributes of the stress response. The definition of pain, according to the International Association for the Study of Pain (Merskey et al., 1979) is

. . . an unpleasant sensory and emotional experience associated with actual or potential tissue damage, or described in terms of such damage. [Note: Pain is always subjective. Each individual learns the application of the word through experiences related to injury early in life . . .] (p. 250).

This definition reflects the multidimensional nature of the concept of acute pain. Acute pain may share most of the defining attributes of the stress response, but it most probably has additional defining attributes that would distinguish it from the stress response. Nursing research has reflected the notion that pain is an antecedent to the stress response. It may be more accurate in many cases to state that tissue damage, rather than pain, is an antecedent to the stress response. Further examination of the defining attributes of acute pain would be required before classifying it as a contrary or model case. Thus, acute pain is classified as a borderline case.

BORDERLINE CASE #2. Gunnar and colleagues have conducted several studies to examine the adrenocortical and behavioral responses of neonates and infants to various stressors including: limb restraints (Malone, Gunnar, & Fisch, 1985), circumcision, blood sampling, weighing, and physical examination (Gunnar et al., 1988), and repeated stressors (Gunnar et al., 1992a). Studies conducted early in this program of research involved the collection procedures and validation that the two sources of cortisol showed acceptable correlation, investigators used only salivary cortisol in subsequent research.

There have been increases in both serum and salivary cortisol that document the infant's response to stressors, specifically to noxious nociceptive and handling stressors. In response to noxious nociceptive stressors (heelsticks and circumcision), the elevation in serum cortisol was also associated with how much a baby cries, but no such association was found with the stress of handling (Gunnar et al., 1988). These cortisol responses showed sensitization to heelsticks and habituation to discharge examinations in healthy newborns (Gunnar et al., 1988, 1992a). However, a different pattern of response was noted in newborns who were considered in "nonoptimal health." Although these newborns showed sensitization to the repeated heelsticks, they failed to show habituation to the discharge exam (Gunnar et al., 1992a). Furthermore, in "nonoptimal health" newborns, crying was associated with an increase in salivary cortisol with both nociceptive stressors and handling stressors (Gunnar, 1992, 1992a).

Studies involving older infants have included examination of salivary cortisol responses to distress-producing events, including separation from mother (Gunnar, Larson, Hertsgaard, Harris, Brodersen, 1992b; Gunnar, Mangelsdorf,

Larson, Hertsgaard, 1989; Larson, Gunnar, & Hertsgaard, 1991). Larson and colleagues (1991) found significant increases in cortisol during separation as compared to a 30-minute play session with the mother. These infants, when separated, were left with a baby-sitter who responded to the infants when they cried, but otherwise interacted minimally with the infants. Interestingly, a recent study (Gunnar et al., 1992b) with a baby sitter who was responsive to the infants when they cried, but also interacted and played with the infants, completely buffered this cortisol response to separation. Gunnar and colleagues (1992b) have proposed that the quality of care received during the mother-infant separation influences the intensity of the stress response.

Although most attributes are present in this borderline case, the measure of a single hormonal response may not be sufficient to document the stress response. The cortisol alone does not represent a composite of interrelated and interdependent neuroendocrine and metabolic responses. Since only one hormone was measured, this program of research best illustrates a borderline case.

IMPLICATIONS TO NURSING RESEARCH

In summary, what is currently known about the pediatric physiologic stress response is derived from numerous studies from various disciplines using different conceptual frameworks and methodologies. It is essential to combine disciplinary resources to capture a broad and comprehensive view of the concept of interest and its short-term and long-term consequences. The continuum of the stress response to medical and operative stressors also requires further investigation. Several studies investigating the concept in response to operative stress captured the initiation and beginning dissipation of the alarm stage of the GAS. Nonetheless, several key questions remain unanswered. Does the stress response continue to dissipate postoperatively? Are three events or nursing interventions that mitigate the stress response postoperatively? How does the stress response to operative stressors compare to that seen with medical stressors? The stress response associated with medical stressors is proposed to differ from operative stressors, given the discrete time frame and degree of control associated with the latter. Which nursing interventions mitigate or exacerbate the stress response associated with medical stressors?

There are several implications of this concept analysis for nursing research. It is imperative that a conceptual framework be included in future research regarding the pediatric physiologic stress response and that there be consistency between the framework and the research hypothesis and methodology. Clarification as to whether the physiologic stress response or an antecedent, empiric referent, or consequence of the physiologic stress response will be the concept of interest in a study is essential.

Implications for nursing research in regard to empirical referents of the physiologic stress response exist as well. How many hormones or metabolic substrates should be measured to consider the data reflective of a composite neuroendocrine and metabolic event? Measuring only one of the hormones or metabolic substrates in isolation is not sufficient to represent the concept and may leave some degree of doubt as to the body's response. Since the stress response is a graded, not an all or none event, it can exist with wide variation in intensity. A baseline assessment of the patient may more accurately determine the existence and degree of intensity of the stress response. The collection of accurate baseline data can verify the existence of the stress response, as well as assist in the identification of factors that may mask (e.g., beta adrenergic blocking agents) or imitate (e.g., exogenous catecholamine administration) the stress response. In addition to using baseline observations, comparisons of the empirical referent to an accepted and a priori standard assist in the accurate interpretation of the value obtained. Although Guzzetta and Forsyth (1979) were interested in determining parameters that were sensitive and clinically useful in the concept of stress rather than the stress response, they developed a priori operational definitions for selected physiological parameters. For instance, the characteristic of the physiological parameter, heart rate, that defined the existence of stress was a rise of greater than 10 beats per minute over three observation periods (Guzzetta & Forsyth, 1979). There is difficulty in determining the level at which the stress response is considered present. The existence and degree of intensity along a continuum is challenging without the use of baseline observations or comparison to an accepted or a priori standard. Of equal importance, the physiologic stress response must be considered in light of statistical as well as clinical significance. It behooves the researcher, as well as the clinician, to determine the criteria for determining presence, clinical, and statistical significance in an a priori fashion.

The implications regarding consequences of the stress response are numerous. There is a need to examine the relationship between the outcome dimension of stress and the consequences of stress response. Little discussion of the consequences of the concept exists in the literature. In addition, minimal distinctions between short- and long-term consequences are found. Whereas sustained activation of the stress response may contribute to some of the clinical states cited in the literature such as the common cold, it most probably does not account for the differences in clinical outcome illustrated by the model cases presented in this analysis.

There appear to be two dichotomous views in the literature regarding the nature of the concept and its consequences: (1) the stress response is benign and the outcomes can range from optimal to pathologic; (2) both the stress response and the outcomes can range from optimal to pathologic. The IOM (1981) report states "[s]tressors, reactions, and mediators are neither 'good' or 'bad'; only consequences can appropriately be qualified as being desirable or undesirable" (p. 22). Although the majority of the literature is consistent with this philosophy, a recent proposition suggests otherwise. It is proposed that stress response dysfunction, characterized by sustained hyperactivity or hypoactivity, leads to pathophysiologic consequences including the presence or the susceptibility to a wide range of psychiatric, endocrine, and inflammatory disorders (i.e., posttraumatic stress disorder) (Chrousos & Gold, 1992; Dorn & Chrousos, 1993). Again, these are long-term consequences, but what, if any, are the short-term consequences of stress response dysfunction?

The elements of the difference between the physiologic and pathophysiologic stress response have plagued the inquisitive nature of many researchers and clinicians. Anand (1993) proposed factors that are associated with the actual or potential risk of a pathologic stress response. These include: (1) patient vulnerability; (2) magnitude of the response; (3) duration of the response; and (4) conditions exacerbating the stress response or its detrimental effects.

The examination of related cases would assist in the identification of the network of concepts of which the concept of interest is a part. It is through this examination that one can understand how the concept is the same and how it is different from those in the same network (Avant, 1993). For this analysis, although related cases were not developed, it should be noted that knowledge of related concepts and creation of related cases can be helpful in analyzing the concept of interest. In particular, the concepts of stability (or instability) and adaptation are most probably in the same network as the concept of interest. Although critical care clinicians commonly refer to patients as stable or unstable, references in the literature to the concept of stability primarily relate to an instrument measuring severity of illness, the Physiologic Stability Index

(Pollack, Ruttiman, Getson, 1988; Ruttiman, Albert, Pollack, & Glass, 1986; Yeh, 1992). Gorski (1983) and other neonatal clinicians use the concept of stability and its contrary term (instability) in discussions of the preterm neonate's neurobehavioral immaturity and disorganization, although the lack of clarity of the concept remains. With regard to the concept of adaptation, Goosen and Bush (1979) reported a concept analysis and viewed adaptation as a 5-step process following the perception of the stimulus that included: (1) cognitive appraisal; (2) coping mechanism; (3) neurophysiological arousal; (4) emotional and physiologic response; and (5) intensification of neurophysiological and psychological response. At each step in the process the individual has the opportunity to continue in the process or to adapt. The conclusions from the concept analysis of adaptation is that this concept encompasses the concept of physiologic stress response. How the concepts of adaptation and stability differ from the physiologic stress response requires further investigation.

Lastly, examination of the pediatric physiologic stress response within a nursing context is integral to the determination of the degree and direction of the child's responses to interpersonal interaction, clinical interventions, and treatment. Investigations must include a clear conceptual-theoretical-empirical structure that accurately defines the role of the concept of interest within that study. It behooves the nurse researcher to maintain an organismic perspective during such investigations, since it is human responses that are of interest and importance to nurses. Wolf (1993) titled a recent editorial "[T]reat the babies, not their stress responses," as a mere reminder of the importance in placing these investigations within the context of patient outcomes. ■

References

Abu-Saad, H. (1984). Assessing children's responses to pain. *Pain, 19,* 163–171.

Abu-Saad, H., & Holzemer, W. L. (1981). Measuring children's self-assessment of pain. *Issues in Comprehensive Pediatric Nursing, 5,* 337–349.

Anand, K. J. S. (1993). Relationships between stress responses and clinical outcome in newborns, infants, and children. *Critical Care Medicine, 21*(9), S358–S359.

Anand, K. J. S., & Hickey, P. R. (1992). Halothane-morphine compared to high dose sufentanil for anesthesia and postoperative analgesia in neonatal cardiac surgery. *New England Journal of Medicine, 326,* 1–9.

Anand, K. J. S., Sippell, W. G., & Aynsley-Green, A. (1987). Randomized trial of fentanyl anaesthesia in preterm babies undergoing surgery: Effects on the stress response. *The Lancet, 1,* 243–248.

Anand, K. S., & Ward-Platt, M. P. (1988). Neonatal and pediatric stress responses to anesthesia and operation. *International Anesthesiology Clinics, 26*(3), 218–225.

Avant, K. C. (1993). The Wilson method of concept analysis. In B. L. Rodgers & K. A. Knafl (Eds.), *Concept development in nursing: Foundations, techniques, and applications* (pp. 51–72). Philadelphia: W. B. Saunders Company.

Cannon, W. B. (1939). *The wisdom of the body.* Philadelphia: W. W. Norton.

Carrieri-Kohlman, V., Lindsey, A. M., & West, C. M. (1993). Alterations in protection. In V. Carrieri-Kohlman, A. M. Lindsey, & C. M. West (Eds.), *Pathophysiological phenomena in nursing: Human responses to illness* (2nd ed., pp. 395–396). Philadelphia: W. B. Saunders Company.

Chrousos, G. P., & Gold, P. W. (1992). The concepts of stress and stress system disorders: Overview of physical and behavioral homeostasis. *Journal of the American Medical Association, 267*(9), 1244–1252.

Cowan, M. J., Heinrich, J., Lucas, M., Sigmon, H., & Hinshaw, A. S. (1993). Integration of biological and nursing sciences: A 10-year plan to enhance research and training. *Research in Nursing & Health, 16,* 3–9.

Craig, K. D., & Grunau, R. V. E. (1993). Neonatal pain perception and behavioral measurement. In K. J. S. Anand & P. J. McGrath (Eds.), *Pain in neonates* (pp. 67–105). Amsterdam: Elsevier.

Dale, J. C. (1986). A multidimensional study of infants' responses to painful stimuli. *Pediatric Nursing, 12,* 31–37.

Dorn, L. D., & Chrousos, G. P. (1993). The endocrinology of stress and stress system disorders in adolescence. *Endocrinology and Metabolism Clinics of North America, 22*(2), 685–700.

Doswell, W. (1989). Physiological responses to stress. *Annual Review of Nursing Research, 7,* 51–69.

Elliot, G., & Eisdorfer, C. (1982). *Stress and human health.* New York: Springer Publishing Company.

Fagin, C. M. (1987). Stress: Implications for nursing research. *Image: Journal of Nursing Scholarship, 19*(1), 4–38.

Fawcett, J. (1993). The structure of contemporary nursing knowledge. In J. Fawcett, *Analysis and evaluation of nursing theories* (pp. 1–3). Philadelphia: F. A. Davis.

Froese-Fretz, A. (1986). The use of transcutaneous electrical nerve stimulators (TENS) during radial arterial blood sampling in newborn infants. Unpublished masters thesis. University of Colorado Health Sciences Center, Denver, CO.

Goosen, G. M. (1989). Concept analysis: An approach to teaching physiologic variables. *Journal of Professional Nursing, 5*(1), 31–38.

Goosen, G. M., & Bush, H. A. (1979). Adaptation: A feedback process. *Advances in Nursing Science, 1*(4), 51–65.

Gorski, P. A. (1983). Premature infant behavioral and physiological responses to caregiving interventions in the intensive care nursery. In J. D. Call, E. Galenson, & R. L. Tyson (Eds.), *Frontiers of infant psychiatry* (pp. 256–263). New York: Basic Books.

Gunnar, M. R. (1992). Reactivity of the hypothalamic-pituitary-adrenocortical system to stressors in normal infants and children. *Pediatrics, 90*(3), 492–497.

Gunnar, M. R., Connors, J., Isensee, J., & Wall, L. (1988). Adrenocortical and behavioral distress in human newborns. *Developmental Psychobiology, 21*(4), 297–310.

Gunnar, M. R., Hertsgaard, L., Larson, M., & Rigatuso, J. (1992a). Cortisol and behavioral responses to repeated stressors in the human newborn. *Developmental Psychobiology, 24*(7), 487–505.

Gunnar, M. R., Larson, M. C., Hertsgaard, I., Harris, M. L., & Brodersen, L. (1992b). The stressfulness of separation among nine-month old infants: Effects of social context variables and infant temperament. *Child Development, 63,* 290–303.

Gunnar, M. R., Mangelsdorf, S., Larson, M., & Hertsgaard, L. (1989). Attachment, temperament, and adrenocortical activity in infancy: A study of psychoendocrine regulation. *Developmental Psychology, 25*(3), 355–363.

Guzzetta, C. E., & Forsyth, G. (1979). Nursing diagnostic pilot study: Psychophysiologic stress. *Advances in Nursing Science, 2*(1), 27–44.

Harris, J. S. (1984). Stressors and stress in critical care. *Critical Care Nurse, 4*(1), 84–97.

Hester, N. O. (1993). Pain in children. *Annual Review of Nursing Research, 11,* 105–142.

Institute of Medicine (IOM) (1981). *Report of a study: Research on stress and human health.* Washington, DC: National Academy Press.

Johnson, C. C., & Strada, M. E. (1986). Acute pain response in infants: As multidimensional description. *Pain, 24,* 373–382.

Kidder, C. (1989). Reestablishing health: Factors influencing the child's recovery in pediatric intensive care. *Journal of Pediatric Nursing, 4*(2), 96–103.

Larson, M. C., Gunnar, M. R., & Hertsgaard, L. (1991). The effects of morning naps, car trips, and maternal separation on adrenocortical activity in human infants. *Child Develpoment, 62,* 362–372.

Levine, S., & Ursin, H. (1991). What is stress? In M. R. Brown, G. F. Koob, & C. Rivier (Eds.), *Stress: Neurobiology and neuroendocrinology* (pp. 3–21). New York: Marcel Dekker, Inc.

Lindsey, A. M., Carrieri-Kohlman, V., & Page, G. G. (1993). Stress response. In V. Carrieri-Kohlman, A. M. Lindsey, & C. M. West (Eds.), *Pathophysiological phenomena in nursing: Human responses to illness* (2nd ed., pp. 397–419). Philadelphia: W. B. Saunders Company.

Lowery, B. J. (1987). Stress research: Some theoretical and methodological issues. *Image: Journal of Nursing Scholarship, 19*(1), 42–46.

Malone, S. M., Gunnar, M. R., & Fisch, R. O. (1985). Adrenocortical and behavioral responses to limb restraint in human neonates. *Developmental Psychobiology, 18*(5), 435–446.

Merskey, H., Albe-Fessard, D. G., Bonica, J. J., Carmon, A., Dubner, R., Kerr, F. W. L., Linblom, U., Mumford, J. M., Nathan, P. W., Noodenbos, W., Pagni, C. A., Renaer, M. J., Sternbach, R. A., & Sunderland, S. (1979). Pain terms: A list with definitions and notes on usage: Recommended by the ISAP subcommittee on taxonomy. *Pain, 6*(3), 249–252.

Mills, N. M. (1989). Pain behaviors in infants and toddlers. *Journal of Pain and Symptom Management, 4,* 184–190.

Norris, S., Campbell, L. A., & Brenkert, S. (1982). Nursing procedures and alterations in transcutaneous oxygen tension in premature infants. *Nursing Research, 31,* 300–336.

Pollack, M. M., Ruttiman, U. E., & Getson, P. R. (1988). Pediatric risk of mortality (PRISM) score. *Critical Care Medicine, 16,* 1110–1116.

Rew, L. (1986). Intuition: Concept analysis of a group phenomenon. *Advances in Nursing Science, 8*(2), 18–21.

Rhoades, R., & Pflanzer, R. (1992). *Human physiology* (2nd ed., pp. 371–529). Philadelphia: Saunders College Publishing.

Ruttiman, U. E., Albert, A., Pollack, M. M., & Glass, N. L. (1986). Dynamic assessment of severity of illness in pediatric intensive care. *Critical Care Medicine, 14*(3), 215–221.

Schmeling, D. J., & Coran, A. G. (1991). Hormonal and metabolic response to operative stress in the neonate. *Journal of Parenteral and Enteral Nutrition, 15*(2), 215–238.

Selye, H. (1946). The general adaptation syndrome and the diseases of adaptation. *The Journal of Clinical Endocrinology, 6*(2), 117–202.

Selye, H. (1993). History of the stress concept. In L. Goldberger & S. Breznitz (Eds.), *Handbook of stress: Theoretical and clinical aspects* (2nd ed., pp. 7–18). New York: The Free Press.

Solomon, S., Bird, C. E., Ling, W., Iwamiya, M., & Young, P. C. M. (1967). Formation and metabolism of steroids in the fetus and placenta. *Recent Progress in Hormone Research, 23,* 297–347.

Stidham, G., & Bugnitz, M. C. (1992). Neuroendocrine response to stress. In M. C. Rogers (Ed.), *Textbook of pediatric intensive care* (2nd ed., pp. 1476–1491).

Thompson, R. H. (1986). Where we stand: Twenty years of research on pediatric hospitalization and health care. *Children's Health Care, 14*(4), 200–210.

Ursin, H., & Olff, M. (1993). The stress response. In S. C. Stanford & P. Salmon (Eds.), *Stress: From synapse to syndrome* (pp. 4–22). London: Academic Press, Harcourt Brace & Company Publishers.

Walker, L. O., & Avant, K. (1988). *Strategies for theory construction in nursing* (2nd ed.). Norwalk, CT: Appleton & Lange.

Weiner, H. (1992). The history of the concept of stress. In H. Weiner (Ed.), *Perturbing the organism: The biology of stressful experiences* (pp. 9–27). Chicago: The University of Chicago Press.

Wilson, T., & Broome, M. E. (1989). Promoting the young child's development in the intensive care unit. *Heart & Lung, 18,* 274–279.

Wolf, A. R. (1993). Treat the babies, not their stress responses (commentary). *The Lancet, 324* (8867), 319–320.

Wolf, A. R., Eyres, R. L., Laussen, P. C., Edwards, J., Stanley, I. J., Rowe, P., & Simon, L. (1993). Effects of extradural analgesia on stress responses to abdominal surgery in infants. *British Journal of Anaesthesia, 70*(6), 654–660.

Yeh, T. S. (1992). The use of scoring systems in the pediatric ICU. *Problems in Critical Care, 3*(4), 599–615.

ANALYSIS OF THE CONCEPTUAL-THEORETICAL-EMPIRICAL STRUCTURE

The stated purpose of Rosenthal-Dichter's (1996) research was to analyze the concept pediatric physiological stress response. The research was designed to generate a middle-range descriptive classification theory of the pediatric physiological stress response using Walker and Avant's (1988) descriptive research method of concept analysis.

IDENTIFICATION OF CONCEPTS

Conceptual Model Concept

Analysis of the research report revealed that the concept analysis was guided by three conceptual models of stress—the Institute of Medicine (1981) model, Levine and Ursin's (1991) model, and Selye's (1993) conceptualization of the General Adaptation Syndrome. The conceptual model concept of interest is stress, which is viewed as a multidimensional concept made up of three dimensions: stressor, mediator, and stress response. The stressor response dimension is of central interest for Rosenthal-Dichter's research.

Middle-Range Theory Concept

Further analysis of the research report revealed that the middle-range descriptive classification theory of the pediatric physiological stress response encompasses just one concept with two dimensions. The concept is pediatric physiological stress response, and its dimensions are neuroendocrine events and metabolic events. The theory is categorized as a descriptive classification theory because the two dimensions of the concept are thought to be interrelated and interdependent.

CLASSIFICATION OF THE MIDDLE-RANGE THEORY CONCEPT

The middle-range theory concept pediatric physiological stress response is classified as a construct in both Kaplan's and Willer and Webster's schemata because it was invented for research purposes and is not immediately accessible to direct sensory observations. Indeed, Rosenthal-Dichter identified several so-called empirical referents that could serve as more observable proxies for the concept, including heart rate, blood pressure, blood volume, central nervous system alertness, and catecholamines.

The concept is classified as a variable because, according to Rosenthal-Dichter, the magnitude and duration of the pediatric physiological stress response can vary from individual to individual, even when the same stressor is present. In particular, Rosenthal-Dichter indicated that the pediatric physiological stress response is a graded, rather than an all or none response. Accordingly, the concept is most appropriately classified as an enumerative unit in Dubin's schema because it always would be present to some degree in studies of responses to stressors.

IDENTIFICATION AND CLASSIFICATION OF PROPOSITIONS

Conceptual Model Propositions

Nonrelational propositions from three conceptual models were used to guide the generation of the middle-range descriptive classification theory of the pediatric physiological stress response. These propositions, which are evident in the research report, are listed in Table A–1.

Conceptual model Propositions 1 and 2 can be formalized as a nonrelational existence proposition:

There is a phenomenon known as stress.

Conceptual model Propositions, 3, 4, 5, 6, and 7 can be formalized as a nonrelational proposition that asserts a constitutive definition:

Stress, which is defined as the nonspecific result of any demand upon the body, encompasses three dimensions: stressor, mediator, and response. The stressor dimension is defined as the demand, challenge, or stimulus that elicits a stress response. The mediator dimension is defined as the process whereby an organism evaluates the stressor. The stress response dimension is defined as the organism's reaction to the stressor.

Middle-Range Theory Propositions

Nonrelational propositions making up the middle-range descriptive classification theory of the pediatric physiological stress response are evident in Rosenthal-Dichter's report. These propositions are listed in Table A–2.

Table A–I ■ CONCEPTUAL MODEL PROPOSITIONS FROM ROSENTHAL-DICTHER'S RESEARCH REPORT

Proposition	Classification
I. Stress is a prevalent topic in today's society.	Nonrelational, Existence
2. Stress also is the subject of voluminous research and an ever-increasing number of professional publications, conferences, and academic courses.	Nonrelational, Existence
3. Stress is the nonspecific result of any demand upon the body.	Nonrelational, Constitutive Definition
4. The multidimensional nature of stress has both facilitated and confounded the process of clarifying the concept of stress.	Nonrelational, Constitutive Definition
5. The term stressor, in contrast to the word stress, is widely accepted and used to refer to the demand, challenge, or stimulus that elicits a stress response.	Nonrelational, Constitutive Definition
6. A mediator or "filter" is the process whereby an organism evaluates the stressor.	Nonrelational, Constitutive Definition
7. The stress response is the organism's reaction to the stressor.	Nonrelational, Constitutive Definition

---

Table A–2 ■ **MIDDLE-RANGE THEORY PROPOSITIONS FROM ROSENTHAL-DICHTER'S RESEARCH REPORT**

Proposition	Classification
1. Attributes of the [pediatric physiological] stress response emerged as consistent themes upon review of the literature.	Nonrelational, Existence Measured Operational Definition
2. The [pediatric physiological] stress response is not an undesirbale or atavistic response, but one that is an integral part of an adaptive biological system. It is considered protective, in fact, the stress response is categorized as a protective life process . . . [that] assists in shielding the organism from stressors and altering the impact of stressors. . . . [It] is necessary to the functioning and survival of the organism in a dynamic, complex environment.	Nonrelational, Constitutive Definition
3. The composite of interrelated and interdependent neuroendocrine and metabolic events that comprise the [pediatric physiological] stress response reflect the coordinating and integrating roles of the brain.	Nonrelational, Constitutive Definition
4. The magnitude and duration of the [pediatric physiological] stress response, even to the same stressor, varies from individual to individual.	Nonrelational, Level of Existence
5. The [pediatric physiological] stress response begins as a normal, protective, and adaptive response to stressors.	Nonrelational, Constitutive Definition
6. The [pediatric physiological] stress response is a graded, not an all or none, response.	Nonrelational, Level of Existence

---

Middle-range theory Proposition 1 can be formalized as a nonrelational existence proposition:

> There is a phenomenon known as the pediatric physiological stress response.

Middle-range theory Propositions 4 and 6 can be formalized as a nonrelational level of existence proposition:

> The phenomenon known as the pediatric physiological stress response can vary in magnitude and duration.

Middle-range theory Propositions 2, 3, and 5 can be formalized as a nonrelational proposition that asserts a constitutive definition:

> The pediatric physiological stress response is defined as an integral part of an adaptive biological system. It is a protective life process that assists in shielding the organism from stressors and altering the impact of stressors, and is necessary to the functioning and survival of the organism in a dynamic, complex environment. The concept pediatric physiological stress response encompasses two interrelated and interdependent dimensions: neuroendocrine events and metabolic events.

A nonrelational proposition that asserts a representational definition was easily extracted from the report. Rosenthal-Dichter pointed out that little had been written about the stress response dimension of stress and that the purpose of her research was to analyze the concept pediatric physiological stress response. Moreover, in Table 1 of the report, she clearly identified the [pediatric physiological] stress response as the "correlate" to the stress response dimension of stress for the concept analysis. The formalized representational definition, which links the conceptual model concept with the middle-range theory concept, is:

> The stress response dimension of the conceptual model concept stress was represented by the middle-range theory concept pediatric physiological stress response.

A nonrelational proposition that asserts a measured operational definition also was extracted from the report. This proposition was extracted from middle-range theory Proposition 1 as well as the list of references at the end of the report. The formalized measured operational definition is:

> The definition and attributes of the pediatric physiological stress response were identified by means of a review of journal articles, books, and book chapters.

The operational definition links the middle-range theory concept with the empirical indicators used to accomplish the concept analysis. In keeping with Walker and Avant's (1988) method of concept analysis and by examination of the list of references used, those empirical indicators were determined to be the literature contained in journal articles, books, and book chapters.

It is important to point out that the operational definition focuses on how the theory concept pediatric physiological stress response was measured for the purposes of the concept analysis. Rosenthal-Dichter identified several empirical referents that could be incorporated into a measured operational definition in future studies of the relation between stressors, mediators, and the pediatric physiological stress response. More specifically, Rosenthal-Dichter stated:

> ■ The classic signs of the "fight or flight" response are empirical referents of the [pediatric] physiological stress response. Other examples of empirical referents abound in the literature and include all hormones and their precursors, metabolic substrates, and other endogenous mediators (i.e., opioids, prostaglandins, cytokines) involved in any aspect of the [pediatric] physiological stress response.

HIERARCHY OF PROPOSITIONS

The formalized nonrelational constitutive definitional propositions for the conceptual model concept stress and the middle-range theory concept pediatric physiological stress response, along with the nonrelational representational definitional proposition, lend themselves to hierarchical arrangement by level of abstraction. The hierarchy is:

> *Abstract proposition:* Stress, which is defined as the nonspecific result of any demand upon the body, encompasses three dimensions: stressor, mediator, and response. The stressor dimension is defined as the demand, challenge, or stimulus that elicits a stress response. The mediator dimension is defined as the process whereby an organism evalu-

ates the stressor. The stress response dimension is defined as the organism's reaction to the stressor.

Somewhat concrete proposition: The stress response dimension of the conceptual model concept stress was represented by the middle-range theory concept pediatric physiological stress response.

More concrete proposition: The pediatric physiological stress response is defined as an integral part of an adaptive biological system. It is a protective life process that assists in shielding the organism from stressors and altering the impact of stressors, and is necessary to the functioning and survival of the organism in a dynamic, complex environment. The concept pediatric physiological stress response encompasses two interrelated and interdependent dimensions: neuroendocrine events and metabolic events.

DIAGRAMS

The conceptual-theoretical-empirical structure for the research is illustrated in Figure A–1. Another diagram was constructed to illustrate the dimensions of the

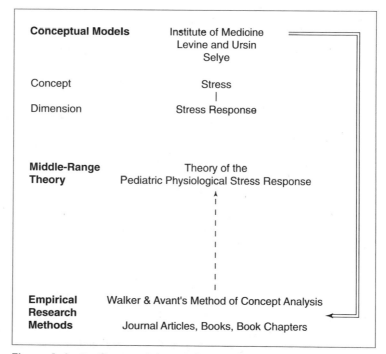

Figure A–I ■ Conceptual-theoretical-empirical structure for Rosenthal-Dichter's research.

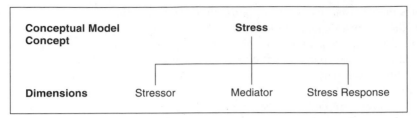

Figure A–2 ■ Diagram of the conceptual-model concept stress and its dimensions.

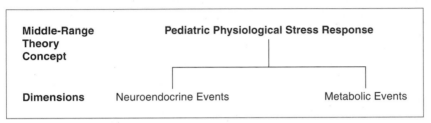

Figure A–3 ■ Diagram of the theory concept pediatric physiological stress response and its dimensions.

conceptual model concept stress (Figure A–2). Still another diagram was constructed to illustrate the dimensions of the theory concept pediatric physiological stress response (Fig. A–3).

EVALUATION OF THE CONCEPTUAL-THEORETICAL-EMPIRICAL STRUCTURE

Analysis of Rosenthal-Dichter's research report revealed that a one-concept middle-range descriptive classification theory was generated. The concept is pediatric physiological stress response. The two dimensions of the concept are neuroendocrine events and metabolic events.

EVALUATION OF THE CONCEPTUAL-THEORETICAL-EMPIRICAL LINKAGES

Specification Adequacy

The criterion of specification adequacy is met. The three conceptual models that guided Rosenthal-Dichter's theory-generating research are explicitly identified and discussed in sufficient breadth and depth so that there is a clear relation of those conceptual models to the middle-range theory and the empirical research method of content analysis of journal articles, books, and book chapters.

Linkage Adequacy

The criterion of linkage adequacy also is met. The linkage between the stress response dimension of the conceptual model concept stress and the middle-range theory concept pediatric physiological stress response was easily extracted from information given in the research report.

Conceptual Model Usage Rating Scale

Evaluation of the criteria of specification adequacy and linkage adequacy is summarized by application of the Conceptual Model Usage Rating Scale. Rosenthal-Dichter's research report earned a score of 3, indicating adequate use of the three conceptual models of stress in the generation of her middle-range theory of the pediatric physiological stress response.

EVALUATION OF THE THEORY

Significance

The middle-range theory of the pediatric physiological stress response meets the criterion of significance. Both social and theoretical significance are addressed in Rosenthal-Dichter's introductory comments. She states, "This impetus to include a biologic or physiologic component in nursing research is expected to continue since the National Institute of Nursing Research has implemented a 10-year program to increase the use of biologic theory and measurements in nursing through a variety of funding mechanisms." Continuing to address social significance, Rosenthal-Dichter added:

> ■ The incorporation of biologic or physiologic components in nursing research is well suited to critical care settings, such as the pediatric or neonatal intensive care unit, given the nature and complexity of the environment and the availability of information derived from the use of invasive monitoring devices. In the pediatric critical care setting, nurses continually assess the physiologic stability of the critically ill child as well as the child's responses to a variety of interpersonal interactions, clinical interventions, and treatments. Clinical parameters, including, but not limited to, heart rate, respiratory rate, and blood pressure, are often used as barometers of physiologic status. This status is continually challenged by a multitude of stressors which induce subsequent responses by the child.

Moreover, later in her article, Rosenthal-Dichter pointed out that various disciplines have an interest in the concept.

Adding to her earlier comments regarding theoretical significance, Rosenthal-Dichter noted:

> ■ Only through a better understanding of the age-appropriate physiologic stress response can nurses accurately confirm its presence and evaluate its potential consequences. In addition, many nursing interventions are evaluated for tolerance or effectiveness using the patient's physiologic stress response as the criterion. Without an understanding of the physiologic stress response of the

neonate, infant, and child, one cannot adequately assess this response in the context of age and clinical condition.

Later, Rosenthal-Dichter pointed out that references to the pediatric physiological stress response are limited to brief descriptions of the concept and brief discussions of proposed differences that might exist at different stages of the patient's development. She went on to note that a previously published seminal review of responses to operative stress was limited to the stressor of surgery and to neonates.

Internal Consistency

The middle-range theory of the pediatric physiological stress response meets the criterion of internal consistency in part. Rosenthal-Dichter uses the terms pediatric physiological stress response and pediatric physiologic stress response interchangeably throughout the report; otherwise, semantic clarity is evident in that the theory concept was constitutively defined in a clear and concise manner. The two dimensions of the concept, however, were not defined. Rosenthal-Dichter uses the terms pediatric physiological stress response and pediatric physiologic stress response interchangeably throughout the report; otherwise, semantic consistency is evident. Indeed, early in the report, Rosenthal-Dichter explicitly stated that the concept pediatric physiological stress response would be referred to as the stress response. Furthermore, the propositions of the theory reflect structural consistency; a hierarchy based on level of abstraction was easily constructed from nonrelational definitional propositions. There are no redundant propositions.

Parsimony

The middle-range theory of the pediatric physiological stress response meets the criterion of parsimony. The analysis revealed that the theory is made up of one concept with two dimensions.

Although dimensions of the more general concept stress response (in contrast to pediatric physiological stress response), as well as other concepts and propositions, are evident in the report, they are not central to the theory. More specifically, Rosenthal-Dichter mentioned that manifestations of stress include psychologic, behavioral, sociocultural, and physiologic responses, which could be considered dimensions of the concept stress response. Other concepts mentioned include physiologic and psychologic stressors, which Rosenthal-Dichter identified as antecedents to the pediatric physiologic stress response, as well as physiologic stability and pathophysiologic clinical states, which she identified as consequences of the pediatric physiological stress response. In addition, Rosenthal-Dichter mentioned the concepts cognitive appraisal and coping, which she identified as mediators of stressors.

Propositions that are not central to the one concept theory of the pediatric physiological stress response include statements that assert relations between stressors, mediators, and the stress response, as well as the statement that "The magnitude and direction of the stress response can be influenced by multidisciplinary interventions." It is not clear whether these concepts and propositions are part of the conceptual models of stress or part of a more elaborate middle-range theory.

Testability

The middle-range theory of the pediatric physiological stress response meets the criterion of testability in that it should be possible to test the theory by reviewing the same literature cited by Rosenthal-Dichter and using Walker and Avant's (1988) method of content analysis.

EVALUATION OF THE RESEARCH DESIGN

Operational Adequacy

The research design meets the criterion of operational adequacy. In particular, Walker and Avant's (1988) method of concept analysis was used appropriately. More precisely, Rosenthal-Dichter appropriately used Walker and Avant's modification of the Wilson (1963) method of concept analysis. In addition, Rosenthal-Dichter explicitly identified her own modifications, which were appropriate. Furthermore, the references cited are representative of the literature on stress, within the context of the three conceptual models Rosenthal-Dichter used to guide her research.

EVALUATION OF THE RESEARCH FINDINGS

Empirical Adequacy

The result of Rosenthal-Dichter's research was the generation of a middle-range descriptive classification theory of the pediatric physiological stress response. The theory, as presented in the report, meets the criterion of empirical adequacy only in part. Rosenthal-Dichter's description of the relevant literature, which represents the data used for the content analysis, clearly supports the definition and attributes of the pediatric physiological stress response.

However, a question about the empirical adequacy of a distinction between the pediatric physiological stress response and the adult physiological stress response must be raised because Rosenthal-Dichter concluded that the attributes of both concepts are the same. Given her conclusion, it may have been more appropriate to label the concept simply as the physiological stress response and eliminate the developmental stage term in the concept name.

EVALUATION OF THE UTILITY OF THE
THEORY FOR PRACTICE

Pragmatic Adequacy

The findings of Rosenthal-Dichter's theory-generating research do not yet meet the criterion of pragmatic adequacy. Given the preliminary nature of the research, it is to Rosenthal-Dichter's credit that she did not discuss the practical or clinical implications of the middle-range theory of the pediatric physiological stress response.

EVALUATION OF THE CONCEPTUAL MODEL

Credibility

The credibility of the three conceptual models of stress used to guide Rosenthal-Dichter's research is not addressed directly in the report. In keeping with theory-generating research, the judgment about credibility is limited to the utility of the conceptual model to guide the selection of empirical research methods and the success of those methods in generating a new theory. Rosenthal-Dichter successfully used a method of content analysis to generate a middle-range theory that was directly linked with a dimension of the conceptual model concept stress. Consequently, it can be inferred that the three conceptual models cited by Rosenthal-Dichter were useful.

Two statements in the implications section of the report indicate that Rosenthal-Dichter recognized the importance of conceptual models as guides for research. She stated, "It is imperative that a conceptual framework be included in future research regarding the pediatric physiological stress response and that there be consistency between the framework and the research hypothesis and methodology." She went on to maintain that "Investigations must include a clear conceptual-theoretical-empirical structure that accurately defines the role of the concept of interest within the study."

References

Institute of Medicine. (1981). *Report of a study: Research on stress and human health.* Washington, DC: National Academy Press.

Levine, S., & Ursin, H. (1991). What is stress? In M. R. Brown, G. F. Koob, & C. Rivier (Eds.), *Stress: Neurobiology and neuroendocrinology* (pp. 3–21). New York: Marcel Dekker.

Rosenthal-Dichter, C. H. (1996). The pediatric physiologic stress response: A concept analysis. *Scholarly Inquiry for Nursing Practice, 10,* 211–234.

Selye, H. (1993). History of the stress concept. In L. Goldberger & S. Breznitz (Eds.), *Handbook of stress: Theoretical and clinical aspects* (2nd ed., pp. 7–18). New York: The Free Press.

Walker, L. O., & Avant, K. (1988). *Strategies for theory construction in nursing* (2nd ed.). Norwalk, CT: Appleton and Lange.

Wilson, J. (1963). *Thinking with concepts.* New York: Cambridge University Press.

Analysis and Evaluation of a Descriptive Theory-Generating Study:
The Case-Study Method

Exploring Music Intervention With Restrained Patients

Linda M. Janelli, RNC, EdD, Genevieve W. Kanski, RN, EdD, Helen M. Jones, RN, MS, and Mary C. Kennedy, RN, MS

Roy's Adaptation Model is used in a case study approach to begin examining the potential of music intervention in hospitalized, restrained patients. Restraints were removed during the time in which the patient listened to a musical tape through a headset. Mr. D, presented in this case study, was one of the 30 medical-surgical patients who participated. His observable positive behaviors increased from 10 during the preintervention period to 12 during the musical intervention. Mr. D displayed no negative behaviors during the entire study period.

If "music hath charms to soothe the savage beast," might it be effective in altering patient behavior and eventually reducing the need for physical restraints? Use of physical restraints continues to be a common practice in many hospital settings. The estimation is that 17–22% of all patients are restrained at some point during their hospitalization (Robbins, Boyko, Lane, Cooper, & Jahnigen, 1987). That statistic is probably conservative in that the authors of this study found patients restrained with no physician's order, making data tracking difficult. In the case study (Robbins et al., 1987) physical restraints are defined as a physical or mechanical device used to restrict the movement of the whole or a portion of a patient's body in order to control physical activities and to protect him, her or others from injury (JCAHO, 1993).

In contrast to hospital settings, nursing homes have had at their disposal a federal mandate to deal with restraint issues. The Omnibus Budget Reconciliation Act of 1990 (OBRA) specifies under what circumstances physical restraints may be

Reprinted from *Nursing Forum*, *30*(4),12–18, 1995, with permission.

employed. OBRA states that nursing home residents have the right to be free from restraints that are not required to treat specific "medical symptoms" (DHHS, 1989). In a recent survey of 159 skilled nursing homes in New York State, 142 (89%) of the facilities acknowledged a decrease in restraint use (Janelli, Kanski, & Neary, 1994). Since 1990 an approximately 47% decrease has been seen in use of restraints across the country (Cassetta, 1993). This reduction would not have been possible without the impetus provided from OBRA.

The potential physical and psychological risks that restraints can impose on patients include, but are not limited to, constipation, decubiti, nosocomial infections, muscle weakness, depression, and social withdrawal (Evans & Strumpf, 1990). If hospitals are interested in maintaining the safety of patients while preserving their dignity and quality of life, then interventions other than physical restraints need to be tried. Although nurses would prefer to use alternatives to restraints, to date no clinical trials of potential strategies have been attempted (Hardin et al., 1994; Scherer, Janelli, Wu, & Kuhn, 1993). Alternatives that are mentioned in the literature—such as Adirondack chairs, reality orientation, and ambulation programs—have been generated from nursing home environments, and are based on anecdotal information, which may not translate to hospital settings.

ROY'S ADAPTATION MODEL

From clinical experience the authors believe that patients, their families, and nursing staffs adapt to the use of physical restraints in different ways. Roy's Adaptation Model (Roy & Roberts, 1981) seems applicable as a framework for examining the issue of restraints and their potential effect on the older patient. Roy's model originated from Selye's Stress Theory, which postulates that human existence is an attempt to cope with the environment. According to Selye, individuals either can adjust to the ever-changing stress in their environment or they can fight back (Wixon, 1978).

Two systems are used within Roy's model—"man" and his environment. Persons are viewed as biopsychosocial beings who interact with the environment. Effective responses that can aid the individual in adapting to the environment are those that promote the integrity of the person in terms of goals of survival, growth, reproduction, and self-mastery (Roy & Roberts, 1981).

Assessment is an important component of the nursing process. Assessment is essential within Roy's model to determine whether the individual is coping with his or her own system and the environment. A first and second level of assessment is required.

FIRST-LEVEL ASSESSMENT. The first-level assessment involves gathering subjective and objective data within the framework of man's four adaptive modes: physiologic needs, role function, interdependence, and self-concept (Riehl & Roy, 1974). Physiologic needs are those factors necessary to regulate the balance of circulation, body temperature, oxygen, fluids, exercise and rest, elimination, and the appetitive system. For example, an older adult who is immobile due to a physical restraint may not achieve a balance between exercise and rest; as a consequence, the gastrointestinal tract might be affected, resulting in constipation.

Role function refers to the part an individual plays within society. Roles either can be ascribed or achieved over a lifetime. As individuals age the number of roles in which they participate decrease due in part to retirement, sickness, and death of friends and/or spouse.

The interdependence mode involves documenting the individual's dependent and independent needs. Individuals who are physically restrained may be dependent on the nursing staff for their basic needs, and yet they may be able to make independent decisions regarding their care and treatment.

The last adaptive mode is self-concept—how one views himself or herself, which usually is related to participation in current roles. An individual may be retired, but feels worthwhile and has a positive self-concept based on past achievements and achievements of children and grandchildren.

SECOND-LEVEL ASSESSMENT. The second-level assessment is associated with examining three types of stimuli or stressors: focal, contextual, and residual. Focal stimuli are those that immediately confront the individual, and the ones to which a person must make an adaptive response. Focal stimuli can be physical, physiological, psychological, or a combination of these forces. Focal stimuli can either be positive—for example, experiencing the birth of a first grandchild—or negative, such as experiencing elder abuse. Contextual or background stimuli involve the environment, which varies in intensity and can be positive or negative. An example of a contextual stimulus is having a grandchild born far from one's own geographical area, making visiting difficult. The third type of stimulus is residual; like contextual, it contributes to focal stimuli. Residual stimuli cannot be validated or measured: they can include such factors as beliefs, attitudes, experiences, or traits. Older adults who have the attitude that they are too young to be considered a grandparent are an example of a residual stimuli. Focal, contextual, and residual stimuli can affect one or all four of the adaptive modes.

GOAL. According to Roy's model, the goal of nursing care is to encourage the patient to adapt in a positive fashion to environmental changes. If the patient is coping ineffectively and consuming energy in this attempt, the nurse's goal would be to change the stimuli to assist the patient's coping mechanisms to bring about adaptation. The end result could be enhancement of the individual's level of wellness.

INTERVENTIONS. The nursing intervention aspect of the nursing process within Roy's model involves the manipulation of the focal, contextual, and residual stimuli so that the patient can cope. The nurse may increase, decrease, or modify internal stimuli (cognator mode) and external stimuli (regulator mode). The nurse also can act as an assistant adaptor by directing energy to or away from the patient. The nurse's intervention approach either can be therapeutic, when the patient responds favorably, or supportive, when the nurse no longer can alter the patient's course of adaptation (Janelli, 1980).

EVALUATION. The final step in the nursing process is evaluation. The patient has either adapted to new behaviors or has been unsuccessful. Reassessment of the influencing stimuli, the goal, and/or the nursing intervention may be necessary if the behavior has not been altered.

APPLYING ROY'S MODEL TO A RESTRAINED PATIENT

A patient who is restrained (as depicted in Figure 1) is affected by the environment in which the restraining takes place. One of man's adaptive mechanisms, in Roy's model, is the cognator mode, which, in this example, refers to how the patient consciously and unconsciously perceives the restraint device. The focal stimuli could be the restraining device; the contextual stimuli could be the patient's hospital environment, the staff patterns and/or nursing tasks that need to be accomplished, and the psychological feelings of being restrained, which could vary between feelings of safety and feelings of humiliation. The residual stimuli refer to the patients, nurses and families' attitudes toward restraints. All three stimuli in turn affect the regulator mode—the patient's reflex response to the restraints—which will impact how the patient copes with the stress of being restrained.

Energy or tension emanates back and forth from Roy's four adaptive modes (self-concept, role function, physiologic needs, interdependence) and the regulator mode. The patient can respond to the stressors of being restrained by using various coping mechanisms, which can be physical (displaying anger), physiological (increased heart rate), and psychological (being depressed). Once the nurse completes the first and second-level assessment, and determines how the patient is cop-

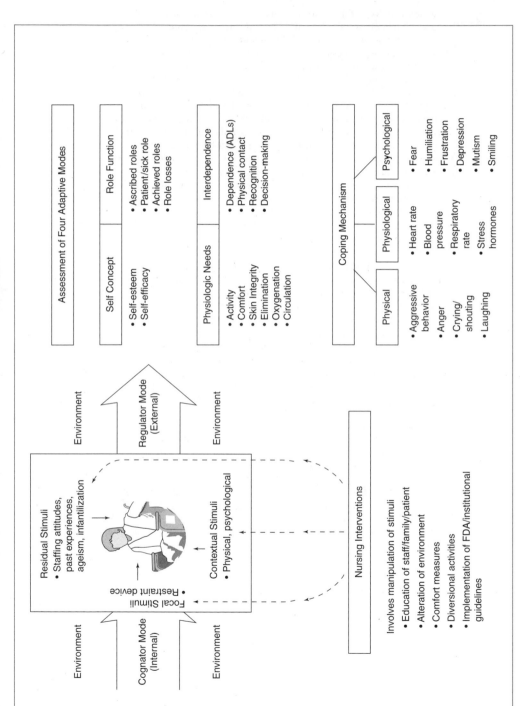

Figure 1 ■ Patient Responses to Physical Restraint Explained Through Roy's Adaptation Model.

ing with being restrained then an appropriate nursing intervention can be formulated. The nursing intervention can be directed toward one or all of the stimuli (focal, contextual, residual).

PATIENT EXAMPLE

Mr. D is a 76-year-old African-American admitted to a tertiary care hospital with a bleeding gastrointestinal tract related to alcohol consumption. Mr. D is one of 30 subjects in a pilot study designed to examine the effect of a music intervention with physically restrained medical-surgical patients. He has a wife and two daughters who requested restraints to prevent Mr. D from pulling at his multiple intravenous lines and Foley catheter. At the time of the intervention, Mr. D was in bed with a Posey vest and bilateral wrist restraints. Prior to the intervention, the Short Portable Mental Status Questionnaire (SPMSQ) was administered to the patient. Mr. D has only 1 error out of 10, which signified that he was alert and mentally intact. Even though the patient was alert, restraints had been applied in response to the family's request and the concern of the nursing staff that Mr. D's treatment could be affected if he pulled out one of his tubes. Table 1 represents an assessment of the patient's four adaptive modes. He stated that being restrained made him feel like a criminal.

MUSIC INTERVENTION

As the authors began exploring potential alternatives to restraints they became aware that many hospitals used piped-in music to decrease patient anxiety and discomfort.

Music as a nursing intervention was chosen also because it is a means of communication, and is considered a universal language that does not require high intellectual ability. Music for therapeutic use has been proven to be of value and is documented throughout history. Music was used as a source of healing by ancient Greeks. Aristotle believed strong emotions and a state of cathartic relief could be aroused by the tones of a flute (Mornhinweg, 1992). It was not, however, until after World War II that music as a therapy became more accepted and was employed in psychiatric and rehabilitation settings. While research studies on the therapeutic effects of music have been increasing, its acceptance and use as a means of therapy have not been evident in general hospital settings (Biley, 1992).

The physiological effects of music have been well-documented (Cook, 1981). They include changes in metabolism, muscular energy, pulse, blood pressure, breathing, and blood volume. Much like a familiar person or cultural medium, music has been shown to decrease anxiety and discomfort. Music has been utilized on a short-term basis as a distractor and as a relaxation technique. Common emotional

Table 1 ■ **THE FOUR ADAPTIVE MODES OF MR. D**

Physiologic Needs	Role Function	Interdependence	Self-Concept
• Bleeding peptic ulcer	Patient has assumed sick role—IV running, Foley catheter in place	In semiprivate room by window	Angry—feels like a criminal in restraints
• ETOH—alcohol abuse	Ascribed roles-patient husband/father	Dependent on staff for basic activities of daily living	Humiliated—no explanation given for restraints
• Mitral valve replacement 2 years prior	Achieved roles-retired worker, friend	Independent in communication of needs	
• Alert—SPMSQ score was 1 error	Social role-smiles, responds appropriately		

reactions of patients to medical treatments and to restraints are anxiety, fear, anger, and depression. If the patient's focus of attention can be directed toward a more pleasant sensory stimulus, such as listening to music, then perhaps it is more easily possible to control reactions such as anxiety (Kaempf & Amodei, 1989). In her work with music, Herth (1978) found that in order for music to have a beneficial influence, the patient had to like the music. She also found that the greater the person's interest in music, the more effectively music could be used to influence his or her behavior.

Mr. D was given a choice of music from four tapes, which included: band, classical, country-western, and popular. He chose popular music—the soundtrack from "Sleepless in Seattle." Mr. D was observed for 10 minutes prior to the intervention with his restraints in place. A Behavior Instrument checklist developed by the investigators was used before, during, and after the intervention. The instrument consisted of 39 items representing both verbal and nonverbal communication such as echolalia, laughing, smiling, and squirming. The checklist required the investigator to place a check next to the behavior if it was observed. The behaviors could be tallied as positive responses such as humming and nodding the head, or as negative responses such as moaning and having a clenched jaw.

During the preintervention period Mr. D demonstrated 10 positive behaviors. He verbalized in an articulate manner the absence of pain, and acknowledged who he was and where he was hospitalized. Mr. D used gestures and smiled while talking. He displayed no negative behaviors during the entire study period.

The restraints were removed, and large, soft headphones were put over Mr. D's ears, and attached to a tape player. Mr. D listened to the music for 50 minutes, during which time the investigator again monitored his behavior. Mr. D's response to the music was very positive in that he laughed appropriately and called out the names of the musicians that he recognized: Jimmy Durante, Louis Armstrong, and Nat King Cole. He smiled and tapped his fingers on the bedrail in time with the music. Even though he was in bed, he tapped his feet. During the intervention period, Mr. D displayed a total of 12 positive behaviors during the intervention. He was one of 18 patients out of 30 who demonstrated an increase in positive responses from preintervention to the intervention. After the tape ended he said he enjoyed the music and thanked the investigators. After the intervention the restraints were replaced, and Mr. D was observed for 10 minutes. During the postintervention, period, Mr. D demonstrated eight positive behaviors. He did not resist when the restraints were reapplied. He yawned and appeared sleepy. The authors noted that the music affected three of Mr. D's four adaptive modes: (a) interdependence, because he was able to make a decision regarding the type of music he wanted to listen to; (b) self-concept, which was enhanced when he accurately identified some of the musicians on the tape; and (c) physiologic needs, in that Mr. D appeared comfortable and relaxed, with his eyes closed periodically.

CLINICAL IMPLICATIONS

Although it is too early to draw conclusions, at least beginning evidence is seen that music is a worthwhile nursing intervention that can be used with hospital patients in an effort to reduce application of restraints. Within the context of Roy's model, music can potentially alter both the patient's focal and contextual stimuli. The possibility exists that music also may alter the staff members' perceptions (residual stimuli) of the patient when they note the change in behavior in response to the music. Nurses generally are willing to try new strategies rather than resort to restraints; the problem, however, is a lack of empirically tested alternatives. This case study demonstrated the effectiveness of music with Mr. D, who overcame his anger and made no attempts to pull out his tubes while listening to music.

Mr. D was one of 13 males and 15 African-Americans who participated in the study. The investigators believe him to be representative of the sample in that he was one of 18 patients who demonstrated an increase in positive behaviors while unrestrained and listening to selected music. Further research is warranted with a larger sample and with the intervention being administered over a period of days. As more data was collected, Roy's model also may require additional transformation in order to explicate better the role of music with the physically restrained. ■

References

Biley, F. (1992). Using music in hospital settings. *Nursing Standard, 6*(35), 37–39.

Cassetta, R. (1993). Restraint use. Still an issue for nurses. *The American Nurse, 25*(7), 16.

Cook, J. (1981). The therapeutic use of music: A literature review. *Nursing Forum, 20*(3), 253–266.

Department of Health and Human Services. (1989). Medicare and medicaid: Regulations for long-term care facilities. *Federal Register, 54,* 5322.

Evans, L., & Strumpf, N. (1990). Myths about elder restraint. *IMAGE, 22,* 124–128.

Hardin, S., Magee, R., Stratmann, D., Vinson, M., Owen, M., & Hyatt, E. (1994). Attitudes toward restraints. *Journal of Gerontological Nursing, 20*(3), 23–31.

Herth, K. (1978). The therapeutic use of music. *Supervisor Nurse, 9*(10), 22–23.

Janelli, L. (1980). Utilizing Roy's adaptation model from a gerontological perspective. *Journal of Gerontological Nursing, 6*(3), 140–150.

Janelli, L., Kanski, G., & Neary, M. (1994). Physical restraints: Has OBRA made a difference? *Journal of Gerontological Nursing, 20*(6), 17–21.

Joint Commission on Accreditation of Healthcare Organizations. (1993). *1994 Accreditation Manual for Hospitals* (Library of Congress Catalog No. 93-78938). Oakbrook Terrace, IL: Author.

Kaempf, G., & Amodei, M. (1989). The effect of music on anxiety. *AORN Journal, 50*(1), 112–118.

Mornhinweg, G. (1992). Effects of music preference and selection on stress reduction. *Journal of Holistic Nursing, 10*(2), 101–109.

Riehl, J., & Roy, C. (1974). *Conceptual models for nursing practice.* New York: Appleton-Century-Crofts.

Robbins, L., Boyko, E., Lane, J., Cooper, D., & Jahnigen, D. (1987). Binding the elderly: A prospective study of the use of mechanical restraints in an acute care hospital. *Journal of American Geriatrics Society, 35,* 290–296.

Roy, C., & Roberts, S. (Eds.). (1981). The Roy adaptation model of nursing. *Theory construction in nursing: An adaptation model* (pp. 42–69). Englewood Cliffs, NJ: Prentice-Hall, Inc.

Scherer, Y., Janelli, L., Wu, Y., & Kuhn, M. (1993). Restrained patients: An important issue for critical care nursing. *Heart & Lung, 22*(1), 77–83.

Wixon, J. (1978). Lesson in living. *Modern Maturity, 21*(6), 10.

ANALYSIS OF THE CONCEPTUAL-THEORETICAL-EMPIRICAL STRUCTURE

The purpose of Janelli, Kanski, Jones, and Kennedy's (1995) research report was to describe the behaviors of a hospitalized patient who was listening to tape-recorded music after his physical restraints had been removed. Janelli et al. explained that the patient example presented in the report was taken from a pilot study that was designed to examine the effect of a music intervention with physically restrained medical-surgical patients. Apparently, the long-range goal of the research was to test a predictive theory of the effects of tape-recorded music on the behaviors of hospitalized patients who were physically restrained. The report, however, was limited to a description of one patient's behaviors. Consequently, the content of the report represents a descriptive naming theory of music-listening behaviors, which was generated by means of the descriptive research method of the case study.

IDENTIFICATION OF CONCEPTS

Conceptual Model Concepts

Analysis of the research report revealed that the research was guided by Roy's Adaptation Model (Roy and Roberts, 1981). The conceptual model concepts of interest are nursing intervention and adaptive modes. The concept nursing intervention has two dimensions: therapeutic nursing intervention and supportive nursing intervention. The concept adaptive modes has four dimensions: physiological mode, self-concept mode, role function mode, and interdependence mode. Janelli et al. used just the physiological mode, self-concept mode, and interdependence mode dimensions in their research.

Middle-Range Theory Concept

Further analysis of the research report revealed that the middle-range descriptive naming theory of music-listening behaviors encompasses just one concept: music-listening behaviors. This label was selected for the theory concept because the major focus of the research report is the behaviors exhibited by a patient while he was out of physical restraints and was listening to tape-recorded music. The theory concept music-listening behaviors is made up of a list of 11 behaviors: making a decision about type of music, laughing, calling out the names of and accurately identifying musicians, smiling, tapping fingers on the bed rail, tapping feet, appearing comfortable, appearing relaxed, closing eyes periodically, stating enjoyment of the music, and thanking the provider of the music.

Although Janelli et al. mentioned other behaviors, repeated readings of the research report indicated that those behaviors were not part of the theory concept music-listening behaviors because they occurred before or after the patient listened to the music and were not specifically associated with the music. For example, Janelli et al. reported that before listening to the music, and while still in restraints, the patient "verbalized in an articulate manner the absence of pain, and acknowledged who he was and where he was hospitalized." In addition, the investigators reported that after the music ended and the restraints were reapplied, the patient "yawned and appeared sleepy."

The theory is categorized as a descriptive naming theory because it is presented as a list of several behaviors, with no indication given of any structural relation between the behaviors. Consideration was given to categorizing the theory as a descriptive classification theory because of Janelli et al.'s reference to positive behaviors and negative behaviors, which could be viewed as two mutually exclusive dimensions of the theory concept music-listening behaviors. Repeated readings of the report, however, led to the decision to categorize the theory as a descriptive naming theory because Janelli et al. emphasized the specific behaviors exhibited by the patient while he was listening to music, and because they reported that the patient displayed no negative behaviors.

CLASSIFICATION OF MIDDLE-RANGE THEORY CONCEPTS

The middle-range theory concept music-listening behaviors is classified as an observational term in Kaplan's schema and as an observable in Willer and Webster's schema because the behaviors may be seen or heard by an observer. The concept is classified as a nonvariable in this report because the case study was of just one patient who exhibited a certain number of behaviors. It is likely that the concept would be a variable in studies of more than one patient because the number of music-listening behaviors might vary from patient to patient. The concept is classified as a relational unit in Dubin's schema because it reflects a combination of music and behaviors.

IDENTIFICATION AND CLASSIFICATION OF PROPOSITIONS

Conceptual Model Propositions

Nonrelational propositions from Roy's Adaptation Model were used to guide the generation of the middle-range descriptive naming theory of music-listening behaviors. The relevant nonrelational propositions are listed in Table B–1.

Table B–1 ■ **CONCEPTUAL MODEL PROPOSITIONS FROM JANELLI, KANSKI, JONES, AND KENNEDY'S RESEARCH REPORT**

Proposition	Classification
1. The first-level assessment involves gathering subjective and objective data within the framework of man's [sic] four adaptive modes: physiological needs, role function, interdependence, and self-concept.	Nonrelational, Existence Constitutive Definition
2. Physiological needs are those factors necessary to regulate the balance of circulation, body temperature, oxygen, fluids, exercise and rest, elimination, and the appetitive system.	Nonrelational, Constitutive Definition
3. The interdependence mode involves documenting the individual's dependent and independent needs.	Nonrelational, Constitutive Definition
4. The . . . self-concept mode [focuses on] how one views himself or herself, which usually is related to participation in current roles.	Nonrelational, Constitutive Definition
5. The nursing intervention aspect of the nursing process within Roy's model involves the manipulation of the focal, contextual, and residual stimuli so that the patient can cope.	Nonrelational, Constitutive Definition
6. The nursing intervention can be directed toward one or all of the stimuli (focal, contextual, residual).	Nonrelational, Constitutive Definition
7. The nurse's intervention approach can be therapeutic, when the patient responds favorably, or supportive, when the nurse no longer can alter the patient's course of adaptation.	Nonrelational, Constitutive Definition

Conceptual model Proposition 1 can be formalized as a nonrelational proposition that asserts the existence of a phenomenon and as a nonrelational proposition that asserts a constitutive definition. The nonrelational existence proposition is:

There is a phenomenon known as adaptive modes.

The constitutive definition is:

Adaptive modes is defined as a multidimensional concept that encompasses four dimensions: physiological mode, self-concept mode, role function mode, and interdependence mode.

Conceptual model Propositions 2, 3, and 4 can be formalized as three nonrelational propositions that assert constitutive definitions for the dimensions of the conceptual model concept adaptive modes that are relevant for the theory of music-listening behaviors. The constitutive definitions are:

The physiological mode dimension of Roy's Adaptation Model concept adaptive modes is defined as physiological needs that are necessary to regulate the balance of circulation, body temperature, oxygen, fluids, exercise and rest, elimination, and the appetitive system.
The interdependence mode dimension of Roy's Adaptation Model concept adaptive modes is defined as the individual's dependent and independent needs.
The self-concept mode dimension of Roy's Adaptation Model concept adaptive modes is defined as one's view of himself or herself, which usually is related to participation in current roles.

Conceptual model Propositions 5, 6, and 7 can be combined into one nonrelational proposition that asserts a constitutive definition. The constitutive definition is:

Nursing intervention is defined as the manipulation of one or all of the focal, contextual, and residual stimuli so that the patient can cope. The concept nursing intervention has two dimensions: therapeutic nursing intervention and supportive nursing intervention.

A portion of conceptual model Proposition 7 can be formalized as a nonrelational proposition that asserts the constitutive definition for the dimension of the conceptual model concept nursing intervention that is relevant for the middle-range theory of music-listening behaviors. The constitutive definition is:

The therapeutic nursing intervention dimension of Roy's Adaptation Model concept nursing intervention is defined as the manipulation of one or all of the focal, contextual, and residual stimuli so that the patient responds favorably.

Middle-Range Theory Propositions

Propositions that are central to the middle-range descriptive naming theory of music-listening behaviors can be extracted from Janelli et al.'s research report. These propositions are listed in Table B–2.

Proposition	Classification
1. Music is a nursing intervention.	Nonrelational, Representational Definition
2. Music . . . is a means of communication, and is considered a universal language that does not require high intellectual ability.	Nonrelational, Existence Constitutive Definition
3. Music for therapeutic use has been proven to be of value and is documented throughout history.	Nonrelational, Representational Definition (Relational)
4. The physiological effects of music have been well-documented. They include changes in metabolism, muscular energy, pulse, blood pressure, breathing, and blood volume.	Nonrelational, Existence Constitutive Definition (Relational)
5. Music has been shown to decrease anxiety and discomfort.	Nonrelational, Existence Constitutive Definition (Relational) Nonrelational, Existence Constitutive Definition (Relational)
6. Music has been used on a short-term basis as a distractor and as a relaxation technique.	Nonrelational, Existence
7. If the patient's focus of attention can be directed toward a more pleasant sensory stimulus, such as listening to music, then perhaps it is more easily possible to control reactions such as anxiety.	(Relational) Nonrelational, Existence
8. In her work with music, Herth found that in order for music to have a beneficial influence, the patient had to like the music. She also found that the greater the person's interest in music, the more effectively music could be used to influence his or her behavior.	Nonrelational, Existence Constitutive Definition
9. The Behavior Instrument checklist . . . consisted of 39 items representing both verbal and nonverbal communication such as echolalia, laughing, smiling, and squirming . . . The behaviors could be tallied as positive responses such as humming and nodding the head, or as negative responses such as moaning and having a clenched jaw.	Nonrelational, Measured Operational Definition Constitutive Definition
10. Mr. D was given a choice of music from four tapes, which included: band, classical, country-western, and popular. He chose popular music—the soundtrack from "Sleepless in Seattle."	Nonrelational, Measured Operational Definition
11. A Behavior Instrument checklist developed by the investigators was used before, during, and after the intervention.	Nonrelational, Measured Operational Definition
12. Large, soft headphones were put over Mr. D's ears, and attached to a tape player.	Nonrelational, Constitutive Definition
13. Mr. D. laughed appropriately and called out the names of the musicians that he recognized.	Nonrelational, Constitutive Definition
14. [Mr. D.] smiled and tapped his fingers on the bed rail in time with the music.	Nonrelational, Constitutive Definition
15. [Mr. D.] tapped his feet.	Nonrelational, Constitutive Definition
16. After the tape ended, [Mr. D.] said he enjoyed the music and thanked the investigators.	Nonrelational, Constitutive Definition Representational Definition
17. The authors noted that the music affected three of Mr. D's four adaptive modes: (a) interdependence, because he was able to make a decision regarding the type of music he wanted to listen to; (b) self-concept, which was enhanced when he accurately identified some of the musicians on the tape; and (c) physiological needs, in that Mr. D. appeared comfortable and relaxed, with his eyes closed periodically.	

Middle-range theory Propositions 2, 4, 5, 6, 7, 8, and 9 can be combined to create a nonrelational proposition that asserts the existence of a phenomenon. Formalized, the nonrelational existence proposition is:

There is a phenomenon known as music-listening behaviors.

In addition, middle-range theory Propositions 2, 4, 5, 6, and 9 can be combined to create a nonrelational proposition that asserts an initial constitutive definition for the theory concept music-listening behaviors. Formalized, the constitutive definition is:

Music-listening behaviors is defined as verbal and nonverbal communication, including echolalia, laughing, smiling, squirming, humming, nodding the head, moaning, and having a clenched jaw; changes in metabolism, muscular energy, pulse, blood pressure, breathing, and blood volume; decreased anxiety and discomfort; and relaxation.

It is important to point out that the analysis revealed that although middle-range theory Propositions 4, 5, 6, 7, and 8 are presented as relational propositions in the research report, they were used to develop the nonrelational existence proposition and the initial constitutive definitional proposition for this case-study report. It is likely that Janelli et al. included the relational propositions as part of their apparent long-range goal of testing a predictive theory of the effects of tape-recorded music on the behaviors of hospitalized patients who were physically restrained.

Middle-range theory Propositions 10, 13, 14, 15, 16, and 17 can be combined to create a nonrelational proposition that asserts another constitutive definition for the theory concept music-listening behaviors. This constitutive definition was extracted from Janelli et al.'s description of the one patient's behaviors. More specifically, it is the constitutive definition that was generated from the case-study research. Formalized, this constitutive definition is:

Music-listening behaviors is defined as the following behaviors: making a decision about type of music, laughing, calling out the names of and accurately identifying musicians, smiling, tapping fingers on the bed rail, tapping feet, appearing comfortable, appearing relaxed, closing eyes periodically, stating enjoyment of the music, and thanking the provider of the music.

Middle-range theory Propositions 1, 3, and 17 contribute to a nonrelational proposition that asserts a representational definition that links dimensions of the two conceptual model concepts (nursing intervention and adaptive modes) with the theory concept (music-listening behaviors). Formalized, the representational definition is:

The therapeutic nursing intervention dimension of Roy's Adaptation Model concept nursing intervention and the interdependence mode, self-concept mode, and physiological mode dimensions of Roy's Adaptation Model concept adaptive modes were represented by music-listening behaviors.

Middle-range theory Propositions 10, 11, and 12 contribute to a measured operational definition. Formalized, the measured operational definition is:

Music-listening behaviors was measured by the Behavior Instrument checklist while the patient was listening to a tape-recorded popular music soundtrack, "Sleepless in Seattle" through large, soft headphones.

This operational definition links the theory concept with its empirical indicators, that is, the tape-recorded music and the Behavior Instrument checklist.

HIERARCHY OF PROPOSITIONS

A hierarchy of propositions based on level of abstraction can be constructed by using the nonrelational constitutive definitional proposition for the relevant dimensions of conceptual model concepts nursing intervention and adaptive modes, the nonrelational constitutive definitional proposition for the middle-range theory concept music-listening behaviors that was generated from the case-study research, the nonrelational representational definitional proposition, and the nonrelational operational definitional proposition. The hierarchy is:

Abstract propositions: The therapeutic nursing intervention dimension of Roy's Adaptation Model concept nursing intervention is defined as the manipulation of one or all of the focal, contextual, and residual stimuli so that the patient responds favorably.

The physiological mode dimension of Roy's Adaptation Model concept adaptive modes is defined as physiological needs that are necessary to regulate the balance of circulation, body temperature, oxygen, fluids, exercise and rest, elimination, and the appetitive system.

The interdependence mode dimension of Roy's Adaptation Model concept adaptive modes is defined as the individual's dependent and independent needs.

The self-concept mode dimension of Roy's Adaptation Model concept adaptive modes is defined as one's view of himself or herself, which usually is related to participation in current roles.

Somewhat concrete proposition: The therapeutic nursing intervention dimension of Roy's Adaptation Model concept nursing intervention and the interdependence mode, self-concept mode, and physiological mode dimensions of Roy's Adaptation Model concept adaptive modes were represented by music-listening behaviors.

More concrete proposition: Music-listening behaviors is defined as the following behaviors: making a decision about type of music, laughing, calling out the names of and accurately identifying musicians, smiling, tapping fingers on the bed rail, tapping feet, appearing comfortable, appearing re-

laxed, closing eyes periodically, stating enjoyment of the
music, and thanking the provider of the music.

Most concrete proposition: Music-listening behaviors was
measured by the Behavior Instrument checklist while the
patient was listening to a tape-recorded popular music
soundtrack, "Sleepless in Seattle" through large, soft headphones.

Furthermore, a hierarchy of propositions based on inductive reasoning can be
constructed from Janelli et al.'s description of the patient's music-listening behaviors. The inductive hierarchy is:

Observation$_1$: Mr. D. was able to make a decision regarding
the type of music he wanted to listen to, and he chose popular music;

Observation$_2$: Mr. D. laughed appropriately;

Observation$_3$: Mr. D. called out the names of the musicians
he recognized;

Observation$_4$: Mr. D. smiled;

Observation$_5$: Mr. D. tapped his fingers on the bed rail in
time with the music;

Observation$_6$: Mr. D. tapped his feet;

Observation$_7$: Mr. D. said he enjoyed the music;

Observation$_8$: Mr. D. thanked the investigators;

Observation$_9$: Mr. D. accurately identified some of the musicians on the tape;

Observation$_{10}$: Mr. D. appeared comfortable;

Observation$_{11}$: Mr. D. appeared relaxed;

Observation$_{12}$: Mr. D. closed his eyes periodically;

Conclusion: Music-listening behaviors is defined as the following behaviors: making a decision about type of music,
laughing, calling out the names of and accurately identifying musicians, smiling, taping fingers on the bed rail, tapping feet, appearing comfortable, appearing relaxed, closing
eyes periodically, stating enjoyment of the music, and
thanking the provider of the music.

DIAGRAMS

The conceptual-theoretical-empirical structure for the research is illustrated in
Figure B–1. Another diagram was constructed to illustrate how Janelli et al. linked
the patient's music-listening behaviors with Roy's Adaptation Model (Fig. B–2).
The question mark (?) seen in Figure B–2 indicates that some music-listening behaviors were not linked to a dimension of Roy's Adaptation Model concept adaptive modes or to any other concept of Roy's model.

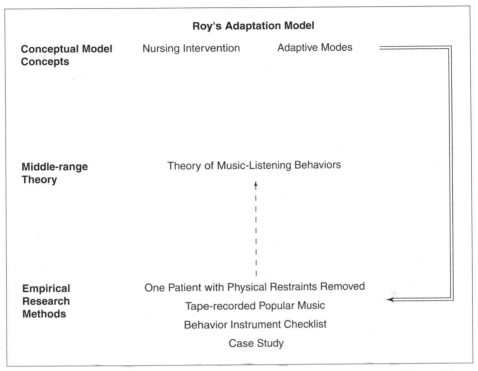

Figure B–I ■ Conceptual-theoretical-empirical structure for Janelli, Kanski, Jones, and Kennedy's research.

EVALUATION OF THE CONCEPTUAL-THEORETICAL-EMPIRICAL STRUCTURE

Analysis of Janelli et al.'s research report revealed that a one-concept middle-range descriptive naming theory of music-listening behaviors was generated. The concept is music-listening behaviors, which is made up of a list of 11 behaviors (Fig. B–2).

EVALUATION OF THE CONCEPTUAL-THEORETICAL-EMPIRICAL LINKAGES

Specification Adequacy

The criterion of specification adequacy is met. The conceptual model that guided Janelli et al.'s theory-generating research is explicitly identified as Roy's Adaptation Model. Roy's model is discussed in considerable detail, and the relation of the conceptual model to the middle-range theory is clear.

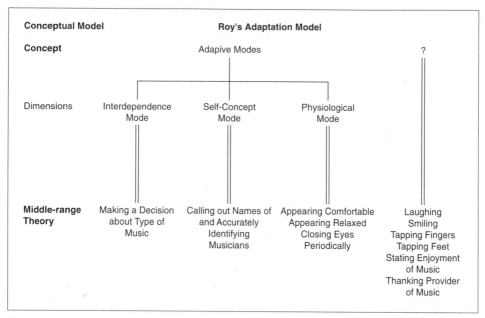

Figure B–2 ■ Incomplete linkage of specific music-listening behaviors with Roy's Adaptation Model concept adaptive modes.

Linkage Adequacy

The criterion of linkage adequacy is met in part. Janelli et al. explicitly identified the nursing intervention as music and linked some music-listening behaviors to dimensions of the conceptual model concept adaptive modes. Other behaviors, however, are not linked to any dimension of adaptive modes or to any other concept of Roy's Adaptation Model (Fig. B–2).

Conceptual Model Usage Rating Scale

Evaluation of the criteria of specification adequacy and linkage adequacy is summarized by application of the Conceptual Model Usage Rating Scale. Janelli et al.'s research report earned a score of 2, indicating minimal use of Roy's Adaptation Model. The rating reflects the incomplete linkage of specific music-listening behaviors to Roy's Adaptation Model.

EVALUATION OF THE THEORY

Significance

The middle-range theory of music-listening behaviors meets the criterion of significance. Janelli et al. addressed the social significance of their research in the introductory section of the report by identifying the extent of physical restraint use in hospitals. They stated:

■ Use of physical restraints continues to be a common practice in many hospital settings. The estimation is that 17–22% of all patients are restrained at some point during their hospitalization. That statistic is probably conservative in that the authors of this study found patients restrained with no physician's order, making data tracking difficult.

Janelli et al. addressed the theoretical significance of their research in the introductory section by stating that:

■ Although nurses would prefer to use alternatives to restraints, to date no clinical trials of potential strategies have been attempted. Alternatives that are mentioned in the literature—such as Adirondack chairs, reality orientation, and ambulation programs—have been generated from nursing home environments, and are based on anecdotal information, which may not translate to hospital settings.

Later in the report, Janelli et al. added to the theoretical significance of their research when they stated, "While research . . . on the therapeutic effects of music [has] been increasing, its acceptance and use as a means of therapy have not been evident in general hospital settings."

Internal Consistency

The middle-range theory of music-listening behaviors meets the criterion of internal consistency in part. Semantic clarity is problematic, in that the precise theory concept of interest is not explicit. The decision to label the concept as music-listening behaviors was made only after repeated readings of the report. Moreover, an explicit definition of music-listening behaviors is not evident, although two constitutive definitions eventually were extracted from the content of the report. One constitutive definition was extracted from the review of the literature and the description of the Behavior Instrument checklist; the other, which is the appropriate constitutive definition for the theory concept in this study, was extracted from Janelli et al.'s description of the patient's behaviors. Semantic consistency is less problematic, in that Janelli et al. consistently used the term "behaviors."

Structural consistency is evident. A hierarchy based on level of abstraction was easily constructed from the formalized nonrelational propositions, and a hierarchy based on inductive reasoning was easily constructed from Janelli et al.'s description of the patient's music-listening behaviors. There are, however, redundant propositions, in that two nonrelational constitutive definitional propositions were extracted from the content of the research report.

Parsimony

Formalization of the middle-range theory of music-listening behaviors indicates that the theory meets the criterion of parsimony. The analysis revealed that the theory is made up of just one concept that encompasses a list of 11 behaviors.

Much of the content of Janelli et al.'s report, however, is not central to the theory. Indeed, repeated readings of the report were required to extract the actual theory that was generated.

Testability

The middle-range theory of music-listening behaviors meets the criterion of testability, inasmuch as it should be possible to test the theory by replicating the study using the methodology employed by Janelli et al. The actual Behavior Instrument checklist would have to be obtained from the investigators for a replication study. Janelli et al. generated no hypotheses, but a falsifiable hypothesis could be developed and tested, asserting that all of the music-listening behaviors exhibited by the one patient in the case study would be exhibited by other patients who were listening to the same tape-recorded music. Another falsifiable hypothesis might be that the same behaviors would be exhibited by patients listening to other types of music.

EVALUATION OF THE RESEARCH DESIGN

Operational Adequacy

The criterion of operational adequacy is met only in part. Although the case-study method of descriptive research was used appropriately, Janelli et al. briefly mentioned the Behavior Instrument checklist scores for other patients included in their pilot study, thereby going beyond the case study. Furthermore, no data are given to support the validity of the instrument. Indeed, Janelli et al. did not discuss the correspondence between music-listening behaviors identified in other studies and the behaviors they included in their instrument. Moreover, Janelli et al. did not indicate whether the behaviors that they reported for the one patient are among those on the instrument. In addition, no data are given to support the intra- or inter-rater reliability of the instrument, both of which are relevant when observation is used as a method of data collection. To their credit, Janelli et al. provided an adequate description of the research procedures.

EVALUATION OF THE RESEARCH FINDINGS

Empirical Adequacy

The result of Janelli et al.'s research was the generation of a middle-range descriptive naming theory of music-listening behaviors. The criterion of empirical adequacy is met, in that the behaviors observed and reported by Janelli et al. were used to develop a constitutive definition for the theory concept music-listening behaviors.

An alternative substantive explanation for the study findings is not offered; indeed, the implication is that the observed behaviors were a direct outcome of substituting music for physical restraints. Moreover, no attempt was made to compare the behaviors exhibited by the one patient (formalized as the constitutive definition that was extracted from the observed patient behaviors) to the music-listening behaviors reported by other investigators (formalized as the initial constitutive definition). For example, no mention was made of such physiological behaviors as changes in metabolism or blood pressure, or of other behaviors such as decreased anxiety (Table B–2, middle-range theory Propositions 4 and 7).

EVALUATION OF THE UTILITY OF THE THEORY FOR PRACTICE

Pragmatic Adequacy

The criterion of pragmatic adequacy was not met. To their credit, Janelli et al. noted that at this stage in their research, "It is too early to draw conclusions." They went beyond their current research, however, with the claim that their findings represent "beginning evidence . . . that music is a worthwhile nursing intervention that can be used with hospitalized patients in an effort to reduce application of restraints." Moreover, Janelli et al. went far beyond the findings of their study when they stated, "The possibility exists that music also may alter the staff members' perceptions . . . of the patient when they note the change in behavior in response to the music."

Janelli et al.'s extensive discussion of Roy's Adaptation Model and their application of Roy's first-level and second-level assessment to hospitalized patients who are physically restrained (Figs. 1 and 2 and narrative in the research report) has clinical merit, although the connection is tenuous between that assessment and the theory of music-listening behaviors. In particular, the inclusion early in the article of guidelines for clinical practice, and a later focus on theory-generating research, led to confusion about the real purpose of the report.

EVALUATION OF THE CONCEPTUAL MODEL

Credibility

The credibility of Roy's Adaptation Model, which Janelli et al. used to guide the generation of the theory of music-listening behaviors, is addressed. In particular, the investigators questioned the credibility of the conceptual model in their statement that "As more data [are] collected, Roy's model also may require additional transformation in order to explicate better the role of music with the physically restrained." Another question regarding credibility arises from the investigators' failure to link some of the music-listening behaviors to Roy's model. It is not known whether their failure to do that was an oversight or a lack of congruence between those music-listening behaviors and some dimensions of Roy's model concept adaptive modes or other concepts of Roy's model.

References

Janelli, L.M., Kanski, G.W., Jones, H.M., & Kennedy, M.C. (1995). Exploring music intervention with restrained patients. *Nursing Forum, 30* (4), 12–18.

Roy, C., & Roberts, S. (1981). *Theory construction in nursing: An adaptation model.* Englewood Cliffs, NJ: Prentice-Hall.

Analysis and Evaluation of a Descriptive Theory-Generating Study: The Interpretive Method of Naturalistic Inquiry

Patient Perceptions of Why, How, and By Whom Dialysis Treatment Modality Was Chosen

Diane M. Breckenridge

Objective: The purpose of this qualitative study was to elicit patients' perceptions of why, how, and by whom their dialysis treatment modality—hemodialysis or continuous ambulatory peritoneal dialysis (CAPD)—was chosen.

Design: The study design utilized a naturalistic method of inquiry employing a qualitative approach. The research was guided by the life-death decisions in health care framework developed by Degner and Beaton and the Neuman Systems Model.

Sample/Setting: Twenty-two informants were recruited from inpatient and outpatient renal dialysis units at a large urban tertiary care center on the east coast of the United States.

Methods: Data were collected by individual, focused, semi-structured in-depth interviews.

Results: A grounded theory, "Patient's Choice of a Treatment Modality versus Selection of Patient's Treatment Modality" emerged from the data provided by the informants. The theory consisted of 11 themes that addressed the why, how, and by whom of decision-making: self decision; access-rationing decision; significant other decision; to live decision; physiologically dictated decision; expert decision; to-be-cared-for decision; independence verses dependence decision; no patient choice in making decision; patient preference/choice; and switching modalities due to patient preference/choice.

Reprinted from *American Nephrology Nurses Association Journal*, 24(3), 313–319, 1997, with permission.

Conclusion: The themes reflected two patterns of decision-making: the patient and/or significant other chose the treatment modality, and the treatment modality was selected because of clinical or practical circumstances.

Since Congress enacted the United States Medicare End-Stage Renal Disease (ESRD) Program in 1973, there has been rapid growth in both the ESRD population and, subsequently, in program costs. This legislation extended financial coverage under Medicare to all United States citizens with renal disease who could benefit from dialysis or transplantation. The program guarantees dialysis to all who want ESRD replacement therapy. In addition, patients can be placed on a renal transplant waiting list but a transplant cannot be guaranteed because of the scarcity of donated organs.

In 1969, 1,000 ESRD patients were treated by dialysis in the United States. In contrast, 16,000 ESRD patients were treated during 1974, one year after the implementation of the ESRD legislation (Health Care Financing Research Report: ESRD, 1991). Today, more than 200,000 ESRD patients are treated, at an annual cost of more than $6 billion (National Kidney Foundation, 1996, telephone communication).

Currently, the United States ESRD program is the only national catastrophic Medicare program that offers universal access regardless of the patients' ability to pay. The typical patient dialyzed in the United States prior to 1973 was a white male under 55 years of age, with a middle income. With the enactment of the ESRD program, access was given to minorities, women, and the economically disadvantaged (Evans, Blagg, & Bryan, 1981).

Prior to the ESRD program, the decision to dialyze a patient was based on a selection process. Dr. Belding Scribner (Fox & Swazey, 1978) gave an opinion that upon review of the national controversy in 1969 regarding the selection criteria, the selection system was probably not going to hold up much longer. The public would become more aware of what the selection process really meant. "In the long run, it's going to be a lot simpler to put everybody who needs it on dialysis. It's the only rational way to solve the selection problems, at least in our culture" (p. 300). Dr. Belding Scribner's opinion in 1969 is what occurred with the passing of the Medicare ESRD Program in 1973.

In the United States, a higher percentage of patients receive incenter hemodialysis (84%) than CAPD (16%) (National Kidney Foundation, 1996, telephone communication; Rettig & Levinsky, 1991). This proportion persists despite research that indicates that CAPD patients report higher quality of life than incenter hemodialysis patients (Bremer, McCauley, Wrona & Johnson, 1989; Deniston, Carpentier-Atling, Kneisley, Hawthorne, & Port, 1989; Evans et al., 1985).

The purpose of this study was to determine patients' perceptions of why, how, and by whom their dialysis treatment—hemodialysis or continuous ambulatory peritoneal dialysis (CAPD)—was chosen. The specific research questions were:

1. How do patients perceive their options regarding dialysis and types of dialysis treatment modalities?
2. What kinds of options do patients perceive to be available to them?
3. To what extent, and in what ways, do patients perceive health care providers or significant others as influencing their decisions?
4. What factors or conditions do patients take into account in choosing a treatment modality?
5. What decision-making processes do patients employ in choosing a treatment modality?
6. What information is available to patients as they make their choices? What are the sources of information?

BACKGROUND

The goal of the study was to enhance understanding of treatment choices, which in turn might help providers to facilitate ESRD patients' informed choice about treatment modality. Most of the research related to the ESRD patient's type of treatment modality has been conducted by asking questions developed from the health care provider's perspective (Deniston et al., 1989; Evans et al., 1985). Wu (1993) stated that there is a great need to study the ESRD patient's dialysis treatment modality from his or her perspective. Furthermore, a basic premise of Nursing's Agenda for Health Care Reform is that:

Consumers must assume more responsibility for their own care and become better informed about the range of providers and potential options for services. Working in a partnership with providers, consumers must actively participate in choices that best meet their needs. (American Nurses Association, 1992, p. 8)

Sadler (1992) stated that in the United States today patients are more involved in making their own decisions in choosing whether they want dialysis, and which modality they prefer. Since the legislated Self-Determination Act to facilitate the patient in making health care decisions was implemented in December 1991, health care professionals at more dialysis units are educating and counseling patients about their choices (Sadler, 1992). Jacox (cited in Bednar, 1993) pointed out that although there are several treatment options for ESRD, little is know about how treatment modalities are chosen.

CONCEPTUAL FRAMEWORK

This study was guided by the Neuman (1995) Systems Model and the life-death decisions framework (Degner & Beaton, 1987). The Neuman Systems Model directs researchers to study patients' perceptions. This study is concerned primarily with perceptions of patients about choice of dialysis treatment modality.

The life-death decisions framework identifies four patterns of controlled decision making: provider-controlled decision making, patient-controlled decision making, family-controlled decision making, and jointly controlled decision making. Degner and Beaton's (1987) conceptualization of controlled decision making was developed from a four year extensive qualitative field study. The results led to the description of the variable "control over the design of therapy" or who actually selected the treatment options after consideration of potential risks and benefits. Degner and Beaton (1987) found preliminary support for the hypothesis that consumers of health care could have systematic preferences about the degree of control they want in treatment decision-making ranging from no control to complete control.

METHOD

The study design utilized a naturalistic method of inquiry employing a qualitative, grounded approach (Glaser & Strauss, 1967).

SAMPLE. The sample was recruited from four renal dialysis units at a large urban tertiary care center on the east coast of the United States. Three of the units provided hemodialysis; one was an outpatient unit, one was an incenter self hemodialysis unit, and one was an in-hospital unit. The fourth was an outpatient CAPD monthly checkup and evaluation unit. Theoretical sampling (see Teaching Sidebar) with sufficient theoretical sensitivity was used to produce the data. Discriminate sampling was used to choose sites, informants, and documents that would maximize opportunities to verify the story line (Sandelowski, 1995a; Strauss & Corbin, 1990). Sample recruitment ceased when data saturation was achieved, that is, when no themes emerged and the themes began to be repetitive.

■ Teaching Sidebar
Research Methodology

Theoretical sampling is one method of selecting participants for qualitative research. Theoretical sampling involves the deliberative selection of research participants who can provide responses to particular questions that emerge as the simultaneous process of data collection and data analysis proceeds.

Sample Size

Although qualitative research frequently involves very small samples (N = 5–10), Sandelowski (1995b) has pointed out that larger samples (N = ± 60) yield "richer," more generalizable results.

The sample consisted of 13 male and 9 female ESRD patients and was identified with the assistance of nurse-managers in the four dialysis units. With two of the patients, the wives always accompanied their husbands to dialysis. Despite the fact that the initial and subsequent questions were directed to the patients, these two wives did most of the storytelling with their husbands (the patients) only making a few comments and agreeing with what their wives said. The informants ranged in age from 29 to 69 years ($M = 53.8$). Length on dialysis ranged from 4 months to 19 years ($M = 5.3$ years). An attempt was made to have a ratio of three black patients to one white patient to mirror the ethnicity of the national population of ESRD patients on dialysis (Eggers, 1992, interview). Due to the large numbers of black patients at the study sites, however, the final sample of 17 black and 5 white informants represented a ratio of approximately 4 black to 1 white patients.

INSTRUMENT. Data were collected through the use of individual, focused, semi-structured, in-depth interviews. The Patient Perception Interview Guide, which contains six open-ended questions, was developed and initially tested in a pilot study (see Table 1). The purpose of this interview guide was to elicit the perceptions of informants about the way their dialysis treatment modality was chosen. Content va-

---

Table 1 ■ THE PATIENT PERCEPTION INTERVIEW GUIDE

1. Please tell me about the way the decision that you would be on (name the dialysis treatment modality, hemodialysis or CAPD) was made.
   Possible Probes:
   a. What optional types of dialysis were presented to you or did you consider? What did you view as the pros and cons?
   b. What kinds of things did you think about or weigh while making your decision?
   c. Please walk me through the way the decision was made.
   d. How important were the doctors'/nurses'/your family members' opinions and/or recommendations?
   e. What kind of information was made available to you? What were the sources? Did you actively seek information about the modalities? If so, what kinds of things did you do? Who did you talk with in order to learn more about the treatment modalities?
2. Have you ever been on another type of dialysis? If yes, for how long?
3. What caused you to switch from one to the other?
4. Which modality do you prefer?
5. What do you like about your preferred choice?
6. Are there any drawbacks to your preferred choice (Dialysis Treatment Modality)?

lidity of the interview guide was assessed by asking nurse-managers of the dialysis units to rate the clarity of the open-ended questions with regard to choice of dialysis modality. Preliminary interviews were then conducted with two nurses who were also patients on dialysis: one on CAPD, the other on hemodialysis. The original Patient Perception Interview Guide was refined based on input from these nurse-patients, as well as pilot study interviews with six dialysis patients.

PROCEDURE. The study protocol was approved by a university medical center human subjects committee. When written permission was received, packets of information regarding the rationale, protocol, risks, pilot study data, and the consent form were submitted to each of the dialysis units prior to implementing the study. All patients asked by the researcher if they had an interest in receiving a consent form and verbal information about the study were interested in participating except one female patient. Approximately fifteen minutes to one half hour was required to discuss the study and consent information with each patient. All aspects of the study were explained, and written informed consent was obtained. If the person gave written informed consent, then the interview took place during the hemodialysis treatment or CAPD evaluation visit that day or at a subsequent visit if the patient could not do the interview that day. Interviews varied in length from 20 minutes to 3 hours ($M = 1.5$ hours).

DATA ANALYSIS. A constant comparative approach was used to analyze the data for themes, patterns, and interrelationships (Glaser & Strauss, 1967). Using this approach, themes were established, and themes were classified into the categories. The software program, Ethnograph, was used to facilitate coding and data management (Tesch, 1990).

RESULTS

The theory of Patient's Choice of a Treatment Modality versus Selection of Patient's Treatment Modality is the substantive grounded theory that emerged from the data. The theory represents the integration of informants' responses to the questions about why, how, and by whom dialysis treatment modality decisions are made.

The theory is made up of 11 themes, which were categorized into two patterns of decision-making (see Table 2). One category, labeled Patient's Choice of Treatment Modality, contained seven themes: self-decision; significant other decision; to live decision; independence versus dependence decision; to be cared for decision; patient preference/choice; and switching modalities due to patient preference/choice. The other category, labeled Selection of Patient's Treatment Modality, contained four themes: access-rationing decision; physiologically dictated decision; no patient choice in making decision; and expert decision.

Each theme is mutually exclusive although, as patients' perceptions were probed, individual patients sometimes expressed more than one theme for the decisions made. The constant comparative method indicated that for these informants, demographics such as gender, age, and race were not directly associated with particular themes. There was overlap in the themes expressed by five patients as to the two categories of Patient's Choice of Treatment Modality and Selection of Patient's Treatment Modality due to clinical and practical circumstances.

The category, Patient's Choice of Treatment Modality, refers to the patients' perception that they and/or significant other had participated in the decision of choice of treatment modality. This pattern is reflected in the following seven themes and informant comments.

The theme, self-decision, is defined as the patient's own choice of modality. This theme, which was mentioned by three informants, is illustrated by a comment from a female informant:

Table 2 ■ **THE THEORY OF PATIENT'S CHOICE OF TREATMENT MODALITY VERSUS SELECTION OF TREATMENT MODALITY FOR THE PATIENT**

Category	Themes and Definitions
Patient's Choice of Treatment Modality	Self-decision—Patient's own choice of modality decision.
	Significant other decision—Patient stated that significant other (family member) had a major influence on modality choice.
	To live decision—Patient stated that dialysis was necessary to live.
	Independence versus dependence decision—Patient stated that she/he wanted to take care of self on modality chosen.
	To be cared for decison—Patient stated that he/she is cared for by another on the modality chosen.
	Patient Preference/Choice—Patient stated that he/she preferred a dialysis modality due to various reasons.
	Switching modality due to patient preference/choice—Patient stated that he/she switched dialysis modality due to preference/own choice.
Selection of Patient's Treatment Modality	Access-rationing decision—Patient stated modality choice decision was based on factors such as availability of space at a center.
	Physiologically dictated decision—Patient's physiological limitations dictated modality choice.
	No patient choice in making decision—Patient stated that he/she had no choice in dialysis modality.
	Expert decision—Patient stated that health care provider (i.e., physician) made modality choice.

■ I am on dialysis because I came to America to visit and I got ill. My cousin was a doctor and she took me to a doctor who told me my kidneys had gone bad. They had to put me right away on dialysis. They explained to me about the other one [CAPD] but this one I liked better. I prefer this one [in-center self hemodialysis].

The theme, significant other decision, was identified by five informants, and is defined as a significant other having a major influence on the choice of a particular dialysis treatment modality. This theme is illustrated by a comment from a male informant who stated that his nephew, also on CAPD, told him about CAPD. This male informant stated that while on hemodialysis his wife had to bring him to the dialysis unit for treatment every other day. He commented:

■ My wife, see, she wouldn't have to come down here and all that, so that gives me the opportunity to stay home [for dialysis].

When another male informant was asked, "Tell about the way the decision was made that you would be on the dialysis treatment modality you are on," his wife, who accompanies her husband to treatments, immediately responded:

■ Peritoneal dialysis is better because I can work all day and my husband can stay at home. Whereas, with hemodialysis you would have to go every other day, a half day to the unit. [She stated that with peritoneal dialysis she only had to bring her husband in once a month for evaluations.] I use my sick time to bring him in.

The theme, to live decision, which was evident in the responses of four informants, is defined as the informants' statement that if they wanted to live, they must be on dialysis. This theme is illustrated by the following comments from three informants:

■ This is the only way that I can live. I always see someone worse off than I. I count my blessings.

■ I am sorry that I have this problem because I have to be on this machine three times a week to live. It is heartbreaking.

■ Don't know how many more years I can live, but I make the best of each day. You all have to go sometime. Nobody stays here forever. And you can't feel sorry for yourself. I don't complain.

The theme, independence versus dependence decision, was mentioned by two informants and is defined as the patient wants to take care of her or himself. A female informant stated:

■ I really don't have any complaints. I had some hard times, but over 18 years I have no complaints. Just to be alive. I can walk around and take care of myself, that is the most important thing.

The theme, to be cared for decision, evident in just one informant's responses, is defined as the patient states that he/she is cared for by another. The informant stated:

■ I had some good doctors, you have to have good doctors and nurses, and the patient can go a long way. I was blessed with that. You can't do it by yourself.

The theme patient preference/choice, was noted in three informants' responses, and is defined as the informants' preference for a certain modality due to various reasons. This theme is illustrated by a male informant's comment:

■ They told me about both [types]. My preference was CAPD... but if it was a situation where I had to go on hemodialysis I would be willing to accept that.

When the informant was asked by the researcher, "Why is your preference CAPD?", his comment revealed that he wanted to be independent:

■ Mainly because it gives me a little bit more freedom. Being able to do it at home I wouldn't have to come to the hospital. It would allow me if I wanted to take a trip, to go somewhere and basically do it myself, instead of having to try to find a facility that could accommodate me.

The theme, switching modalities due to patient preference/choice, which was identified by six informants, is defined as the informant switches dialysis modality due to own preference or choice. This theme is illustrated by the following comment from a female informant:

■ When I went on dialysis, I was automatically put on hemodialysis. I was not even told about CAPD. The doctor might have mentioned it, but I was so sick at the time I didn't catch on to it. My response was that if I had been told about something like that, I would have wanted to go with it.

The researcher then asked, "How did you get on CAPD?" This female informant replied:

■ Another woman was at the unit where I was on dialysis, and she was on CAPD. She told me about it, and I knew this was something I wanted to do. So when they came to show the film, I was immediately drawn to it [CAPD], and I knew that was what I wanted to do. I told them I wanted someone from the CAPD center to talk to me about CAPD. I had to call myself to set up an appointment.

When the researcher asked, "Do you like CAPD?," the informant replied:

■ "If I had a choice, it would be CAPD."

The category, Selection of Patient's Treatment Modality, refers to the patients' perception that they and/or their significant others had not participated in the decision of the treatment modality. This pattern is shown in the following four themes and informant comments.

The theme, access-rationing decision, was identified by two informants. This theme is defined as the decision was based on factors such as availability of space at a center and or reimbursement of services. Availability of space is illustrated by the following statement by a male informant:

■ I tried first to get into G.S. (another facility) but they were booked up and there were no openings, but there was an opening here. I would like to go back to G.S., where I am on the waiting list and because of the excellent physical therapy. They don't have physical therapy here. I am supposed to be on therapy. I had three fingers amputated on my left hand and both legs are amputated below the knee.

When the researcher asked the informant, "Why is there no physical therapy?" he stated,

■ "I keep asking."

The factor of reimbursement of services was evident in the response from the wife of another patient, when asked the question, "Tell about the way the decision was made that you would be on the dialysis treatment modality you are on":

■ I heard that the Kidney Disease Program of this state is one of the best. We wanted to move to Texas. My sister is there and two of my husband's sons. We checked into the financial portion that Medicare does not take care of and Texas has no state plan for the 20% that Medicare does not take care of. The last time we investigated private health insurance was probably 7 or 8 years ago. It was half our income. It was $2,400 a quarter. I don't know what we'll do if we go to Texas.

The theme, physiologically dictated decision, which was noted by five informants, is defined as a decision in which physiological limitations dictate the decision as to modality type. This theme is illustrated by the following comment from a male informant:

■ Every time I get a fistula [for hemodialysis] my blood clots and I have to get another one. Sometimes I get another fistula, and before I get well it [a blood clot] would break loose, and they would have to operate on it [the fistula]. I lost a lot of blood. So then I found out about this [CAPD] [Note: the patient is now on CAPD].

The theme, no patient choice, was mentioned by two informants, and is defined as the patient had no choice in the type of modality. This theme as well as the theme, expert decision, that was mentioned by six informants and is defined as an expert (e.g., physician) made the decision are illustrated in the following comments of a female informant:

■ I wanted to be on hemodialysis. I didn't want to be on this [CAPD]. When I was in the hospital, the doctor in charge over there wanted to put the catheter in my stomach [for CAPD]. I said I wanted something in my arm [for hemodialysis]. He said, "No." They were saying I could put this in my stomach until all the infection goes away in my arm. Then when the infection goes I can get something in my arm. Right now I have no access. So I said go ahead and put it in my stomach. He [physician] said the decision is yours to make but I felt the decision wasn't mine to make. Because he wanted me to say that I wanted peritoneal dialysis. You have to agree to be on peritoneal dialysis, you have to agree to whatever they want to. If you don't agree to what they want you to agree to, they won't accept your answer until you agree to what they want to hear. That's the way that works.

The theme, expert decision, was also illustrated in this comment from a female informant on hemodialysis:

■ The only thing the Doctor said was that I was going to be on dialysis. I didn't know it was like this. I didn't have a choice. He didn't say you have choices of dialysis, which would you like? I was told the one. I was going to be on this machine. That's it.

When the informant was asked by the researcher if she wanted to learn about the other types of dialysis, she replied:

■ No, it don't make sense. There are scars on me now. Terrible— scarred for life. No scars at all until this.

DISCUSSION

The informants' stories indicated that the way the decision was made unfolded into why, how, and/or by whom they were on the type of dialysis that they were on. Responses dealing with the why of the decision focused on such clinical circumstances as poor vascular access or such practical circumstances as lack of transportation to a dialysis center. The how of decision-making focused on situations in which information received by patients from other patients influenced their reasons to want to switch modality type. The by whom of decision-making focused on the fact that the decision regarding the type of dialysis was made by self, by a significant other (e.g., nephew; wife), or by an expert (e.g., physician). Some informants stated that the physician made the decisions and implied that their physician was the expert. A few informants were upset that they had no choice in the decision but others clearly deferred the decision to the physician.

Evidence suggests that even though the United States health care delivery system implies the availability of choice through the Self Determination Act, there is diversity among patients regarding their value of choice. In the Degner and Sloan (1992) study, a high proportion (80%) of cancer patients preferred to delegate decisional responsibility about type of treatment to their physician. This is in marked contrast to findings of previous studies, which revealed that patients preferred to make the decisions (Blanchard, Labrecque, Ruckdeschel & Blanchard, 1988; Cassileth, Zupkis, Sutton-Smith, & March, 1980). Further studies to understand who participates in life-death decisions are recommended (Breckenridge, 1995b).

Hypotheses generated from the present study findings can be tested to establish the validity of this generated theory, "Patient's Choice of Treatment Modality verses Selection of Patient's Treatment Modality", as well as its generalizability (Fawcett & Downs, 1992). The hypothesis recommended for further testing is that patient choice alone is inadequate because other factors have an impact on the decision for the type of treatment chosen or selected. The applicability of this theory to other clinical populations to determine patients' perceptions of why, how, and by whom the decision for the choice of treatment should also be explored. Further research is needed to identify patterns of decision making by patients who have other clinical conditions that are associated with various treatment options.

IMPLICATIONS FOR PRACTICE

The application of theory in practice can also test its validity (Fawcett & Downs, 1992). When interviewing patients, nurses can assess decision making according to the theory's categories and themes (see Table 2). This framework can assist nurses in understanding decision making patterns. Interventions can be designed to enhance a patient's preference as to choice and selection of a treatment. Nurses can also use this theory as a basis for including a patient's perspective in effecting health policy in developing Clinical Practice Guidelines (Breckenridge, 1995a). ■

References

American Nurses Association. (1992). *Nursing's agenda for health care reform.* Washington, DC: Author

Bednar, B. (1993). Developing clinical practice guidelines: An interview with Ada Jacox. *ANNA Journal, 20*(2), 121–126.

Blanchard, C.G., Labrecque, M.S., Ruckdeschel, J.C., & Blanchard, E.B. (1988). Information and decision making preferences of hospitalized adult cancer patients. *Social Science Medicine, 27,* 1139–1145.

Breckenridge, D.M. (1995a). ANNA's participation in the future development of clinical practice guidelines. *Contemporary Dialysis and Nephrology, 16*(6), 36–38,44.

Breckenridge, D.M. (1995b). Patients' choice . . . is it? A qualitative study of patients' perceptions of why, how, and by whom dialysis treatment modality was chosen. Doctoral dissertation, University of Maryland.

Bremer, B.A., McCauley, C.R., Wrona, R.M., & Johnson, J.P. (1989). Quality of life in end-stage renal disease: A reexamination. *American Journal of Kidney Diseases, 13*(3), 200–209.

Cassileth, B.R., Zupkis, R.V., Sutton-Smith, K., & March, V. (1980). Information and participation preferences among cancer patients. *Annals of Internal Medicine. 92,* 832–835.

Degner, L.F., & Beaton, J.I. (1987). *Life-death decisions in health care.* New York: Hemisphere Publishing Corporation.

Degner, L.F., & Sloan, J.A. (1992). Decision making during serious illness: What role do patients really want to play? *Journal of Clinical Epidemiology, 45*(9), 941–950.

Deniston, O.L., Carpentier-Atling, P., Kneisley, J., Hawthorne, V.M., & Port, F.K. (1989). Assessment of quality of life in end-stage renal disease. *Health Services Research, 24*(4), 555–578.

Eggers, P.W. (1992, April 1). Interview with Eggers, Chief, Program Evaluation Branch, Office of Research and Demonstration, Health Care Financing Administration (HCFA). National Kidney Foundation (October 29, 1996). Telephone communication. New York.

Evans, R.W., Blagg, C.R., & Bryan, F. (1981). Implications for health care policy: A social and demographic profile of hemodialysis patients in the United States. *Journal of the American Medical Association, 245*(5), 487–491.

Evans, R.W., Manninen, D.L., Garrison, L.P., Hart, G., Blagg, C.R., Gutman, R.A., Hull, A.R., & Lowrie, E.G. (1985). The quality of life of patients with end-stage renal disease. *The New England Journal of Medicine, 213*(9), 553–559.

Fawcett, J. & Downs, F.S. (1992). *The relationship of theory and research.* Second Edition. Philadelphia: F.A. Davis Company.

Fox, R.C. & Swazey, J.P. (1978). *The courage to fail: A social view of organ transplants and dialysis.* Chicago: The University of Chicago Press.

Glaser, R. & Strauss, A.L. (1967). *The discovery of grounded theory: Strategies for qualitative research.* New York: Aldine Publishing Company.

Neuman, B. (1995). *The Neuman Systems Model.* (3rd ed). East Norwalk, CT: Appleton and Lange, Inc.

Rettig, R.A., & Levinsky, N.G. (Eds.). (1991) *Kidney failure and the federal government,* (Institute of Medicine, Committee for the Study of the Medicare End-Stage Renal Disease Program). Washington, DC: National Academy Press.

Sadler, J. (1992, March 11). Interview with J. Sadler, M.D., Associate Professor of Medicine, Head, Division of Nephrology, Department of Medicine, University of Maryland.

Sandelowski, M. (1995a). Qualitative analysis: What it is and how to begin. *Research in Nursing and Health, 18*, 371–375.

Sandelowski, M. (1995b). Focus on qualitative methods: Sample size in qualitative research. *Research in Nursing and Health, 18*, 179–183.

Strauss, A., & Corbin, J. (1990). *Basics of qualitative research: Grounded theory procedures and techniques.* Newbury Park, CA: Sage Publications.

Tesch, R. (1990). *Qualitative research: Analysis type and software tools.* New York: Falmer Press.

U.S. Department of Health and Human Services. (1991). *Health care financing report: End-stage renal disease* (HCFA Publication No. 03319). Rockville, MD: Author.

Wu, A.W. (1993, March). Paper presented at the *Quality of Life Conference.* Cosponsored by Johns Hopkins University and University of Maryland, Baltimore, MD.

ANALYSIS OF THE CONCEPTUAL-THEORETICAL-EMPIRICAL STRUCTURE

The stated purpose of Breckenridge's (1997) research was to determine patients' perceptions of why, how, and by whom their dialysis treatment—hemodialysis or continuous ambulatory peritoneal dialysis (CAPD)—was chosen. The research was designed to generate a middle-range descriptive classification theory, which Breckenridge called patient's choice of a treatment modality versus selection of patient's treatment modality, by means of the descriptive interpretative research method of naturalistic inquiry, using a qualitative, grounded approach.

IDENTIFICATION OF CONCEPTS

Conceptual Model Concepts

Analysis of the research report revealed that the research was guided by Neuman's (1995) Systems Model and Degner and Beaton's (1987) life-death decisions framework. The conceptual model concepts of interest are patients' perceptions, from Neuman's model, and control over the design of therapy, from Degner and Beaton's framework.

Middle-Range Theory Concepts

Further analysis of the research report revealed that the middle-range descriptive classification theory of patient's choice of treatment modality versus selection of patient's treatment modality encompasses two multidimensional concepts. The two concepts and their dimensions are listed in Table C–1. It should be noted that the concepts are what Breckenridge called "patterns of decision-making" and "categories." The dimensions of each concept are what she called "themes."

The theory of patient's choice of treatment modality versus selection of patient's treatment modality is categorized as a descriptive classification theory because although there is some overlap between the two concepts, they are treated as separate phenomena, and because the dimensions of each concept are mutually exclusive. More specifically, Breckenridge explained that although some study informants identified themes that reflected dimensions for each of the two concepts, "each theme [i.e., dimension] is mutually exclusive."

CLASSIFICATION OF MIDDLE-RANGE THEORY CONCEPTS

Both middle-range theory concepts—patient's choice of treatment modality and selection of the patient's treatment modality—are classified as theoretical terms in Kaplan's schema, as constructs in Willer and Webster's schema, and as summative units in Dubin's schema because they refer to complex, global phenomena that can be interpreted only through their dimensions.

Table C–I ■ THE THEORY OF PATIENT'S CHOICE OF A TREATMENT MODALITY VERSUS SELECTION OF PATIENT'S TREATMENT MODALITY: CONCEPTS AND THEIR DIMENSIONS

Concepts
  Dimensions
Patient's Chioce of Treatment Modality
  Self-Decision
  Significant Other Decision
  To Live Decision
  Independence Versus Dependence Decision
  To Be Cared For Decision
  Patient Preference/Choice
  Switching Modalities Due to Patient Preference/Choice
Selection of the Patient's Treatment Modality
  Access-Rationing Decision
  Physiologically Dictated Decision
  No Patient Choice in Making Decision
  Expert Decision

Both concepts are classified as variables because a different number of study informants' responses reflected each concept. Indeed, Breckenridge reported the exact number of informants whose responses reflected each dimension of each concept.

IDENTIFICATION AND CLASSIFICATION OF PROPOSITIONS

Conceptual Model Propositions

Nonrelational propositions from Neuman's Systems Model and Degner and Beaton's life-death decisions framework were used to guide the generation of the middle-range descriptive classification theory of patient's choice of treatment modality versus selection of patient's treatment modality. The nonrelational propositions are listed in Table C–2.

Conceptual model Propositions 1 and 3 can be formalized as nonrelational propositions that assert the existence of phenomena:

There is a phenomenon known as patients' perceptions.

There is a phenomenon known as control over the design of therapy.

Conceptual model Proposition 4 can be formalized as a nonrelational proposition that asserts the level of existence of a phenomenon:

The phenomenon known as control over the design of therapy can vary from preference for no control to preference for complete control.

Conceptual model Propositions 2 and 3 can be formalized as a nonrelational proposition that asserts a constitutive definition:

Control over the design of therapy is defined as who actually selected the treatment options after consideration of potential risks and benefits. The concept con-

---

Table C–2 ■ **CONCEPTUAL MODEL PROPOSITIONS FROM BRECKENRIDGE'S RESEARCH REPORT**

Proposition	Classification
1. The Neuman Systems Model directs researchers to study patients' perceptions.	Nonrelational, Existence
2. The life-death decisions framework identifies four patterns of controlled decision making: provider-controlled decision making, patient-controlled decision making, family-controlled decision making, and jointly-controlled decision making.	Nonrelational, Constitutive Definition
3. [Degner and Beaton's research] results led to the description of the variable "control over the design of therapy" or who actually selected the treatment options after consideration of potential risks and benefits.	Nonrelational, Existence Constitutive Definition
4. Consumers of health care could have systematic preferences about the degree of control they want in treatment decision making ranging from no control to complete control.	Nonrelational, Level of Existence

trol over the design of therapy encompasses four dimensions: provider-controlled decision making, patient-controlled decision making, family-controlled decision making, and jointly-controlled decision making.

Middle-Range Theory Propositions

Nonrelational propositions that are central to the middle-range descriptive classification theory of patient's choice of treatment modality versus selection of patient's treatment modality are evident in the research report. The nonrelational propositions are listed in Table C–3.

Middle-range theory Propositions 1 and 9 can be formalized as nonrelational propositions that assert the existence of phenomena:

There is a phenomenon known as patient's choice of treatment modality.

There is a phenomenon known as selection of patient's treatment modality.

Table C–3 ■ **MIDDLE-RANGE THEORY PROPOSITIONS FROM BRECKENRIDGE'S RESEARCH REPORT**

Proposition	Classification
1. Patient's choice of treatment modality refers to the patients' perception that they and/or [their] significant other[s] had participated in the decision of choice of treatment modality.	Nonrelational, Existence Constitutive Definition
2. Self-decision is defined as the patient's own choice of modality.	Nonrelational, Constitutive Definition
3. Significant other decision . . . is defined as a significant other having a major influence on the choice of a particular dialysis treatment modality.	Nonrelational, Constitutive Definition
4. To live decision . . . is defined as the informants' statement that if they wanted to live, they must be on dialysis.	Nonrelational, Constitutive Definition
5. Independence versus dependence decision . . . is defined as the patient wants to take care of her or himself.	Nonrelational, Constitutive Definition
6. To be cared for decision . . . is defined as the patient states that he/she is cared for by another.	Nonrelational, Constitutive Definition
7. Patient preference/choice . . . is defined as the informants' preference for a certain modality due to various reasons.	Nonrelational, Constitutive Definition
8. Switching modalities due to patient preference/choice . . . is defined as the informant switches dialysis modality due to own preference or choice.	Nonrelational, Constitutive Definition
9. Selection of patient's treatment modality refers to the patients' perception that they and/or their significant others had not participated in the decision of the treatment modality.	Nonrelational, Existence Constitutive Definition
10. Access-rationing decision . . . is defined as the decision was based on factors such as availability of space at a center and/or reimbursement of services.	Nonrelational, Constitutive Definition
11. Physiologically dictated decision . . . is defined as a decision in which physiological limitations dictate the decision as to modality type.	Nonrelational, Constitutive Definition
12. No patient choice . . . is defined as the patient had no choice in the type of modality.	Nonrelational, Constitutive Definition
13. Expert decision . . . is defined as an expert (e.g., physician) made the decision.	Nonrelational, Constitutive Definition

Middle-range theory Propositions 1, 2, 3, 4, 5, 6, 7, and 8 can be formalized as a nonrelational proposition that asserts a constitutive definition for the theory concept patient's choice of treatment modality:

> Patient's choice of treatment modality is defined as the patient's perception that they and/or their significant others had participated in the decision of choice of treatment modality. The concept patient's choice of treatment modality encompasses seven dimensions: self-decision, significant other decision, to live decision, independence versus dependence decision, to be cared for decision, patient preference/choice, and switching modalities due to patient preference/choice.

Middle-range theory Propositions 2, 3, 4, 5, 6, 7, and 8 address the seven dimensions of the theory concept patient's choice of treatment modality and already are stated in the formal manner of nonrelational propositions that assert constitutive definitions (Table C–3).

Middle-range theory Propositions 9, 10, 11, 12, and 13 can be formalized as a nonrelational proposition that asserts a constitutive definition for the theory concept selection of patient's treatment modality:

> Selection of patient's treatment modality is defined as the patients' perception that they and/or their significant others had not participated in the decision of the treatment modality. The concept selection of patient's treatment modality encompasses four dimensions: access-rationing decision, physiologically dictated decision, no patient choice in making decision, and expert decision.

Middle-range theory Propositions 10, 11, 12, and 13 address the four dimensions of the theory concept selection of patient's treatment modality, and already are stated in the formal manner of nonrelational propositions that assert constitutive definitions (Table C–3).

A nonrelational proposition asserting a representational definition was extracted from the research report. Breckenridge linked the Neuman's Systems Model concept patients' perceptions to the middle-range theory concepts when she stated, "This study is concerned primarily with perceptions of patients about choice of dialysis treatment modality," and when she later explained that the theory "represents the integration of informants' responses to questions about why, how, and by whom dialysis treatment modality decisions are made," which were based on interviews designed to "elicit the perceptions of informants about the way their dialysis treatment modality was chosen." The formalized nonrelational representational definitional proposition is:

> The Neuman's Systems Model concept patients' perceptions was represented by the middle-range theory concepts patient's choice of treatment modality and selection of patient's treatment modality.

This representational definitional proposition links Neuman's Systems Model concept patients' perceptions to the two middle-range theory concepts. No proposition was found for the linkage of Degner and Beaton's life-death decisions framework concept control over the design of therapy to the middle-range theory concepts.

A nonrelational proposition asserting a measured operational definition was easily extracted from the report. Breckenridge explicitly stated that "Data were collected through the use of individual, focused, semistructured, in-depth interviews." In addition, she explained that the Patient Perception Interview Guide was used, and that the data were analyzed for "themes, patterns, and interrelationships." The formalized measured operational definition is:

> The concepts and dimensions of the theory of patient's choice of treatment modality versus selection of patient's treatment modality were measured by informants' responses to individual, focused, semistructured, in-depth interviews, using the Patient Perception Interview Guide.

This operational definition links the concepts of the theory with the empirical indicator, that is, the Patient Perception Interview Guide.

HIERARCHY OF PROPOSITIONS

Given the incomplete linkage of the conceptual models with the middle-range theory, a hierarchy based on level of abstraction cannot be constructed. However, the report contained sufficient raw data, in the form of examples of informants' verbatim responses, to construct hierarchies based on inductive reasoning for some dimensions of each theory concept. More specifically, for the theory concept patient's choice of treatment modality, sufficient data were provided for the dimensions significant other decision and to live decision. For the theory concept selection of patient's treatment modality, sufficient data were provided for the dimensions access-rationing decision and expert decision. Journal space limitations most likely prevented inclusion of enough raw data to develop inductive hierarchies for all dimensions of each theory concept.

Construction of hierarchies by inductive reasoning is exemplified by two hierarchies. The first hierarchy is for the to live decision dimension of the theory concept patient's choice of treatment modality. The verbatim responses for the dimension are the observations, and the nonrelational constitutive definitional proposition for the dimension is the conclusion.

Observation₁: This is the only way that I can live. I always see someone worse off than I. I count my blessings.

Observation₂: I am sorry that I have this problem because I have to be on this machine three times a week to live. It is heartbreaking.

Observation₃: Don't know how many more years I can live, but I make the best of each day. You all have to go sometime. Nobody stays here forever. And you can't feel sorry for yourself. I don't complain.

Conclusion: To live decision is defined as the informants' statement that if they wanted to live, they must be on dialysis.

The second hierarchy is for the access-rationing dimension of the theory concept selection of patient's treatment modality. Once again, the verbatim responses for the dimension are the observations, and the nonrelational constitutive definitional proposition for the dimension is the conclusion.

> **Observation$_1$:** I tried first to get into G.S. (another facility) but they were booked up and there were no openings, but there was an opening here. I would like to go back to G.S., where I am on the waiting list and because of the excellent physical therapy. They don't have physical therapy here. I am supposed to be on therapy. I had three fingers amputated on my left hand and both legs are amputated below the knee.
>
> **Observation$_2$:** I heard that the Kidney Disease Program of this state is one of the best. We wanted to move to Texas. My sister is there and two of my husband's sons. We checked into the financial portion that Medicare does not take care of and Texas has no state plan for the 20% that Medicare does not take care of. The last time we investigated private health insurance was probably 7 or 8 years ago. It was half our income. It was $2,400 a quarter. I don't know what we'll do if we go to Texas.
>
> **Conclusion:** Access-rationing decision is defined as the decision was based on factors such as availability of space at a center and/or reimbursement of services.

DIAGRAMS

The conceptual-theoretical-empirical structure for the research is illustrated in Figure C–1. Another diagram was constructed to illustrate the dimensions of the two concepts making up the middle-range descriptive classification theory of patient's choice of treatment modality versus selection of patient's treatment modality (Fig. C–2).

EVALUATION OF THE CONCEPTUAL-THEORETICAL-EMPIRICAL STRUCTURE

Analysis of Breckenridge's research report revealed that a middle-range descriptive classification theory of patient's choice of treatment modality versus selection of patient's treatment modality was generated. The theory is made up of two multidimensional concepts (Table C–1).

EVALUATION OF THE CONCEPTUAL-THEORETICAL-EMPIRICAL LINKAGES

Specification Adequacy

The criterion of specification adequacy is met only in part. The conceptual models that guided Breckenridge's theory-generating research are explicitly identified as Neuman's Systems Model and Degner and Beaton's life-death decisions

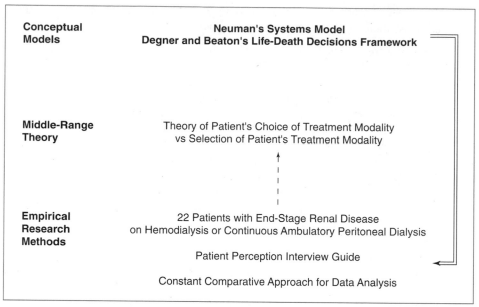

Figure C–1 ■ Conceptual-theoretical-empirical structure for Breckenridge's research.

framework. However, although Breckenridge included an adequate overview of the Degner and Beaton life-death decisions framework, she provided very little content about the Neuman Systems Model. Consequently, the relation of the two conceptual models to the middle-range theory and the empirical research methods is not as clear as it should be.

Linkage Adequacy

The criterion of linkage adequacy is met in part. The linkage between Neuman's Systems Model emphasis on patient perceptions and the purpose of the study is evident, and a representational definition was extracted from the report. In contrast, the linkage between Degner and Beaton's life-death framework and the study purpose and findings is not explicit, and a representational definition could not be extracted from the report.

Conceptual Model Usage Rating Scale

Evaluation of the criteria of specification adequacy and linkage adequacy is summarized by application of the Conceptual Model Usage Rating Scale. Breckenridge's research report earned a score of 1, indicating insufficient use of the two conceptual models. The score is based on the paucity of information given about

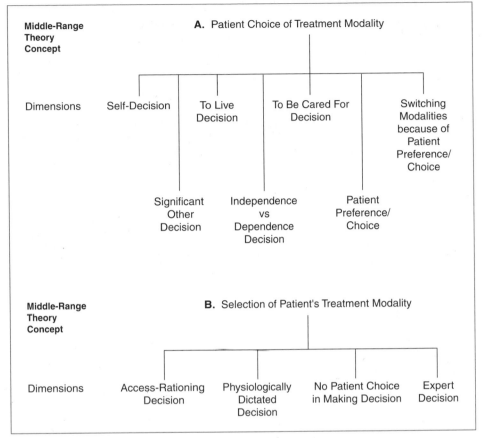

Figure C–2 ■ Concepts of the theory of patient's choice of treatment (A) versus selection of treatment modality (B) and their dimensions.

the Neuman Systems Model and the lack of a linkage between the study purpose or findings and Degner and Beaton's life-death decisions framework.

EVALUATION OF THE THEORY

Significance

The middle-range theory of patient's choice of treatment modality versus selection of patient's treatment modality meets the criterion of significance. Breckenridge discussed the social significance of her research in the introductory section of the report. She explained that the federally funded United States Medicare End Stage Renal Disease (ESRD) Program provides financial coverage to all citizens with renal disease who can benefit from dialysis. She also cited statistics for the number of patients who received dialysis before and since the funding legislation was passed in 1973, as well as the number of patients who receive in-center hemodialysis versus those who receive CAPD. Breckenridge further explained that "Prior to the ESRD program, the decision to dialyze a patient was based on a selection process," whereas at the current time, all eligible ESRD patients are dialyzed.

Breckenridge discussed the theoretical significance of her research in the background section of the report. She commented:

■ Most of the research related to the ESRD patient's type of treatment modality has been conducted by asking questions developed from the health care provider's perspective. Wu stated that there is a great need to study the ESRD patient's dialysis treatment modality from his or her perspective. . . . Sadler stated that in the United States today patients are more involved in making their own decisions in choosing whether they want dialysis, and which modality they prefer. Since the legislated Self-Determination Act to facilitate the patient in making health care decisions was implemented in December 1991, health care professionals at more dialysis units are educating and counseling patients about their choices. Jacox pointed out that although there are several treatment options for ESRD, little is known about how treatment modalities are chosen.

Internal Consistency

The middle-range theory of patient's choice of treatment modality versus selection of patient's treatment modality meets the criterion of internal consistency. Semantic clarity and consistency are evident. The two theory concepts and their respective dimensions are constitutively defined in a clear and concise manner, there are no redundancies in the concepts or dimensions, and no other terms were introduced in the report.

The propositions of the theory reflect structural consistency. Hierarchies based on inductive reasoning could be constructed for 4 of the 11 dimensions. The data presented for the remaining 7 dimensions, for which hierarchies cannot be constructed, support the conclusions represented by their constitutive definitions. There are no redundant propositions.

Parsimony

The middle-range theory of patient's choice of treatment modality versus selection of patient's treatment modality meets the criterion of parsimony. The theory, which is made up of two concepts, each of which includes several mutually exclusive dimensions, is neither oversimplified nor excessively verbose.

Testability

The middle-range theory of patient's choice of treatment modality versus selection of patient's treatment modality meets the criterion of testability. It should be possible to replicate Breckenridge's study with the same methods. Furthermore, the hypothesis proposed by Breckenridge that "patient choice alone is inadequate because other factors have an impact on the decision for the type of treatment chosen or selected" is falsifiable.

EVALUATION OF THE RESEARCH DESIGN

Operational Adequacy

The research design meets the criterion of operational adequacy. The sampling technique, the empirical indicator, the data-collection procedure, and the data-analysis approach all are in keeping with the interpretive method of naturalistic inquiry.

EVALUATION OF THE RESEARCH FINDINGS

Empirical Adequacy

The result of Breckenridge's research was the generation of a middle-range descriptive classification theory of patient's choice of treatment modality versus selection of patient's treatment modality. The theory, as presented in the report, meets the criterion of empirical adequacy for descriptive research using an interpretative method. The data presented in the form of verbatim responses from informants support the constitutive definitions for the respective dimensions of the two concepts, and the data for the several dimensions of each concept, in turn, support the constitutive definitions for the two concepts.

EVALUATION OF THE UTILITY OF THE THEORY FOR PRACTICE

Pragmatic Adequacy

The middle-range theory of patient's choice of treatment modality versus selection of patient's treatment modality meets the criterion of pragmatic adequacy. Indeed, Breckenridge identified guidelines for nursing care and pointed out that the theory could serve as the basis for health policy. She stated:

> ■ When interviewing patients, nurses can assess decision making according to the theory's categories [concepts] and themes [dimensions]. This [theory] can assist nurses in understanding decision making patterns. Interventions can be designed to enhance a patient's preference as to choice and selection of a treatment. Nurses can also use this theory as a basis for including a patient's perspective in effecting health policy in developing Clinical Practice Guidelines.

Assessment of End Stage Renal Disease patients' decision making with regard to dialysis modality certainly is feasible and clinicians have the legal ability to carry out such assessments. Moreover, given the legislation regarding patient self-determination, such assessments should meet their expectations.

EVALUATION OF THE CONCEPTUAL MODEL

Credibility

The credibility of Neuman's Systems Model and Degner and Beaton's life-death decisions framework, which Breckenridge used to guide the generation of the middle-range theory of patient's choice of treatment modality versus selection of patient's treatment modality, is not addressed explicitly in the report. It can only be inferred that the two conceptual models provided a useful guide for the selection of the empirical research methods.

References

Breckenridge, D.M. (1997). Patients' perceptions of why, how, and by whom dialysis treatment modality was chosen. *American Nephrology Nurses Association Journal, 24,* 313–319.

Degner, L.F., & Beaton, J.I. (1987). *Life-death decisions in health care.* New York: Hemisphere.

Neuman, B. (1995). *The Neuman systems model* (3rd ed.). Norwalk, CT: Appleton and Lange.

Analysis and Evaluation of a Descriptive Theory-Testing Study: The Method of Psychometric Analysis

The Inventory of Functional Status-Caregiver of a Child in a Body Cast

Diana M.L. Newman, RN, EdD

The Inventory of Functional Status-Caregiver of a Child in a Body Cast (IFSCCBC), which was derived from the Roy Adaptation Model, includes subscales measuring the extent to which parental caregivers or their surrogates continue their usual household, social and community, childcare, personal care, and occupational activities while caring for a child in a body cast. Content validity was established at 90%. Internal consistency reliability ranged from 0.63 to 0.88, using item to subscale correlations. Subscale to total IFSCCBC score correlations ranged from 0.14 to 0.75. Initial construct validity testing was accomplished by examination of subscale to subscale correlations. The IFSCCBC may be used in research and clinical practice to assess the functional status of parents or their surrogates while they are caring for a child in a body cast.

Mothers, fathers, and others who care for young children in body casts face challenges that disrupt their usual pattern of daily living. The developmental needs of the child, the specific care requirements related to the body cast, and the changes in usual caregiver activities imposed by the child's special care requirements comprise the typical challenges that must be faced. The Inventory of Functional Status-Caregiver of a Child in a Body Cast (IFSCCBC) was designed to measure the extent to which maternal or paternal caregivers or parental surrogates continue their usual household, social and community, childcare, personal care, occupational, and

Reprinted from *Journal of Pediatric Nursing, 12*(3), 142–147, 1997, with permission.

educational activities while caring for a child in a body cast. This article reports the development and initial psychometric testing of the IFSCCBC.

BACKGROUND

Little is known about the impact of caring for a child in a body cast on the caregiver's functional status. Cuddy (1986) noted that parents are not prepared for the challenges of caring for an immobile child in a body cast. McHale and Corbett (1988) reported considerable emotional upheaval in parents whose child was placed in a Pavlik harness, which is a body brace used to treat developmentally dislocated hips. Corbett (1989) found that information about the Pavlik harness enhanced parents' cooperation with the treatment regimen.

The investigator's clinical experiences suggested that a parent's performance of his or her usual daily activities may be altered during the time that the child is at home in a body cast. The lack of any literature dealing directly with parental functional status while caring for a child in a body cast led to an exploratory qualitative study (Newman & Fawcett, 1995). The study sample consisted of 35 mothers who identified themselves as the primary caregiver of a young child at home in a body cast. The findings revealed that the inability of mothers to obtain adequate babysitters severely limited their participation in usual social, community, occupational, and educational activities. The mothers reported that the care of the child frequently was physically exhausting. Although a routine for care typically was established, the burden of providing this care did not lessen over time and, in fact, frequently increased. The mothers stated that child-care activities were difficult, especially dressing the child and keeping the cast clean. Positioning the child was a constant challenge, and lifting the child frequently created back strain and back aches for the mothers. Transportation of the child for follow-up care was often hindered because of the lack of an appropriate car seat.

The mothers also reported that the child's emotional reactions to the cast and the interruption of normal growth and development patterns had a substantial impact on all of their own usual activities. For example, the mothers' personal care activities and conjugal sexual activities were frequently compromised because of fatigue, as well as the fact that the child slept in the same room as the parents and was awake periodically during the night. Mothers also experienced sleeping problems because they had to get up with the child at night or get up earlier than usual to get ready for the demands of the next day. The IFSCCBC built on the findings of the qualitative study, and was specifically designed to quantify the functional status of parents or their surrogates while caring for a child in a body cast.

Conceptual Framework

The IFSCCBC was adapted from other measures of functional status, including the Inventory of Functional Status-Antepartum Period (IFSAP) (Tulman et al., 1991) and the Inventory of Functional Status After Childbirth (IFSAC) (Fawcett, Tulman, & Myers, 1988). All of the instruments were derived from the role function response mode of the Roy Adaptation Model of Nursing (Roy & Andrews, 1991). The Roy model proposes that people are challenged to adapt to constantly changing environmental stimuli. Responses to stimuli are observed in four modes: physiological, self-concept, role function, and interdependence. The role function response mode, of central interest in the development of the instruments, emphasizes the need for social integrity and deals with primary, secondary, and tertiary role activities. Role, according to Roy and Andrews (1991), is a "set of expectations about how a person occupying one position behaves toward a person occupying the complementary position" (p. 348). According to Roy and Andrews (1991), one's primary role "determines the majority of behaviors engaged in by the person during a particular period of life" (p. 349), and is exemplified by a 25-year-old adult woman. One's secondary roles are those that are assumed to complete the tasks associated with developmental stage and primary role, such as a 28-year-old adult woman who is a mother and a teacher. One's tertiary roles are "related primarily to secondary roles and represent ways in which individuals meet their role associated obligations" (p. 349), such as a 35-year-old woman who is a Girl Scout leader in association with her secondary role as mother. Within the context of the Roy Adaptation Model, the actual performance of primary, secondary and tertiary role activities is regarded as functional status. Figure 1 depicts the linkages between the Roy Adaptation Model role function mode and the IFSCCBC subscales.

It is important to point out that the IFSCCBC is limited to assessment of actual role performance. The instrument does not measure feelings or attitudes about roles, such as role conflict, overload, or ambiguity. The instrument also does not measure the caregiver's ability to perform activities, that is, functional ability. In fact, it was assumed that the caregivers were capable of performing all activities included on the IFSCCBC.

INSTRUMENT DEVELOPMENT

The IFSCCBC items were drawn from the IFSAP (Tulman et al., 1991), the IFSAC (Fawcett et al., 1988), and the findings of the previous qualitative study (Newman & Fawcett, 1995). Seventy-one items were originally identified. As the result of reliability testing, the final form of the IFSCCBC is a 49-item paper-and-pencil questionnaire that has an eighth grade reading level (Dale & O'Rourke, 1976). Items are arranged in six subscales and the instrument contains space for comments at the end of each subscale. The 9-item Household Activities subscale, the 6-item Social and Community Activities subscale, Part A (3 items) of the 8-item Care of Child in Body Cast Activities subscale, and the 9-item Care of Other Child(ren) Activities subscales are rated on 4-point scales of 1 = "not at all," 2 = "partially," 3 = "fully," and 4 = "more than before." Part B (5 items) of the Care of Child in Body Cast Activities subscale, the 10-item Personal Care Activities subscale, and the 7-item Occupational Activities subscale are rated on 4-point scales of 1 = "not at all," 2 = "sometimes," 3 = "most of the time," and 4 = "all of the time." The entire Educational Activities subscale was dropped as the result of reliability testing.

Caregivers are instructed to rate the extent to which activities performed before the child's casting are being continued during the time the child is in a body cast, as well as to indicate and rate which activities they have begun since the child

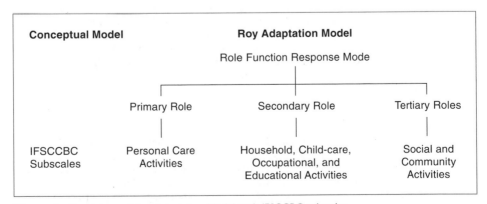

Figure 1 ■ Linkage of Roy Adaptation Model with IFSCCBC subscales.

was placed in the body cast. A "not applicable" code, which is excluded from the score calculations, is used for items not performed by a caregiver.

Inasmuch as each caregiver has an individual repertoire of role activities, not all IFSCCBC items may be applicable to his or her situation. For example, a caregiver who is not employed would not respond to any of the items on the Occupational Activities subscale. Similarly, a caregiver who did not participate in community service organizations would not respond to that particular item on the Social and Community Activities subscale, although he or she would respond to other Social and Community Activities subscale items that are relevant. Therefore, a mean score is calculated for each subscale and the total IFSCCBC for each caregiver, and it is used as the raw score for analyses. The mean score is the sum of item scores divided by the number of items to which the individual responded for each subscale and the total IFSCCBC. The possible range of individual mean scores for each subscale and the total IFSCCBC is 1 to 4. The higher the score, the greater the functional status.

The instrument development protocol was approved by a university human subjects committee and the cooperating hospital institutional review boards. Completion of the questionnaires by subjects constituted informed consent. Written informed consent was obtained when required by the hospital institutional review board.

CONTENT VALIDITY

Content validity was assessed to ascertain that the items originally selected for the IFSCCBC represented those items that are relevant to the specific situation of caregivers of children in body casts. Popham's (1978) average congruency procedure was used to determine content validity. This procedure is a measure of the average percentage of agreement for all questionnaire items across all judges. Parents or parental surrogates of children from birth to 3 years, in body casts because of developmentally dislocated hips or acquired trauma, served as content validity judges. The actual caregivers of children in body casts were selected as judges because they, rather than the conceptual model, the literature, other instruments, or health care providers, were regarded as the experts with regard to particular activities that comprised the IFSCCBC items.

The judges were asked to compare the items on each subscale of the IFSCCBC with the definition of that subscale and then rate each item as relevant, undecided, or not relevant. In round one of the content validity procedure, 71 IFSCCBC items were submitted to 12 parents or parental surrogates. The average congruency score was 86%. As a result, the wording of four items was refined. The round two content validity procedure involved eight parents, none of whom had participated in round one. The average congruency score was 78%. Inasmuch as the low congruency score in round two was caused by the parents' inability to understand the rating procedure, the instructions were clarified for round three. Round three used five parents, none of whom had participated in rounds one or two. The average congruency score was 90%, which meets Popham's (1978) criterion for acceptable content validity.

RELIABILITY

Sample

The reliability testing sample consisted of 105 parents or parental surrogates caring for a child at home in a body cast. The subjects represent a convenience sample that was recruited from orthopaedic clinics in children's hospitals in Connecticut, Delaware, Indiana, Massachusetts, Michigan, Ohio, and Pennsylvania. The demographic characteristics of the sample are given in Table 1. The typical

Table I ■ **CHARACTERISTICS OF THE SAMPLE (N = 105)**

	n	%
Primary caregiver		
Mother	95	90%
Father	6	6%
Grandmother	3	3%
Friend	I	<1%

	M	Range
Age of caregiver	30.6 yrs	17–46 yrs

	n	%
Education of caregiver		
Less than high school	8	8%
High school	40	38%
Attended college	47	45%
Attended graduate school	9	9%
Unknown	I	<1%
Employment status of caregiver		
Employed	51	49%
Unemployed	47	45%
On leave from work	5	5%
Looking for work	I	<1%
Unknown	I	<1%
Occupation of the caregiver		
Homemaker	37	36%
Professional/managerial	31	30%
Sales/clerical	13	13%
Skilled craftsman	6	6%
Students	5	5%
Retired	3	3%
Homemaker/employed	6	6%
Unknown	4	1%
Residence		
City	47	45%
Suburbs	38	36%
Rural areas	17	16%
Unknown	3	3%
Adults living in household		
Spouse	85	83%
Other family members (grandparents, sisters, brothers, aunts, uncles)	16	16%
Unknown	4	1%

	M	Range
Number of children in household	2	2–11
I Child	n = 44	
>I Child	n = 61	

	M	SD
Age of youngest child	18.5 mo	12.41
Age of child in body cast	20.01 mo	12.35
Time spent in body cast	8.66 wk	3.29

(*continued on page 288*)

Table I ■ **CHARACTERISTICS OF THE SAMPLE (N = 105)** (*Continued*)

	n	%
Reason for body cast		
Developmentally dislocated hip	95	91%
Fractured femur	10	9%
Gender of child in body cast		
Female	78	74%
Male	27	26%

caregiver was an employed mother who was approximately 30-years-old. The children in the body casts were predominantly girls (78%) and, on average, 20.6 months old. Most of the children (91%) were in body casts because of developmentally dislocated hip. The children had, on average, been in a body cast for 2 months at the time of administration of the IFSCCBC (Table 1). The subjects completed the IFSCCBC as a self-administered questionnaire while they were at the clinic.

Internal Consistency Reliability Testing

The means and standard deviations for each subscale and the total 49-item IFSCCBC are presented in Table 2. Internal consistency reliability was determined by correlating each subscale item score with its respective subscale total score and calculating the average correlation for each subscale. This analysis excluded the "not applicable" code. Initial inspection of the data for the original 71-item instrument, which included an Educational Activities subscale, revealed that several items did not meet the criterion of a correlation of ≥.40 established for this study. More specifically, several items on the Household Activities subscale, the Care of Child in Body Cast subscale, the Care of Other Children subscale, the Personal Care Activities subscale, as well as all of the items on the Educational Activities subscale had item to subscale correlations below 0.40 and were deleted. Subsequently, the item to subscale correlations were recomputed.

The average correlation for each subscale was then calculated using Fisher's z′ transformation (Cohen & Cohen, 1975). The average correlation replaced the more traditional Cronbach's alpha procedure because it takes into account individual differences in types of activities performed. Such individual differences preclude the effective use of Cronbach's alpha because of the fact that few if any sub-

Table 2 ■ **INTERNAL CONSISTENCY SAMPLE: MEANS AND STANDARD DEVIATIONS FOR THE INVENTORY OF FUNCTIONAL STATUS-CAREGIVER OF A CHILD IN A BODY CAST (N = 105)**

Subscale	Number of Items	M	SD
Household activities	9	2.5	.43
Social and community activities	6	2.0	.62
Childcare for child in body cast activities	8	3.1	.58
Childcare for other children activities	9	2.6	.63
Personal care activities	10	1.9	.65
Occupational activities	7	2.1	.87
Total IFSCCBC	49	2.4	.33

jects respond to every IFSCCBC item. More specifically, in the calculation of Cronbach's alpha, items coded as "not applicable" because the subject does not perform those activities are treated as missing data and cause the entire subscale to be eliminated from the calculations. As can be seen in Table 3, the average item to subscale correlation ranged from 0.63 for the Care of Child in Body Cast subscale to 0.88 for the Occupational Activities subscale.

Internal consistency reliability also was assessed by correlating each subscale score with the total IFSCCBC score. As reported in Table 3, the correlations ranged from 0.14 for the Care of Child In Body Cast subscale to 0.75 for the Personal Care Activities subscale.

Construct Validity

Initial assessment of the construct validity of the IFSCCBC was undertaken by examining its subscale structure. Factor analysis could not be used in this study because of the approach to measuring functional status used and as explained previously, all subjects do not respond to all of the IFSCCBC items. Therefore, empirical testing of the subscale structure was accomplished by calculating Pearson correlations between the IFSCCBC subscales. As expected, the magnitude of most of the correlations between the subscales was low, ranging from 0.10 to 0.31 (see Table 4). However, the relatively greater magnitude of the correlation between Personal Care Activities and Occupational Activities ($r = .79$) suggests an overlap between these subscales.

DISCUSSION

The content validity of the IFSCCBC was accomplished using a quantitative approach. The level of agreement achieved among the judges (90%) indicates that the items reflect the definition of the subscale for which they were written.

Internal consistency reliability was determined by examination of subscale item to subscale total and subscale to total instrument correlations. The subscale item to subscale total correlations indicate a modest level of internal consistency reliability. Although a reliability coefficient of at least 0.70 is required when using the Cronbach's alpha procedure, the procedures used for this study typically yield more conservative estimates of reliability than the Cronbach's alpha procedure (Nunnally & Bernstein, 1994). Consequently, the magnitude of coefficients obtained for the subscale item to subscale totals (0.63 to 0.88) may be considered satisfactory.

The generally low magnitude of the subscale to total correlations, along with the low subscale to subscale correlations, suggest that the instrument is composed

---

Table 3 ■ **INTERNAL CONSISTENCY RELIABILITY COEFFICIENTS FOR THE INVENTORY OF FUNCTIONAL STATUS-CAREGIVER OF CHILD IN BODY CAST (IFSCCBC) ($N = 105$)**

Subscale	Item to Subscale*	Subscale to Total
Household activities	.63	.53
Social and community activities	.70	.53
Childcare for the child in a body cast activities	.63	.14
Childcare for the other children activities	.75	.49
Personal care activities	.73	.75
Occupational activities	.88	.73

*Average correlation using Fisher's z' transformation.

Table 4 ■ **SUBSCALE CORRELATIONS FOR THE INVENTORY OF FUNCTIONAL STATUS-CAREGIVER OF CHILD IN BODY CAST**

	Social and Community	Childcare For Child in Body Cast	Childcare Other Children	Personal Care	Occupational
Household	.30 (n = 105)	−.10 (n = 105)	.14 (n = 59)	.23 (n = 104)	.10 (n = 56)
Social and community		.15 (n = 105)	.23 (n = 59)	.22 (n = 104)	−.03 (n = 56)
Childcare child in body cast			−.13 (n = 59)	−.20 (n = 104)	−.31 (n = 56)
Childcare other children				.19 (n = 58)	.29 (n = 32)
Personal care					.79 (n = 56)

of distinct subscales and that subscale scores, rather than the total IFSCCBC score, are more reliable and informative measures of caregiver functional status while caring for a child in a body cast.

The data indicate that caregiver's performance of activities related to the care of the child in a body cast has a substantial and potentially detrimental impact on the performance of all other activities. As can be seen in Table 2, activities related to the care of the child in the body cast are performed at a higher level than any other activities. Furthermore, the negative subscale to subscale correlations for the Care of Child in Body Cast subscale and the Household, Childcare of Other Children, Personal Care, and Occupational Activities subscales (Table 4) reflect the impact of caring for the child in a cast on the performance of other role activities. The sign of these correlations clearly indicate that as the performance of activities related to care of the child in the body cast increases, the performance of all other activities decreases. Further research to investigate the full effect, or burden, of caring for a child in a body cast is recommended.

Implications for Clinical Practice

Nurses working with children recognize the need to provide comprehensive care for the child and his or her caregivers. The IFSCCBC provides a mechanism to assess the functional status of the caregiver, typically the mother, during the time the child is in a body cast. It is recommended that the IFSCCBC be administered to the primary caregiver immediately after the child is placed in the body cast to establish a baseline measure of functional status and periodically thereafter to assess the effect of caring for the child.

The IFSCCBC may be completed either by caregiver self-administration or by interviews conducted by the clinician in person or by telephone. It can be given to the primary caregiver to complete during the clinic visit or at home, with return by mail or at the time of the next clinic visit. Advantages of the IFSCCBC include the insight it provides into activities not typically addressed by nurses who work with children in body casts and their caregivers, as well as assessment of activities that are particularly important for safe and effective care of the child.

Furthermore, the IFSCCBC facilitates a match between a broad spectrum of caregiver needs and specific nursing interventions. For example, nurses may refer caregivers to trained babysitters to facilitate the caregivers' performance of household, social and community, childcare, personal care, and occupational activities. In addition, the establishment of telephone support groups for the caregivers could provide a way to share specific information that might lessen the burden of caring for children in body casts.

In conclusion, data obtained from the IFSCCBC can be used to identify the need for specific interventions that would enhance caregiver functional status. These interventions would be based on the individual caregiver's usual activities rather than the clinician's judgements about the importance of activities that may not be consistent with the caregiver's activities. ■

References

Cohen, J., & Cohen, P. (1975). *Applied multiple regression/correlational analysis for the behavioral sciences.* Hillsdale, NJ: Lawrence Erlbaum.

Corbett, D. (1989). Information needs of parents of a child in a Pavlik harness. *Orthopaedic Nursing, 8*(1), 20–23.

Cuddy, C.M. (1986). Caring for the child in a spica cast: A parent's perspective. *Orthopaedic Nursing, 5*(3), 17–21.

Dale, E., & O'Rourke, J. (1976). *Living word vocabulary.* Elgin, Il.: Dome.

Fawcett, J., Tulman, L., & Myers, S. (1988). Development of the Inventory of Functional Status After Childbirth. *Journal of Nurse-Midwifery, 33*(6), 252–260.

McHale, K.A., & Corbett, D. (1988). Parental noncompliance with a Pavlik harness. *Journal of Pediatric Orthopaedics, 9*(6), 649–652.

Newman, D.M.L., & Fawcett, J. (1995). Caring for a young child at home in a body cast: Impact on the caregiver. *Orthopaedic Nursing, 14*(1), 41–46.

Nunnally, J.C., & Bernstein, I.H. (1994). *Psychometric theory* (3rd ed). New York: McGraw-Hill.

Popham, W.J. (1978). *Criterion-referenced measurement.* Englewood Cliffs, NJ: Prentice-Hall.

Roy, C., & Andrews, H.A. (1991). *The Roy adaptation model. The definitive statement.* Norwalk, CT: Appleton & Lange.

Tulman, L., Higgins, K., Fawcett, J., Nunno, C., Van Sickel, C., Haas, M.B., & Speca, M.M. (1991). The Inventory of Functional Status-Antepartum Period: Development and testing. *Journal of Nurse Midwifery, 36*(2), 117–123.

ANALYSIS OF THE CONCEPTUAL-THEORETICAL-EMPIRICAL STRUCTURE

The stated purpose of Newman's (1997) research was to develop and determine the psychometric properties of the Inventory of Functional Status–Caregiver of a Child in a Body Cast (IFSCCBC). The research was designed to test a middle-range descriptive classification theory of the functional status of caregivers of children in body casts, using the descriptive research method of psychometric analysis.

IDENTIFICATION OF CONCEPTS

Conceptual Model Concept

Analysis of the research report revealed that the research was guided by Roy's Adaptation Model (Roy and Andrews, 1991). The conceptual model concept of interest is response mode, which is a multidimensional concept made up of four dimensions: physiological mode, self-concept mode, role function mode, and interdependence mode. Newman used only the role function mode dimension to guide the development of the IFSCCBC.

Middle Range Theory Concept

Further analysis of the research report revealed that the middle-range descriptive classification theory of the functional status of caregivers of children in body casts encompasses one multidimensional concept: functional status of a caregiver of a child in a body cast. The dimensions of the concept are personal-care activities, household activities, child-care activities, occupational activities, educational activities, and social and community activities. The theory is categorized as a descriptive classification theory because the caregiver's activities were grouped into six dimensions, and those dimensions were thought to be mutually exclusive.

CLASSIFICATION OF THE MIDDLE-RANGE THEORY CONCEPT

The middle-range theory concept functional status of a caregiver of a child in a body cast is classified as a construct in both Kaplan's and Willer and Webster's schemata because it was invented for research purposes and is not immediately accessible to direct sensory observations. Indeed, the research was directed toward the development of a valid and reliable instrument that could be used to measure an observable proxy for the construct, that is, the caregiver's report of his or her functional status while caring for a child in a body cast.

The concept is classified as a variable because functional status can vary between caregivers. Indeed, the standard deviations given in Table 2 of the research report indicate variability in the IFSCCBC subscales. The concept is classified as a statistical unit in Dubin's schema because the raw score for each caregiver is a mean. Newman explained:

> ■ Inasmuch as each caregiver has an individual repertoire of role activities, not all IFSCCBC items may be applicable to his or her situation. . . . Therefore, a mean score is calculated for each subscale and the total IFSCCBC for each caregiver, and it is used as the raw score for analyses. The mean score is the sum of item scores divided by the number of items to which the individual responded for each subscale and the total IFSCCBC.

IDENTIFICATION AND CLASSIFICATION OF PROPOSITIONS

Conceptual Model Propositions

Nonrelational propositions from Roy's Adaptation Model were used to guide the development of the middle-range descriptive classification theory of the functional status of caregivers of children in body casts. The nonrelational propositions are listed in Table D–1.

Table D–I ■ **CONCEPTUAL MODEL PROPOSITIONS FROM NEWMAN'S RESEARCH REPORT**

Proposition	Classification
1. Responses to stimuli are observed in four modes: physiological, self-concept, role function, and interdependence.	Nonrelational, Existence Constitutive Definition
2. The role function response mode, of central interest in the development of the [IFSCCBC], emphasizes the need for social integrity and deals with primary-, secondary-, and tertiary-role activities.	Nonrelational, Constitutive Definition
3. One's primary role determines the majority of behaviors engaged in by the person during a particular period of life.	Nonrelational, Constitutive Definition
4. One's secondary roles are those that are assumed to complete the tasks associated with developmental stage and primary role.	Nonrelational, Constitutive Definitions
5. One's tertiary roles are related primarily to secondary roles and represent ways in which individuals meet their role associated obligations.	Nonrelational, Constitutive Definition

---

Conceptual model Proposition 1 can be formalized as a nonrelational proposition that asserts the existence of a phenomenon and as a nonrelational proposition that asserts a constitutive definition. The nonrelational existence proposition is:

There is a phenomenon known as response mode.

The constitutive definition is:

Response mode is defined as a multidimensional concept that encompasses four dimensions: physiological mode responses, self-concept mode responses, role function mode responses, and interdependence mode responses.

Conceptual model Propositions 2, 3, 4, and 5 can be formalized as a nonrelational proposition that asserts a constitutive definition. The proposition is:

The role function mode dimension of Roy's Adaptation Model concept response mode is defined as the need for social integrity within primary-, secondary-, and tertiary-role activities. The role function mode dimension encompasses three subdimensions: primary role, secondary roles, and tertiary roles. The primary-role subdimension is defined as the majority of behaviors engaged in by the person during a particular period of life. The secondary-roles subdimension is defined as roles that are assumed to complete the tasks associated with developmental stage and the primary role. The tertiary-roles subdimension is defined as roles that are related primarily to secondary roles and represent ways in which individuals meet their role associated obligations.

Middle-Range Theory Propositions

Nonrelational propositions that are central to the middle-range descriptive classification theory of the functional status of caregivers of children in body casts are evident in Newman's report. Those propositions are listed in Table D–2.

Table D–2 ■ **MIDDLE-RANGE THEORY PROPOSITIONS FROM NEWMAN'S RESEARCH REPORT**

Proposition	Classification
1. The Inventory of Functional Status-Caregiver of a Child in a Body Cast was designed to measure the extent to which maternal or paternal caregivers or parental surrogates continue their usual household, social and community, child-care, personal-care, occupational, and educational activities while caring for a child in a body cast.	Nonrelational, Existence Constitutive Definition
2. The investigator's clinical experiences suggested that a parent's performance of his or her usual daily activities may be altered during the time that the child is at home in a body cast.	Nonrelational, Level of Existence
3. An exploratory qualitative study . . . revealed that the inability of mothers to obtain adequate baby sitters severely limited their participation in usual social, community, occupational, and educational activities.	Nonrelational, Level of Existence
4. The mothers reported that the care of the child frequently was physically exhausting. The mothers stated that child-care activities were difficult, especially dressing the child and keeping the cast clean. Positioning the child was a constant challenge, and lifting the child frequently created back strain and back aches for the mothers. Transportation of the child for follow-up care was often hindered because of the lack of an appropriate car seat.	Nonrelational, Level of Existence
5. The mothers also reported that the child's emotional reactions to the cast and the interruption of normal growth and development patterns had a substantial impact on all of their own usual activities. For example, the mothers' personal-care activities and conjugal sexual activities were frequently compromised because of fatigue, as well as the fact that the child slept in the same room as the parents and was awake periodically during the night. Mothers also experienced sleeping problems because they had to get up with the child at night or get up earlier than usual to get ready for the demands of the next day.	Nonrelational, Level of Existence
6. The [IFSCCBC was] derived from the role function response mode of Roy's Adaptation Model of Nursing.	Nonrelational, Representational Definition
7. Within the context of Roy's Adaptation Model, the actual performance of primary-, secondary-, and tertiary-role activities is regarded as functional status.	Nonrelational, Representational Definition
8. Figure 1 depicts the linkages between Roy's Adaptation Model and the IFSCCBC subscales.	Nonrelational, Representational Definition
9. The IFSCCBC is limited to assessment of actual role performance.	Nonrelational, Measured Operational Definition
10. Seventy-one items were originally identified. As a result of reliability testing, the final form of the IFSCCBC is a 49-item paper-and-pencil questionnaire . . . The 9-item Household Activities subscale, the 6-item Social and Community Activities subscale, Part A (3 items) of the 8-item Care of Child in Body Cast Activities Subscale, and the 9-item Care of Other Child(ren) Activities subscales . . . Part B (5 items) of the Care of Child in Body Cast Activities subscale, the 10-item Personal-Care Activities subscale, and the 7-item Occupational Activities subscale.	Nonrelational, Constitutive Definition Results of testing implicit hypothesis
11. The entire Educational Activities subscale was dropped as the result of reliability testing.	Nonrelational, Constitutive Definition Result of testing implicit hypothesis

---

Table D–2 ■ **MIDDLE-RANGE THEORY PROPOSITIONS FROM NEWMAN'S RESEARCH REPORT**   (*Conitinued*)

Proposition	Classification
12. As expected, the magnitude of most of the correlations between the subscales was low, ranging from 0.10 to 0.31. However, the relatively greater magnitude of the correlation between Personal-Care Activities and Occupational Activities ($r = .79$) suggests an overlap between these subscales.	Nonrelational, Result of testing implicit hypothesis

---

Middle-range theory Proposition 1 can be formalized as a nonrelational proposition that asserts the existence of a phenomenon. The nonrelational existence proposition is:

> There is a phenomenon known as functional status of a caregiver of a child in a body cast.

Middle-range theory Propositions 2, 3, 4, and 5 can be formalized as a nonrelational proposition that asserts level of existence. The formalized proposition is:

> A parent experiences alterations in the performance of usual role activities when he or she is the caregiver of a child in a body cast.

Middle-range theory Proposition 1 also can be formalized as a nonrelational proposition that asserts the constitutive definition for the theory concept that was tested by means of the development and psychometric analysis of the IFSCCBC. This constitutive definition is:

> Functional status of a caregiver of a child in a body cast is defined as the extent to which maternal or paternal caregivers or parental surrogates continue their usual household, social and community, child-care, personal-care, occupational, and educational activities while caring for a child in a body cast.

Middle-range theory Propositions 6, 7, and 8, along with the content of Figure 1 in the research report, can be formalized as the following nonrelational proposition that asserts a representational definition:

> The primary-, secondary-, and tertiary-role subdimensions of the role function mode dimension of Roy's Adaptation Model concept response mode were represented by the middle-range theory concept functional status of a caregiver of a child in a body cast. The primary-role subdimension was represented by the theory concept dimension personal-care activities. The secondary-roles subdimension was represented by the theory concept dimensions household activities, child-care activities, occupational activities, and educational activities. The tertiary-roles subdimension was represented by the theory concept dimension social and community activities.

This representational definition clearly links the dimension and subdimensions of the conceptual model concept with the middle-range theory concept and its dimensions.

Middle-range theory Proposition 9 asserts a measured operational definition. Formalized, the measured operational definition is:

> Functional status of a caregiver of a child in a body cast was measured by the Inventory of Functional Status-Caregiver of a Child in a Body Cast (IFSCCBC).

The operational definition links the middle-range theory concept with the empirical indicator, that is, the IFSCCBC. It should be noted that the formalized measured operational definition requires recognition that Newman equates role performance with functional status.

Middle-range theory Propositions 10 and 11 represent an implicit hypothesis, which was tested by means of the psychometric analysis of the IFSCCBC. Formalized, and stated in empirical indicator terms, the hypothesis is:

> The IFSCCBC contains 71 items that encompass seven subscales: the Personal-Care Activities Subscale, the Household Activities Subscale, the Care of Child in Body Cast Activities subscale, the Care of Other Child(ren) Activities subscale, the Occupational Activities subscale, the Educational Activities subscale, and the Social and Community Activities subscale.

Middle-range theory Propositions 10 and 11 also can be formalized as a nonrelational proposition that asserts the constitutive definition for the theory concept that emerged from the psychometric analysis of the IFSCCBC. This constitutive definition is:

> Functional status of a caregiver of a child in a body cast is defined as the extent to which maternal or paternal caregivers or parental surrogates continue their usual household, social and community, child-care, personal-care, and occupational activities while caring for a child in a body cast.

Middle-range theory Proposition 12 represents another implicit hypothesis tested by means of the psychometric analysis of the IFSCCBC. Stated in terms of the empirical indicator, this hypothesis, which asserts a relation between the dimensions of the theory concept functional status of a caregiver of a child in a body cast, is:

> The correlations between the IFSCCBC subscales will be of low magnitude.

HIERARCHY OF PROPOSITIONS

A hierarchy of propositions based on level of abstraction can be constructed by using the nonrelational constitutive definitional propositions for the conceptual model concept dimension role function mode, the nonrelational constitutive definitional proposition for the middle-range theory concept functional status of a caregiver of a child in a body cast that was tested by the psychometric analysis, the nonrelational representational definitional proposition, and the nonrelational operational definitional proposition. The hierarchy is:

> **Abstract proposition:** The role function mode dimension of Roy's Adaptation Model concept response mode is defined as the need for social integrity within primary-, secondary-,

and tertiary-role activities. The role function mode dimension encompasses three subdimensions: primary role, secondary roles, and tertiary roles. The primary-role subdimension is defined as the majority of behaviors engaged in by the person during a particular period of life. The secondary-roles subdimension is defined as roles that are assumed to complete the tasks associated with developmental stage and the primary role. The tertiary-roles subdimension is defined as roles that are related primarily to secondary roles and represent ways in which individuals meet their role associated obligations.

Somewhat concrete propositions: The primary-, secondary-, and tertiary-role subdimensions of the role function mode dimension of Roy's Adaptation Model concept response mode were represented by the middle-range theory concept functional status of a caregiver of a child in a body cast. The primary-role subdimension was represented by the theory concept dimension personal-care activities. The secondary-roles subdimension was represented by the theory concept dimensions household activities, child-care activities, occupational activities, and educational activities. The tertiary-roles subdimension was represented by the theory concept dimension social and community activities.

More concrete proposition: Functional status of a caregiver of a child in a body cast is defined as the extent to which maternal or paternal caregivers or parental surrogates continue their usual household, social and community, child-care, personal-care, occupational, and educational activities while caring for a child in a body cast.

Most concrete proposition: Functional status of a caregiver of a child in a body cast was measured by the Inventory of Functional and Status-Caregiver of a Child in a Body Cast (IFSCCBC).

In addition, a hierarchy of propositions based on deductive reasoning can be constructed using the formalized version of nonrelational theory Propositions 2, 3, 4, and 5 and nonrelational theory Proposition 7. The deductive hierarchy is:

Axiom$_1$: If a parent experiences alterations in the performance of usual role activities when he or she is the caregiver of a child in a body cast, and

Axiom$_2$: if within the context of Roy's Adaptation Model, the actual performance of primary-, secondary-, and tertiary-role activities is regarded as functional status, then

Theorem: a parent experiences alterations in functional status when he or she is the caregiver of a child in a body cast.

The theorem is the formal proposition that supports the formalization of the measured operational definition given earlier.

DIAGRAMS

The conceptual-theoretical-empirical structure for the research is illustrated in Figure D–1. Two other diagrams were constructed to illustrate the one concept middle-range theory before and after testing (Fig. D–2). As can be seen in Figure D–2, the educational activities dimension of the concept functional status of a caregiver of a child in a body cast was not retained after psychometric analysis of the IFSCCBC.

EVALUATION OF THE CONCEPTUAL-THEORETICAL-EMPIRICAL STRUCTURE

Analysis of Newman's research report revealed that a one-concept middle-range descriptive classification theory was tested. The concept is functional status of a care-giver of a child in a body cast. The six dimensions of the theory that was tested are personal-care activities, household activities, child-care activities, occupational activities, educational activities, and social and community activities (Fig. D–2).

EVALUATION OF CONCEPTUAL-THEORETICAL-EMPIRICAL LINKAGES

Specification Adequacy

The criterion of specification adequacy is met. The conceptual model that guided Newman's theory-testing research is explicitly identified as Roy's Adaptation Model. Roy's model is discussed in sufficient breadth and depth so that its relation to the middle-range theory and the empirical research method of psychometric analysis of the IFSCCBC is clear.

Linkage Adequacy

The criterion of linkage adequacy also is met. The linkage between the role function mode dimension and subdimensions of the conceptual model concept response mode and the middle-range theory concept functional status of a caregiver of a child in a body cast and its dimensions is stated explicitly in the research report.

Conceptual Model Usage Rating Scale

Evaluation of the criteria of specification adequacy and linkage adequacy is summarized by application of the Conceptual Model Usage Rating Scale. Newman's research report earned a score of 3, indicating adequate use of Roy's Adaptation Model in the development of the middle-range theory of the functional status of caregivers of children in body casts.

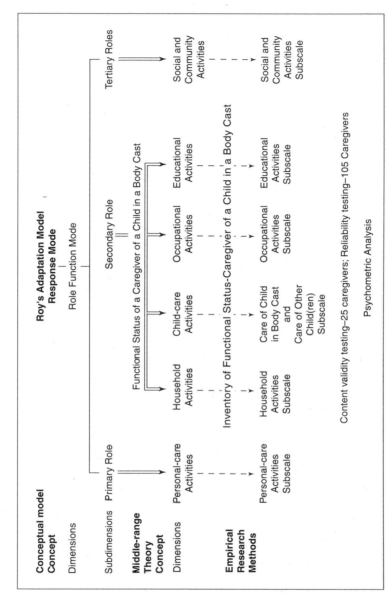

Figure D–I ■ Conceptual-theoretical-empirical structure for Newman's research.

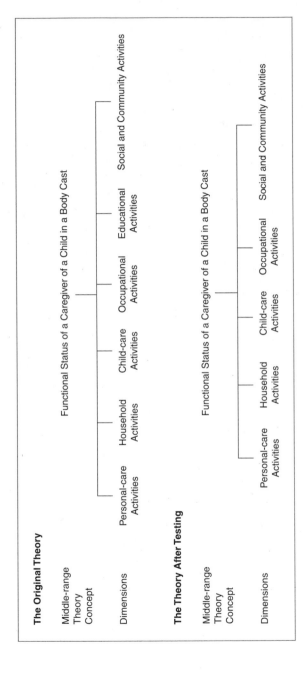

Figure D–2 ■ The theory before and after testing.

EVALUATION OF THE THEORY

Significance

The middle-range theory of the functional status of caregivers of children in body casts meets the criterion of significance. Newman addressed social significance in the introductory section of the report. She stated:

■ Mothers, fathers, and others who care for young children in body casts face challenges that disrupt their usual pattern of daily living. The developmental needs of the child, the specific care requirements related to the body cast, and the changes in usual caregiver activities imposed by the child's special care requirements comprise the typical challenges that must be faced.

Newman addressed theoretical significance in the background section of the report. She pointed out that "Little is known about the impact of caring for a child in a body cast on the caregiver's functional status." After reviewing the existing research, including a qualitative study she conducted, she explained, "The IFSCCBC built on the findings of the qualitative study, and was specifically designed to quantify the functional status of parents or their surrogates while caring for a child in a body cast."

Internal Consistency

The middle-range theory of the functional status of caregivers of children in body casts meets the criterion of internal consistency in part. Semantic clarity is evident in that the theory concept is constitutively defined initially in a clear and concise manner, and the constitutive definition that emerged from the psychometric analysis is easily extracted from the research report. The dimensions of the theory concept, however, are not defined. Semantic consistency is generally evident. Although Newman uses the term "functional status" interchangeably with the phrase "actual role performance" and "performance of usual activities," the various terms do not create much confusion because Newman tells the reader that "actual performance of primary-, secondary-, and tertiary-role activities is regarded as functional status."

The propositions of the theory reflect structural consistency. A hierarchy based on level of abstraction and a hierarchy based on deductive reasoning were easily constructed from nonrelational propositions that were given in the report. There are no redundant propositions.

Parsimony

The middle-range theory of the functional status of caregivers of children in body casts meets the criterion of parsimony. The analysis revealed that the theory that was tested was made up of one concept with six dimensions (Fig. D–2). Psychometric analysis yielded an even more parsimonious theory made up of one concept with just five dimensions. In addition, Newman reported that the number of items on the IFSCCBC was reduced from 71 to 49 as a result of reliability testing (Table D–2, middle-range theory Proposition 10). Inasmuch as each item was a specific activity that might be performed by caregivers of children in body casts, the reliability testing yielded a much more parsimonious list of activities.

Testability

The middle-range theory of the functional status of caregivers of children in body casts meets the criterion of testability. The original theory of the functional status of caregivers of children in body casts was tested through development and psychometric analysis of the IFSCCBC. The implicit hypothesis that 71 IFSCCBC items were required to capture the full domain of activities comprising functional status of a caregiver of a child in a body cast was falsified, as was the implicit hypothesis that the correlations between the IFSCCBC subscales would be of low magnitude.

Furthermore, the theory that emerged from the psychometric testing also is testable. The nonrelational proposition to be tested is:

> The phenomenon known as functional status of a caregiver of a child in a body cast encompasses the dimensions of personal-care activities, household activities, child-care activities, occupational activities, and social and community activities; the dimension of child-care activities encompasses the two subdimensions of care of child in body cast and care of other child(ren).

That proposition could be empirically tested by means of psychometric analysis to test the following falsifiable hypothesis:

> The 49 items of the Inventory of Functional Status-Caregiver of a Child in a Body Cast are categorized into six subscales: Personal-Care Activities, 10 items; Household Activities, 9 items; Care of Child in Body Cast Activities, 8 items; Care of Other Child(ren) Activities, 9 items; Occupational Activities, 7 items; and Social and Community Activities, 6 items.

EVALUATION OF THE RESEARCH DESIGN

Operational Adequacy

The research design meets the criterion of operational adequacy. The sample used for content validity testing was representative of the clinical population of interest, as was the sample used for reliability and construct validity testing. Indeed, Newman pointed out that she selected actual caregivers of children in body casts as the content validity judges "because they, rather than the conceptual model, the literature, other instruments, or health care providers, were regarded as the experts with regard to particular activities that comprised the IFSCCBC items." Moreover, the reliability and construct validity testing sample was recruited from orthopedic clinics located in a relatively wide geographic area and all subjects were the primary caregivers of children who had been in body casts for an average of 2 months.

The size of the content validity sample was adequate but a question might be raised about the size of the sample for reliability and construct validity testing. In particular, some researchers might regard 105 subjects as too few for the psychometric analysis of a 71-item instrument. However, experts do not agree on the number of subjects needed for psychometric studies. Moreover, Guadagnoli and Velicer (1988) pointed out that "rules of thumb" for the number of subjects per item lack any theoretical rationale and demonstrated that such rules also lack empirical support.

The IFSCCBC was directly derived from the theory, with clear correspondence between the dimensions of the concept functional status of a caregiver of a child in a body cast and the instrument subscales. Furthermore, the data-collection procedure was appropriate and the statistical techniques associated with the descriptive research method of psychometric analysis were used in an appropriate manner.

EVALUATION OF THE RESEARCH FINDINGS
Empirical Adequacy

The middle-range theory of the functional status of caregivers of children in body casts does not meet the criterion of empirical adequacy. Psychometric analysis revealed that the implicit hypothesis of 71 IFSCCBC items was not supported (Table D–2, middle-range theory Proposition 10). The results of the psychometric analysis yielded just 49 IFSCCBC items, which measure the personal-care activities, household activities, occupational activities, child-care activities, and social and community activities dimensions of the theory concept functional status of a caregiver of a child in a body cast. The educational activities dimension of the theory concept could not be retained due to very low reliability of the items comprising the IFSCCBC educational activities subscale (Table D–2, middle-range theory Proposition 11; Fig. D–2). It is possible that the educational activities subscale was not reliable because just five percent of the sample were students at the time of data collection. Further research is needed to determine if the original theory would meet the empirical adequacy criterion if administered to a sample that included a larger subsample of caregivers who were students. Further research also is needed to determine if the more parsimonious theory meets the empirical adequacy criterion when tested with a different sample. Furthermore, the implicit hypothesis that the correlations between the IFSCCBC subscales would be of low magnitude was not supported (Table D–2, middle-range theory Proposition 12).

EVALUATION OF THE UTILITY OF THE THEORY FOR PRACTICE
Pragmatic Adequacy

The findings of Newman's theory-testing research meet the criterion of pragmatic adequacy. The theory of the functional status of caregivers of children in body casts is relevant for the parents or parental surrogates who care for a child during the time that the child is in a body cast. Newman suggested clinical practice guidelines when she pointed out that "Nurses working with children recognize the need to provide comprehensive care for the child and his or her caregivers. The IFSCCBC provides a mechanism to assess the functional status of the caregiver, . . . during the time that the child is in a body cast." Furthermore, Newman provided a recommendation for timing of administration of the IFSCCBC and pointed out diverse methods of its administration.

The feasibility of the use of the IFSCCBC in clinical situations is supported, inasmuch as data for psychometric testing were collected in typical clinical settings. Minimal training is required to use the IFSCCBC, and the cost of duplicating the instrument should be minimal. Moreover, the use of the IFSCCBC should be congruent with caregivers' expectations. Indeed, attention to the impact of caring for a child in a body cast on their own performance of usual activities may even exceed the caregivers' expectations. In addition, nurses and other health care providers have the legal ability to use the IFSCCBC as an assessment tool.

It is anticipated that the results of the assessment would lead to nursing interventions. Indeed, Newman identified some nursing interventions that might follow from the assessment of the caregiver's functional status. Research is, of course, required to determine the efficacy of those interventions.

EVALUATION OF THE CONCEPTUAL MODEL

Credibility

The credibility of Roy's Adaptation Model, which Newman used to guide the development of the IFSCCBC, is not addressed explicitly in the report. Examination of the findings of the psychometric analysis of the IFSCCBC revealed some support for the credibility of Roy's model. In particular, the subscales measuring activities linked to the three subdimensions of the role function mode (i.e., primary-, secondary-, and tertiary-roles) were retained, and the item-to-subscale internal consistency reliability coefficients were satisfactory. A question about the credibility of the Roy model is raised, however, by the finding of a relatively high correlation ($r = .79$) between the IFSCCBC subscale measuring primary-role activities (the personal-care activities subscale) and one of the subscales measuring secondary-role activities (the occupational activities subscale). Additional research is needed to determine whether caregivers of children in body casts view personal-care activities and occupational activities as the same or different dimensions of functional status. Because at the time of Newman's study approximately one-half of the caregivers who participated were unemployed, on leave from work, or looking for work, in future research an attempt should be made to increase the number of caregivers who are employed during the time that the child is in a body cast.

References

Guadagnoli, E., & Velicer, W.F. (1988). Relation of sample size to the stability of component patterns. *Psychological Bulletin, 103,* 265–275.

Newman, D.M.L. (1997). The Inventory of Functional Status-Caregiver of a Child in a Body Cast. *Journal of Pediatric Nursing, 12,* 142–147.

Roy, C., & Andrews, H.A. (1991). *The Roy adaptation model: The definitive statement.* Norwalk, CT: Appleton and Lange.

Analysis and Evaluation of a Descriptive Theory-Testing Study:
The Survey Method

Stress Experience of Spouses of Patients Having Coronary Artery Bypass During Hospitalization and 6 Weeks After Discharge

Nancy Trygar Artinian, PhD, RN

The purpose of this study was to describe stress process variables in spouses of patients having coronary artery bypass surgery during hospitalization (T_1) and 6 weeks after discharge (T_2). Problems and concerns of spouses at T_1 and T_2 and spouse perceptions of nurse support were also addressed. Eighty-six women participated in the study at T_1 and 67 women participated at T_2. Data were collected by self-report instruments and open-ended questions. Women reported an average number of family life changes and high levels of social support at T_1 and T_2. Women perceived their husband's illness severity at the extreme end of the continuum at T_1 and T_2. Physical and mental symptoms of stress were high at T_1 but significantly less at T_2. Marital quality was average at T_1 but significantly less at T_2. Hospital environment, lack of information, and family members were frequently reported to make hospitalization more difficult. Husband's self-care activities, uncertainty, and husband's physical and mental symptoms were concerns that spouses frequently reported at T_2.

The family is the usual context in which illness occurs. Because the family is an interdependent system, illness or change in one member of the system is followed by change in other members. Not only does the patient's illness affect the family but also the family's ability to deal in an optimal manner with its ill member has a significant impact on the patient's physical and emotional adaptation to the illness.[1-3]

Reprinted from *Heart and Lung*, 20(1), 52–59, 1991, with permission.

Although the need for coronary artery bypass graft (CABG) surgery may occur during any one of the family developmental stages, the spouse often remains the primary member in the family to weather the impact of the surgery. Researchers have found that spouses of the patient having CABG need to have questions answered honestly during the intraoperative period and to be called at home if the patient's condition changes after surgery.[4,5] Gilliss[6] found that spouses of patients undergoing cardiac surgery had more subjective stress than patients had, and that families encountered the following stressors: waiting for surgery, lack of control of hospital events, lack of privacy, feeling uninformed, and receiving misinformation from well-meaning friends. In a previous study,[7,8] I identified insensitivity and impersonalization from hospital staff, disrupted family life, financial strain, family member distress, lack of intrafamily support, and waiting for surgery as concerns among family members of patients hospitalized for CABG. Stanley[9] found social activity, role changes, sexual functioning, vigilance, and economic adequacy as problem areas of adjustment 4 to 10 weeks after the mate's bypass surgery.

The stress of surgery may have a deleterious effect on the spouse's health, as well as impairing the spouse's ability to relate effectively with the patient. More research is needed to address the entire stress process of the spouse of the patient having CABG. Although problems and concerns of the spouse of the patient having CABG have been addressed, studies have not documented changes in stress process variables over time or investigated spouse perceptions of illness severity or of nurse support. In this study some of those gaps are addressed.

Information was obtained from female spouses about their stress experience during hospitalization (T_1) and 6 weeks after discharge (T_2). The following research questions were addressed:

1. What levels of hardships and demands, social support, perception of illness severity, coping responses, and stress responses do spouses of patients having CABG experience at T_1 and T_2?
2. Is there a significant change between T_1 and T_2 for the identified stress process variables?
3. What situation-specific hardships and demands do spouses of patients having CABG experience during hospitalization?
4. What situation-specific hardships and demands do spouses of patients having CABG have after their husband's return home?
5. What support do spouses of patients having CABG receive from nurses?

CONCEPTUAL FRAMEWORK AND DEFINITIONS

The Spouse Stress Theoretical Model that I deduced from Roy's[10] conceptual model provided the overall framework for this study (Fig. 1). In the Roy nursing model, the person is an adaptive system with stimuli input, mediating internal processes, and behavioral output. The advantage of using the Roy nursing model over other stress models such as Lazarus's is that it directs assessment of multiple dimensions of stress response.

For the purpose of this study the following definitions were used:

Hardships and demands refers to major life changes that may have occurred before the critical illness event that result in continuing strains on family life.[11]

Social support is an interpersonal transaction involving one or more of the following: affect, affirmation, or aid.[12]

Perception of illness severity refers to spouses' subjective definitions of the seriousness of their partner's illness.

Active coping includes cognitive or behavioral attempts to manage one's appraisal of the stressfulness of the event or deal directly with the problem and its effects.[13]

Avoidance coping refers to attempts to avoid actively confronting the problem.[13]

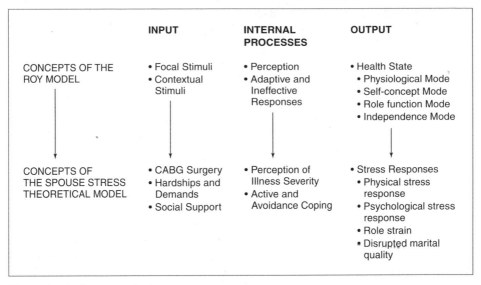

Figure 1 ■ Person as adaptive system.

Stress responses refer to dysfunctional or disrupted behavior in the physical, psychologic, and social dimensions of spouses in response to a critical illness event.

METHOD

DESIGN AND SAMPLE. A descriptive design was used to conduct this longitudinal study. The sample was a convenience sample of spouses of patients having CABG admitted to three Midwestern hospitals. All spouses who met the following criteria were admitted to the sample: (1) female (to control for sex differences only women were used), (2) husband undergoing his "first" CABG surgery, (3) lives with husband, (4) able to read and understand English, (5) in the intensive care unit (ICU) waiting room on the day of surgery, and (6) agrees to a second contact by mail 6 weeks after discharge.

The sample consisted of 86 women between the ages of 32 years and 74 years with a mean of 56 years. Educational level of the women ranged from 8 to 19 years with a mean of 13 years. The average family income of this sample was $40,000 to $49,999. Sixty-seven respondents remained in the study at T_2, representing a 22% attrition rate.

PROCEDURE. Spouses were initially contacted on the day of surgery in the ICU waiting room. The study was explained very briefly through a personal encounter accompanied by introductory letters from the investigator and cardiac surgeon. A time was arranged to meet the spouse on the first or second postoperative day. During the second meeting spouses were given a detailed explanation of the study and also provided with a consent form. Women who consented to participate were given an instrument packet and were asked to return it as instructed within 48 hours. Respondents were given 48 hours to complete the instruments to minimize the possibility that answering a large number of questions would cause more stress. Many respondents stated that the instrument gave them something to do while they were in the waiting room. Six weeks later women received the second instrument packet in the mail.

INSTRUMENTS. *Family Inventory of Life Events and Changes* (FILE) was one of the tools to measure hardships and demands.[11] FILE is a 71-item self-report of all life events experienced by the family. The overall Cronbach's alpha has been reported as 0.71 and was 0.86 in this sample (N = 86). Satisfactory validity assessments have been reported.[11]

The *Spouse Stressor Scale* (SSS) was developed for this study as a situation-specific measure of hardships and demands. The SSS contains 33 items on a Likert-type scale, which describe possible stressors associated with hospitalization to a critical care unit. Content validity was established through a panel of seven expert clinicians. Cronbach's alpha reliability was 0.93 in this sample.

The *Norbeck Social Support Questionnaire* (NSSQ) was used to measure social support.[14] The NSSQ measures affect, affirmation, and aid as functional components of social support. Satisfactory concurrent and construct validity and reliability have been reported.[14]

The *Indices of Coping Responses*[13] measured active and avoidance coping by asking respondents to rate their frequency of use of 32 different coping responses on a 0 to 3 scale (changed from 1 to 4 on original instrument to increase conceptual clarity). Satisfactory levels of reliability and validity have been reported.[13]

A *Cantril Self-Anchoring Ladder* was used to obtain respondents' perceptions of the severity of their husbands' condition.[15] A ladder device with rungs numbered 0 to 10 was used to represent spouses' definitions of the two extremes of severity on a scale measuring "minimal severity" (0) to "extreme severity" (10).

The *Strain Questionnaire* (SQ) was used to measure physical and psychologic stress responses.[16] The SQ is a 48-item scale designed to measure self-report levels of behavioral, cognitive, and physical stress complaints. For this study a 44-item scale was used. Four of the original items were dropped because of their overlap with items on the tool to measure coping. The scale range was changed from 1 to 5 to 0 to 4 to increase conceptual clarity. Reliability and validity have been reported for the SQ.[16]

The *Role Strain Scale* was designed for this study to measure disrupted or dysfunctional behavior in the role-function mode. The Role Strain Scale, a 10-item scale, was adapted from a role strain measurement developed by Katz and Piotrkowski.[17] Cronbach's alpha for this sample was 0.95. Respondents rate on a Likert-type scale how easy or difficult it is to arrange time to do various role activities. The possible Role Strain Scale range is from 0 to 40, 40 reflecting extreme difficulty in arranging time to do various role-related activities.

The *Dyadic Adjustment Scale*, a 32-item scale, was used to measure marital quality.[18] The possible score range is from 0 to 151 with the highest score indicating the best marital quality. Evidence for reliability and validity has been reported in the literature.[18] Cronbach's alpha for this sample was 0.91.

DATA ANALYSIS. Descriptive statistics were used to assess all study variables. Matched-pairs *t*-tests were used to compare mean scores on the main study variables at T_1 and T_2. Qualitative data from open-ended questions were analyzed by content analysis.

RESULTS

DESCRIPTION OF MAIN STUDY VARIABLES. The first two research questions addressed levels of stress process variables experienced by spouses and whether changes between T_1 and T_2 were significant (Table I). There was not a significant difference between hardships and demands experienced at T_1 and T_2. The FILE mean was slightly lower than 9.21, the norm, although the norm reflected family life changes occurring during and before the 12 months in relation to the time of measurement.[11] The FILE mean for this study reflected family life changes that occurred only during the 12 months before cardiac surgery.

Table I ■ **DIFFERENCES BETWEEN T_1 AND T_2 FOR EACH STUDY VARIABLE**

Variable	Mean	SD	t value*	Two-tailed probability
Hardships and demands (FILE)				
T_1	7.94	5.83	0.62	0.539
T_2	7.61	5.74		
Social support (NSSQ)				
T_1	66.24	8.08	1.65	0.103
T_2	65.09	8.84		
Perception of illness severity (Ladder Scale)				
T_1	8.62	1.93	5.36	0.000
T_2	6.83	2.91		
Active coping (Indices of Coping Responses)				
T_1	66.70	11.32	−0.54	0.589
T_2	67.32	10.03		
Avoidance coping (Indices of Coping Responses)				
T_1	11.76	2.64	−0.32	0.747
T_2	11.88	2.73		
Physical and psychological stress response (SQ)				
T_1	38.72	28.76	5.01	0.000
T_2	27.00	28.07		
Role strain (Role Strain Scale)				
T_1	10.52	8.07	0.79	0.432
T_2	9.84	8.11		
Marital quality stress response (Dyadic Adjustment Scale)				
T_1	106.19	16.09	2.13	0.037
T_2	102.13	19.85		

*Paired t test.

Women had fairly high levels of social support, and no significant difference was found between T_1 and T_2. The social support scores reported reflect a modification of Norbeck's[19] directions for scoring. The mean network size was 11.41, and in this sample the size of the network was positively related to a composite stress response score ($r = 0.24$, $p < 0.015$). Women in this sample who had larger networks had more stress response; thus functional support scores for this study were modified by controlling for network size. Under revised scoring procedures the total possible support score was 72.

Women had fairly high levels of perception of illness severity at T_1 with levels significantly less at T_2. Taking the instrument modifications into account, this sample used active coping more frequently than the normed community sample (mean 36.99) of adults, and there was not a significant difference between T_1 and

T_2. Avoidance coping methods were also used more frequently than the normed community sample (mean 3.55), and there was not a significant difference between T_1 and T_2.

Adjusting for instrument modifications, the physical and mental stress response score was the norm at T_1 and slightly below the norm at T_2. The change in physical and mental stress response between T_1 and T_2 was significant. Respondents had low to moderate levels of role strain, and the difference between the T_1 and T_2 was not significant. The marital quality score at T_1 was 106.19 and at T_2 was 102.13. As a basis of comparison, a study by Spanier[18] yielded a mean marital quality score of 114.8 in a community sample of 218 married persons. This study's sample had a lower mean dyadic adjustment score at T_1 than the comparison community sample and the score was significantly less at T_2.

STRESSORS ENCOUNTERED BY SPOUSES DURING HOSPITALIZATION. The SSS supplemented FILE as a measure of hardships and demands specific to hospitalization. The range of scores in this study was from 0 to 103, out of a total of 132, with a mean of 36.51 and an SD of 28.81. On the whole this study's sample reported a low to moderate amount of hospital-related stressors.

Specific items from the SSS that were rated fairly to extremely stressful by 40% or more of the respondents included: (1) inability to discuss my partner's progress with the physician every day, (2) not knowing the specific facts concerning my spouse's progress, (3) not knowing my spouse's chances for a satisfactory recovery, (4) not knowing exactly what is being done for my spouse, (5) having to travel long distances to get to and from the hospital, (6) inability to see my spouse as often as I would like, (7) uncomfortable furniture in the waiting room, and (8) not knowing which hospital staff members to approach for information.

The qualitative data provided further information about what exacerbates the stressfulness of hospitalization. Several different categories of answers came forth from the open-ended question, "Is there anything or anyone that has been unpleasant or made this situation more difficult for you to cope with?" (Table II). The majority of spouses responded that there was no one or nothing that made their situation more difficult for them. However, 20% described the hospital environment or hospital personnel as being unpleasant. Typical responses mentioned that the volunteer in the waiting room was insensitive, the waiting room was too small, the waiting room chairs were too hard, or the visiting hours were unreasonable. Twelve percent answered that other family members made their situation more difficult. One women stated, "My children have made this time difficult; they are angry at me, like it is my fault." Only a small number of respondents reported that "other responsibilities" or "their spouse" made coping with their situation difficult.

PROBLEMS AND CONCERNS OF SPOUSES AFTER DISCHARGE. The qualitative data also enhanced insight into the stressfulness of the immediate postdischarge period (Table III). At T_2, several categories of answers emerged in response to the question, "What

Table II ■ **SPOUSES' DESCRIPTIONS OF FACTORS THAT MADE THEIR HOSPITALIZATION EXPERIENCE MORE DIFFICULT (N = 86)**

Factor	No.	%
Nothing	52	60
Hospital environment or hospital personnel	17	20
Family members	10	12
Other responsibilities	3	3
Husband	2	2

Table III ■ **SPOUSES' DESCRIPTIONS OF PROBLEMS AND CONCERNS THAT MADE ADJUSTMENT CONTINUE TO BE DIFFICULT 6 WEEKS AFTER SURGERY (N = 67)**

Problem/concern	No.	%
Most frequently reported		
Husband's eating and exercise habits and activity level	26	39
Uncertainty about husband's future or about what to expect	23	34
Husband's mental state/depression	16	24
Taking on new and/or additional responbilities	16	24
Husband's physical symptoms	13	19
Life not back to "normal"	8	12
Preparing special diet	7	10
Least frequently reported		
Uncertainty re: "doing all the right things for him"	5	7
Getting time to myself	5	7
Husband has not returned to work	4	6
Husband insensitive to their needs	3	4
Fear of leaving husband alone	2	3
Depleted finances	2	3
Family arguments	1	1

concerns have you had since your husband has been home?" Thirty-nine percent referred to their husband's activity level or eating and exercise habits as a concern. "My biggest problem is keeping him from overdoing it," "My husband isn't walking enough," or "My husband is not watching his diet" were typical responses.

Thirty-four percent stated that uncertainty about their husband's future or about what to expect was a concern. One women stated, "Will my husband have another heart attack? I really don't know what to expect, which makes me feel very confused at times." Another spouse stated, "I am always wondering: Is this how he should feel? Is he progressing normally? Is there something I should be doing to help him?"

Twenty-four percent discussed their husband's mental state as a concern. Some examples were, "It has been difficult coping with my husband's irritability," "Trying to cheer him up hasn't been easy," "Coping with his depression has been tough," and "I think I have had the most difficulty with his mood swings."

Taking on new additional responsibilities was also cited as a concern by 24%. Sample responses in this category were, "It's been tough going back to work full-time after not working outside the home in 17 years," or "It is not easy learning how to drive when you are 60, but I am trying."

Physical symptoms that their husbands experienced such as inability to sleep, pain, breathing problems, or high blood pressure, were concerns for 19%. Twelve percent stated that "life isn't back to normal" or "having to make so many changes in routine" has been difficult. Preparing the special diet was difficult for 10%. For example, one woman said, "Making meals and reading labels on everything I buy hasn't been easy."

Several categories of answers had only a few respondents. Concerns least frequently reported were fear about "doing the right things" for their husband, not having time to themselves, husband still off work, husband insensitive to their needs, leaving their husband alone, depleted finances, and an increase in family arguments. SPOUSE PERCEPTIONS OF SUPPORT FROM NURSES DURING HOSPITALIZATION. Several categories of answers emerged in response to the question, "Describe an incident in which you thought you received support from a nurse" (Table IV). Thirty per-

Table IV ■ SPOUSES' PERCEPTIONS OF SUPPORT FROM NURSES
DURING HOSPITALIZATION (N = 67)

Supportive behavior	No.	%
Giving explanations	20	30
Giving reassurance	11	16
Permitting flexible visiting hours	5	7
Making an "extra effort" or displaying kindness and thoughtfulness	5	7
Giving encouragement to call hospital at any time	2	3
Providing competent care to husband	2	3

cent thought nurses were supportive when they gave explanations. Typical responses were, "I found the nurses helpful when they answered all our questions honestly," or "Nurses were great when they explained what they were doing and why they were doing it." Sixteen percent found nurses supportive when they gave reassurance. Women described the following nursing actions as reassuring: "She reassured me that my husband's confusion was not unusual and that it would disappear," "It was reassuring to have the nurse call me each night to let me know how he was doing," or "One nurse told me she would care for my husband as if he were her own father."

Seven percent found nurses who permitted flexible visiting hours supportive. Seven percent also found nurses supportive when they displayed certain behavioral manifestations such as (1) making an extra effort: "My husband lost his rosary and he was so upset when he couldn't find it [that] his nurse went down to the laundry and found it," or (2) having an "excellent bedside manner" such as displaying "kindness and thoughtfulness." A small number of women found nurses supportive when "they encouraged me to call the hospital at any time," or when they provided competent care to their husbands such as "giving pain medication promptly" or "suctioning and assisting husband to breathe easier."

SPOUSE PERCEPTIONS OF NONSUPPORT FROM NURSES DURING HOSPITALIZATION.
The majority of respondents were unable to describe any situations in which nurses had been nonsupportive (Table V). However, there were a few nursing actions that spouses perceived as not helpful. Twelve percent described certain nonsupportive behavioral manifestations, such as answering questions abruptly, unwillingness to answer a request, making light of their concerns, "being in a rush," or "acting businesslike and distant."

Twelve percent believed nurses were nonsupportive when they did not provide competent care. Spouses' perceptions of noncompetent care related to "waiting forever for the nurse to answer my husband's light," "not giving my husband pain medication when he requested it," or "not giving explanations to me, only to my husband." Three percent thought nurses were nonsupportive when they did not

Table V ■ SPOUSES' PERCEPTION OF NONSUPPORT FROM NURSES
DURING HOSPITALIZATION (N = 67)

Nonsupportive behavior	No.	%
No nonsupportive behaviors	43	64
Behavioral manifestations	8	12
Did not provide care that husband needed	8	12
Did not answer questions	2	3
Felt alone	2	3

answer questions, and 3% described the feeling of being "completely alone" in the hospital and thought that this feeling somehow related to activities of nurses.

LIMITATIONS

Certain limitations to this study need to be taken into account as the findings of this sample are interpreted. First, the use of a nonprobability sample carries the risk that subjects who agreed to participate differed in some meaningful way from subjects who were not willing to participate. Twenty-seven percent refused to participate, stating that they were "too nervous," "ill," or "stressed." In addition, the method of selection leaves open the questions: Are spouses who are not in the waiting room on the day of surgery different from those who are? Do they use more avoidance coping strategies? Do they have more life stresses? Second, there was a 22% attrition rate between T_1 and T_2. Furthermore, the sample was limited to female spouses. All of the factors mentioned above limit the representatives of the sample.

DISCUSSION

On the basis of the study findings, it was evident that women had had an average amount of family life change within the 12 months before their husband's surgery, which suggests that the women were adjusting simultaneously to multiple life changes rather than solely to their husband's surgery and recovery. Most women were fortunate to have high levels of social support, which remained consistent between T_1 and T_2. This finding is consistent with Stanley's[9] finding that the level of spouse satisfaction with social support was high 4 to 10 weeks after bypass surgery. It is interesting to note that at T_1, women listed fairly large numbers in their social network, perhaps because of the crisis nature of cardiac surgery. The number in the network was positively related to stress response, which is consistent with the literature that states that there are costs to maintaining social support relationships.[20]

The majority of women in the study perceived their husband's condition at the time of surgery to be at the extreme severity end of the scale with the level of severity perceived as significantly less at T_2. However, 60% of the sample still perceived their husband's condition to be serious 6 weeks after discharge; that is, they perceived their husband's condition to be at level 7 or above on the ladder scale of severity. There were no significant differences between the frequency of use of coping methods at T_1 and T_2. This finding is consistent with the finding that levels of stressors were the same during hospitalization and at home 6 weeks after discharge.

Although women continued to have physical and mental symptoms of stress at T_2, they were significantly less than at T_1, which is often considered to be a time of crisis. Women had low but consistent levels of role strain at T_1 and T_2. At T_1 wives had slightly lower levels of marital quality than average, and the level was significantly lower at T_2. The findings suggest that worry, fear, anxiety, and perceived caretaking responsibilities affected the marital relationship. However, these findings need to be interpreted with caution because the status of the preoperative marital relationships is unknown.

Fortunately, the majority of women could not describe factors that made their hospital experience more difficult; however, the reliability of those responses and whether women felt free to share their true responses may be questioned. Factors that were stressful for some women related to lack of information about their husband's status and treatment. Other factors such as standardized hospital regulations, for example, waiting room policies and visiting hours, and intrafamily problems were also seen as problematic. Although taking on other responsibilities was infrequently reported as a problem at T_1, it became a greater concern at T_2.

Many factors were identified that made adjustment at home difficult and that help explain why at T_2 levels of marital quality were lower and perceptions of illness severity still remained at the extreme end of the scale. Women were bothered by their husbands' self-care activities such as poor eating habits, lack of exercise, or overextended activity levels. It was very difficult for women to cope with uncertainty either related to their husbands' life expectancy, their husbands' projected course of recovery, or how they could best help their husbands. Women seemed unprepared for their husbands' irritability or depression. Physical symptoms were worrisome, and feeling that life was not back to normal at 6 weeks further compounded the stressfulness experienced at 6 weeks. It was also difficult for some women to adjust to preparing foods differently.

Nurses were not identified in spouses' network lists; however, when spouses were asked about support from nurses, giving explanations and reassurance, showing thoughtfulness and understanding, and permitting flexible visiting hours were important factors. It is positive to note that the majority of women could not discuss nurses as nonsupportive. A few cited hurried, abrupt, or distant behavior, not providing the care they thought their husbands needed, or not answering questions as nonsupportive nurse behavior.

IMPLICATIONS

The results of this study have several implications for nursing practice. The first implication is that nurses and other health professionals need to be attentive to the stress process experience of spouses after hospital discharge as well as during hospitalization. The stress experience is not confined to hospitalization but lingers until 6 weeks after surgery, if not longer. Follow-up home care should be incorporated into the total plan of care. Nurses and other health care providers need to make provisions for *planned* attempts at offering informational and emotional support during hospitalization as well as after discharge.

The findings suggest that women with larger social networks had a more difficult time with their husband's surgery. Because the size of the network does not equal the quality of support offered, nurses cannot assume that spouses surrounded by family and friends have all the help they need. It may be more important to target these women in nursing assessments.

Spouses' identifying lack of information as stressful indicates an important area for nursing intervention. Planned regular conferences with the spouse, nurse, and physician are needed. Many of the plans and aids used for cardiac preoperative and postoperative teaching are designed for the patient alone. Specific content relevant to spouses needs to be included in teaching plans. Other researchers have come to a similar conclusion, that is, that the spouse should be included in the rehabilitation program as early as possible.[21]

Reassessment of the hospital environment and hospital regulations needs to occur. Is an untrained volunteer the best person to supervise the intensive care waiting room? Can ICU policies and regulations be changed so that the needs of both nurses and spouses are met?

Problems and concerns reported by spouses after hospital discharge provide suggestions about how to prepare spouses for discharge. Nurses can help relieve some uncertainty. Preparing women to expect their husbands' possibly altered mental state and rehearsing with spouses how they might deal with it may prove to be a useful nursing intervention. Reviewing what physical symptoms husbands may exhibit at home, and helping spouses distinguish between "normal" and "abnormal" may help relieve anxiety. Developing a plan to follow if abnormal symptoms do occur may help spouses achieve a sense of competence. Arranging for the dietitian to provide meal preparation tips may also be helpful.

Levin[22] discussed "right responsibility," "overresponsibility," "caring," and "caretaking." Overresponsibility refers to the spouses assuming too much responsibility for their husbands' actions. Caretaking refers to spouses' attempts to control their husbands' activities. Right responsibility means basing actions on an accurate perception of reality. Caring, motivated by love, involves letting go and encouraging independence. Discussing these issues with the spouse before discharge may lessen spouses' concerns related to their husbands' self-care activities.

In summary, the findings suggest that cardiac surgery is a prolonged stressful experience for spouses. The findings help explain why spouses of patients having cardiac surgery might have more subjective stress than patients, as found by Gilliss.[6] Fortunately the findings also suggest many ways that nurses can intervene to help spouses cope with their husbands' cardiac surgery. ■

References

1. Bedsworth J, Molen M. Psychological stress in spouses with myocardial infarction. Heart Lung 1982;11:450–6.
2. Chatham MA. The effect of family involvement on patients' manifestations of postcardiotomy psychosis. Heart Lung 1978;7:995–9.
3. Radley A, Green R. Bearing illness: study of couples where the husband awaits coronary graft surgery. Soc Sci Med 1986;23:577–85.
4. Norheim C. Family needs of patients having coronary artery bypass graft surgery during the intraoperative period. Heart Lung 1989;18:622–6.
5. Rodgers CD. Needs of relatives of cardiac surgery patients during the critical care phase. Focus Crit Care 1983;10(5):50–5.
6. Gillis CL. Reducing family stress during and after coronary artery bypass surgery. Nurs Clin North Am 1984;19:103–12.
7. Artinian NT. Bypass surgery: families' perceptions. Applied Nursing Research 1988;1;43–4.
8. Artinian NT. Family member perceptions of a cardiac surgery events. Focus Crit Care 1989;16:301–8.
9. Stanley MJB. Adjustment problems of spouses of patients undergoing coronary artery bypass graft surgery during early convalescence. Heart Lung 1988;17:677–82.
10. Roy C. Introduction to nursing: an adaptation model. 2nd ed. Englewood Cliffs, New Jersey: Prentice-Hall, 1984.
11. McCubbin HI, Patterson JM. FILE family inventory life events and changes. In: McCubbin HI, Thompson AJ, eds. Family assessment inventories for research and practice. Madison, Wisconsin: University of Wisconsin-Madison, 1987;21–39.
12. Kahn RI, Antonucci TC. Convoys over the life course; attachment, roles and social support. In: Baltes P, Brim O, eds. Life-span development behavior. New York: Academic Press, 1980;253–86.
13. Moos RH, Cronkite RC, Billings AG, Finney IW. Health and daily living form manual. Palo Alto, California: Social Ecology Laboratory, Department of Psychiatry and Behavioral Sciences, Veterans Administration and Stanford University Medical Centers, 1986.
14. Norbeck JS, Lindsey AM, Carrieri VL. The development of an instrument to measure social support. Nurs Res 1981;30:264–9.
15. Cantril H. The pattern of human concerns. New Brunswick, New Jersey: Rutgers University Press, 1965.
16. Lefebvre RC, Standford SL. A multi-model questionnaire for stress. J Human Stress 1985;11:69–75.
17. Katz MH, Piotrkowski CS. Correlates of role strain among employed black women. Family Relations 1983;32:331–9.
18. Spanier GB. Measuring dyadic adjustment: new scales for assessing the quality of marriage and similar dyads. J Marriage Fam 1976;38:15–28.
19. Norbeck J. Revised scoring instructions for the Norbeck social support questionnaire (NSSQ). San Francisco: University of California, 1984.
20. Tilden VP, Galyen RD. Cost and conflict: the darker side of social support. West J Nurs Res 1987;9:9–18.

21. Miller P, Wikoff R, McMahon M, Garrett MJ, Ringel K. Marital functioning after cardiac surgery. Heart Lung 1990;19:55–61.

22. Levin RF. Heartmates: a survival guide for the cardiac spouse. New York: Prentice-Hall, 1987.

ANALYSIS OF THE CONCEPTUAL-THEORETICAL-EMPIRICAL STRUCTURE

The stated purpose of Artinian's (1991) research was to describe stress process variables in spouses of patients having coronary artery bypass graft (CABG) surgery during hospitalization and 6 weeks after discharge. The research was designed to test a middle-range descriptive classification theory of spouses' CABG-related stress experiences by means of descriptive research, using the survey method. Although Artinian referred to the theory as "the spouse stress theoretical model," the decision was made to use the label "spouses' CABG-related stress experiences" to avoid confusion with the conceptual model and to bring the label for the theory closer to the clinical population of interest.

IDENTIFICATION OF CONCEPTS

Conceptual Model Concepts

Analysis of the research report revealed that the research was guided by Roy's (1984) Adaptation Model. The particular conceptual model concepts employed in the research are stimuli input, mediating internal processes, and behavioral output. The concept stimuli input encompasses two dimensions: focal stimuli and contextual stimuli. The concept mediating internal processes encompasses three dimensions: perception, adaptive responses, and ineffective responses. The concept behavioral output encompasses one dimension and four subdimensions. The dimension is health state, and the subdimensions are physiological mode, self-concept mode, role function mode, and interdependence mode.

Middle-Range Theory Concepts

Further analysis of the research report revealed that the middle-range descriptive classification theory of spouses' CABG-related stress experiences encompasses six concepts, five of which are multidimensional. All concepts and dimensions are listed in Table E–1.

The decision to include time as a concept was based on the centrality to the theory of the two time periods for data collection. The theory is categorized as a descriptive classification theory because the six concepts and the various dimensions are treated as mutually exclusive.

CLASSIFICATION OF MIDDLE-RANGE THEORY CONCEPTS

The classification of each middle-range theory concept is given in Table E–1. The theory concepts hardships and demands, social support, perception of illness severity, and coping responses are classified as constructs in both Kaplan's and Willer and Webster's schemata because the terms were invented for research purposes and can be inferred only through study participants' responses to questionnaires.

The theory concept hardships and demands is classified as a relational unit in Dubin's schema because it represents an interaction between the study participant and external events and stressors. The theory concept social support is classified as a relational unit in Dubin's schema because it involves an interaction between an individual and others who provide support.

The theory concept perception of illness severity is classified as an enumerative unit in Dubin's schema because, as measured in this study by the Cantril Self-Anchoring Ladder, a value representing no illness severity was not possible. Indeed, even though 0 was the lowest score on the scale, the descriptor for that score was "minimal severity." The theory concept coping responses is tentatively classified as an enumerative unit in Dubin's schema because the study participants' scores on the Indices of Coping Responses suggest that they used at least one coping response.

Table E–1 ■ THE THEORY OF SPOUSES' CABG-RELATED STRESS EXPERIENCES: CONCEPTS, THEIR DIMENSIONS, AND CLASSIFICATION

Concept Dimensions	Kaplan	Willer and Webster	Nonvariable or Variable	Dubin
Hardships and Demands Life Events Hospital-related Stressors Postdischarge Stressors	Construct	Construct	Variable	Relational Unit
Social Support Functional Support Social Network Nurse Support	Construct	Construct	Variable	Relational Unit
Perception of Illness Severity	Construct	Construct	Variable	Enumerative Unit
Coping Responses Active Coping Avoidance Coping	Construct	Construct	Variable	Enumerative Unit
Stress Responses Physical Psychologic Role Strain Marital Quality	Theoretical Term	Construct	Variable	Summative Unit
Time During Husband's Hospitalization for CABG 6 Weeks after Husband's Discharge	Observational Term	Observable	Variable	Enumerative Unit

The theory concept stress responses is classified as a theoretical term in Kaplan's schema, as a construct in Willer and Webster's schema, and as a summative unit in Dubin's schema because it refers to a complex, global phenomenon.

The theory concept time is classified as an observational term in Kaplan's schema and as an observable in Willer and Webster's schema because it most likely can be seen in a record kept by the investigator for each study participant. It is classified as an enumerative unit in Dubin's schema because it is always present.

All of the concepts are classified as variables because the scores for each one varied in this study. The concept time is classified as a variable because there are two time periods: during hospitalization and 6 weeks after discharge.

IDENTIFICATION AND CLASSIFICATION OF PROPOSITIONS

Conceptual Model Propositions

Just one nonrelational proposition addressing the concepts of Roy's Adaptation Model was evident in the report:

> In the Roy nursing model, the person is an adaptive system with stimuli input, mediating internal processes, and behavioral output.

That proposition can be formalized as three nonrelational propositions asserting the existence of phenomena:

> There is a phenomenon known as stimuli input.

> There is a phenomenon known as mediating internal processes.

> There is a phenomenon known as behavioral output.

In addition, nonrelational propositions asserting rudimentary constitutive definitions were extracted by combining the one nonrelational proposition found in the research report with the content of Figure 1 in the report. The constitutive definitions are:

> Stimuli input is defined as having two dimensions: focal stimuli and contextual stimuli.

> Mediating internal processes is defined as having three dimensions: perception, adaptive responses, and ineffective responses.

> Behavioral output is defined as having one dimension and four subdimensions. The dimension is health state, and the subdimensions are physiological mode, self-concept mode, role function mode, and interdependence mode.

Middle-Range Theory Propositions

Nonrelational and relational propositions that are central to the middle-range descriptive classification theory of spouses' CABG-related stress experiences are evident or can be extracted from the research report. The propositions that were stated explicitly in the report are listed in Table E–2.

Text continues on page 321

Table E–2 ■ **MIDDLE-RANGE THEORY PROPOSITIONS FROM ARTINIAN'S RESEARCH REPORT**

Proposition	Classification
1. Hardships and demands refers to major life changes that may have occurred before the critical illness that result in continuing strains on family life.	Nonrelational, Existence Constitutive Definition
2. Social support is an interpersonal transaction involving one or more of the following: affect, affirmation, or aid.	Nonrelational, Existence Constitutive Definition
3. Perception of illness severity refers to spouses' subjective definitions of the seriousness of their partner's illness.	Nonrelational, Existence Constitutive Definition
4. Active coping includes cognitive or behavioral attempts to manage one's appraisal of the stressfulness of the event or deal directly with the problem and its effects.	Nonrelational, Existence Constitutive Definition
5. Avoidance coping refers to attempts to avoid actively confronting the problem.	Nonrelational, Existence Constitutive Definition
6. Stress responses refer to dysfunctional or disrupted behavior in the physical, psychologic, and social dimensions of spouses in response to a critical illness event.	Nonrelational, Existence Constitutive Definition
7. [The] Family Inventory of Life Events and Changes (FILE) was one of the tools used to measure hardships and demands.	Nonrelational, Measured Operational Definition
8. The Spouse Stressor Scale (SSS) was developed for this study as a situation-specific measure of hardships and demands.	Nonrelational, Measured Operational Definition
9. Hardships and demands . . . [include] possible stressors associated with hospitalization to a critical care unit.	Nonrelational, Constitutive Definition
10. The Norbeck Social Support Questionnaire was used to measure social support.	Nonrelational, Measured Operational Definition
11. The Indices of Coping Responses measured active and avoidance coping.	Nonrelational, Measured Operational Definition
12. A Cantril Self-Anchoring Ladder was used to obtain respondents' perceptions of the severity of their husbands' condition.	Nonrelational, Measured Operational Definition
13. The Strain Questionnaire was used to measure physical and psychologic stress responses.	Nonrelational, Measured Operational Definition
14. The Role Strain Scale was designed for this study to measure disrupted or dysfunctional behavior in the role-function mode.	Nonrelational, Measured Operational Definition
15. Role strain [refers to] disrupted or dysfunctional behavior . . . [focusing on] arranging time to do various role-related activities.	Nonrelational, Constitutive Definition
16. The Dyadic Adjustment Scale was used to measure marital quality.	Nonrelational, Measured Operational Definition
17. There was not a significant difference between hardships and demands experienced at T_1 and T_2.	Relational, Existence Hypothesis
18. The FILE mean was slightly lower than 9.21, the norm.	Nonrelational, Level of Existence
19. Women had fairly high levels of social support.	Nonrelational, Level of Existence

(continued on page 320)

Table E–2 ■ **MIDDLE-RANGE THEORY PROPOSITIONS FROM ARTINIAN'S RESEARCH REPORT** (*Continued*)

Proposition	Classification
20. No significant difference [in the functional support dimension of social support] was found between T_1 and T_2.	Relational, Existence
21. In this sample the size of the [social] network was positively related to a composite stress response score ($r = 0.24$, $p < 0.015$). Women in this sample who had larger networks had more stress response.	Relational, Existence
22. Women had fairly high levels of perception of illness severity at T_1 with levels significantly less at T_2.	Nonrelational, Level of Existence Relational, Existence
23. This sample used active coping more frequently than the normed community sample of adults.	Nonrelational, Level of Existence
24. There was not a significant difference [in active coping] between T_1 and T_2.	Relational, Existence
25. Avoidance coping methods were also used more frequently than the normed community sample.	Nonrelational, Level of Existence
26. There was not a significant difference [in avoidance coping] between T_1 and T_2.	Relational, Existence
27. The physical and mental stress response score was the norm at T_1 and slightly below the norm at T_2.	Nonrelational, Level of Existence
28. The change in physical and mental stress response between T_1 and T_2 was significant.	Relational, Existence
29. Respondents had low to moderate levels of role strain.	Nonrelational, Level of Existence
30. The difference [in role strain] between T_1 and T_2 was not significant.	Relational, Existence
31. The marital quality score at T_1 was 106.19 and at T_2 was 102.13. The study's sample had a lower mean dyadic adjustment score at T_1 than the comparison community sample.	Nonrelational, Level of Existence
32. The score [for marital quality] was significantly less at T_2.	Relational, Existence
33. On the whole, this study's sample reported a low to moderate amount of hospital-related stressors.	Nonrelational, Level of Existence
34. [Hardships and demands include] stressors encountered by spouses during hospitalization.	Nonrelational, Consitutive Definition
35. [Stressors encountered by spouses during hospitalization was measured by the open-ended question,] "Is there anything or anyone that has been unpleasant or made this situation more difficult for you to cope with?"	Nonrelational, Measured Operational Definition
36. Several different categories of answers came forth from the open-ended question . . . The majority of spouses responded that there was no one or nothing that made their situation more difficult for them. However, 20% described the hospital environment or hospital personnel as unpleasant . . . Twelve percent answered that other family members made their situation more difficult . . . Only a small number of respondents reported that "other responsibilities" or "their spouse" made coping with the situation difficult.	Nonrelational, Level of existence
37. [Hardships and demands includes] the stressfulness of the immediate postdischarge period . . . [expressed as] problems and concerns of spouses after discharge.	Nonrelational, Constitutive Definition
38. Problems and concerns of spouses after discharge was measured by the open-ended question, "What concerns have you had since your husband has been home?"	Nonrelational, Measured Operational Definition
39. At T_2, several categories of answers emerged in response to the [open-ended] question [measuring the post-discharge stressors dimension of hardships and demands]. Thirty-nine percent referred	Nonrelational, Level of Existence

(*continued on page 321*)

Proposition	Classification
to their husband's activity level or eating and exercise. . . . Thirty-four percent stated that uncertainty about their husband's future or about what to expect was a concern. . . Twenty-four percent discussed their husband's mental state as a concern . . . Taking on new or additional responsibilities was also cited as a concern by 24% . . . Physical symptoms that their husbands experienced . . . were concerns for 19%. Twelve percent stated that "life isn't back to normal" or "having to make so many changes in routine" has been difficult. Preparing the special diet was difficult for 10%. Several categories of answers had only a few respondents. Concerns least frequently reported were fear about "doing the right things" for their husband, not having time to themselves, husband still off work, husband insensitive to their needs, leaving their husband alone, depleted finances, and an increase in family arguments.	
40. [Social support includes] spouse perceptions of support or nonsupport from nurses during hospitalization.	Nonrelational, Constitutive Definition
41. Spouse perceptions of support or nonsupport from nurses during hospitalization was measured by the open-ended question, "Describe an incident in which you thought you received support from a nurse."	Nonrelational, Measured Operational Definition
42. Several categories of answers emerged in response to the [open-ended] question [that measured the nurse support dimension of social support]. Thirty percent thought nurses were supportive when they gave explanations . . . Sixteen percent found nurses supportive when they gave reassurance . . . Seven percent found nurses who permitted flexible visiting hours supportive. Seven percent also found nurses supportive when they displayed certain behavioral manifestations . . . A small number of women found nurses supportive when "they encouraged me to call the hospital at any time," or when they provided competent care to their husbands . . . The majority of respondents were unable to describe any situations in which nurses had been nonsupportive. However, there were a few nursing actions that spouses perceived as not helpful. Twelve percent described certain nonsupportive behavioral manifestations . . . Twelve percent believed nurses were nonsupportive when they did not provide competent care . . . Three percent thought nurses were nonsupportive when they did not answer questions, and 3% described the feeling of being "completely alone" in the hospital and thought that this feeling somehow related to activities of nurses.	Nonrelational, Level of Existence

NONRELATIONAL PROPOSITIONS. Middle-range theory Propositions 1, 2, 3, 4, 5, and 6, combined with information extracted from the introductory section of the report, can be formalized as nonrelational existence propositions:

There is a phenomenon known as hardships and demands.

There is a phenomenon known as social support.

There is a phenomenon known as perception of illness severity.

There is a phenomenon known as coping responses.

There is a phenomenon known as stress responses.

Middle-range theory Propositions 1, 9, 34, and 37 can be combined into a nonrelational proposition asserting a constitutive definition for the concept hardships and demands. Formalized, the constitutive definition is:

> Hardships and demands is defined as having three dimensions: life events, hospital-related stressors, and postdischarge stressors. The dimension life events is defined as major life changes that may have occured before the critical illness that results in continuing strains on family life. The dimension hospital-related stressors is defined as possible stressors associated with hospitalization to a critical care unit, as well as other stressors encountered by spouses during hospitalization. The dimension postdischarge stressors is defined as problems and concerns experienced by spouses during the immediate postdischarge period.

Middle-range theory Propositions 2 and 40, along with information extracted from the instruments, results, and discussion sections of the report, can be formalized as a nonrelational proposition asserting a constitutive definition for the concept social support:

> Social support is defined as an interpersonal transaction and encompasses three dimensions: functional support, social network, and nurse support. The functional support dimension is defined as the level of affect, affirmation, and aid. The social network dimension is defined as the size of the spouses' social networks. The nurse support dimension is defined as spouses' perceptions of support or nonsupport from nurses during hospitalization.

Middle-range theory Proposition 3 can be formalized as a nonrelational proposition that asserts a constitutive definition for the concept perception of illness severity:

> Perception of illness severity is defined as spouses' subjective definitions of the seriousness of their partner's illness.

Middle-range theory Propositions 4 and 5 can be formalized as a nonrelational proposition that asserts a constitutive definition for the concept coping responses:

> Coping responses is defined as having two dimensions: active coping and avoidance coping. The active coping dimension is defined as cognitive or behavioral attempts to manage one's appraisal of the stressfulness of the event or deal directly with the problem and its effects. The avoidance coping dimension is defined as attempts to avoid actively confronting the problem.

Middle-range theory Propositions 6 and 15, along with information extracted from the description of the instruments and the content of Figure 1 in the report, can be formalized as a nonrelational proposition that asserts a constitutive definition for the concept stress responses:

> Stress responses is defined as spouses' dysfunctional or disrupted behavior in response to a critical illness event within four dimensions: physical, psychologic, role strain, and marital quality. The physical dimension is defined as physical stress complaints. The psychologic dimension is defined as behavioral and cognitive complaints. The role strain dimension is defined as disrupted or dysfunctional behavior dealing with arranging time to do various role-related activities. The martial quality dimension is defined as disrupted dyadic adjustment.

A nonrelational proposition that asserts a rudimentary constitutive definition for the concept time can be extracted from information given in the introductory section of the research report. Formalized, the constitutive definition is:

> Time is defined as having two dimensions: during the spouse's husband's hospitalization and 6 weeks after his discharge.

Nonrelational propositions that assert representational definitions can be extracted from information given in the narrative and especially from Figure 1 in the report. These representational propositions link Roy's Adaptation Model concepts with the middle-range theory concepts. Formalized, the representational definitions are:

> Roy's Adaptation Model concept stimuli input is represented by middle-range theory concepts hardships and demands and social support.

> Roy's Adaptation Model concept mediating internal processes is represented by middle-range theory concepts perception of illness severity and coping responses.

> Roy's Adaptation Model concept behavioral output is represented by the middle-range theory concept stress responses.

> The role function mode subdimension of Roy's Adaptation Model concept behavioral output is represented by the role strain dimension of middle-range theory concept stress responses.

Middle-range theory Propositions 7, 8, 10, 11, 12, 13, 14, 16, 35, 38, and 41, along with information extracted from the description of the instruments, can be formalized as nonrelational propositions that assert measured operational definitions. These measured operational definitions link the middle-range theory concepts with their respective empirical indicators. Formalized, the measured operational definitions are:

> The life events dimension of hardships and demands was measured by the Family Inventory of Life Events and Changes.

> The hospital-related stressors dimension of hardships and demands was measured by the Spouse Stressor Scale, and the open-ended question asking: "Is there anything or anyone that has been unpleasant or made this situation more difficult for you to cope with?"

> The postdischarge stressors dimension of hardships and demands was measured by the open-ended question asking: "What concerns have you had since your husband has been home?" The functional support and social network dimensions of social support were measured by the Norbeck Social Support Questionnaire.

> The nurse support dimension of social support was measured by an open-ended question asking the study participant to: "Describe an incident in which you thought you received support from a nurse."

> Perception of illness severity was measured by a Cantril Self-Anchoring Ladder.

> The active coping and avoidance coping dimensions of coping responses were measured by the Indices of Coping Responses.

The physical and psychologic dimensions of stress responses were measured by the Strain Questionnaire.

The role strain dimension of stress responses was measured by the Role Strain Scale.

The marital quality dimension of stress responses was measured by the Dyadic Adjustment Scale.

No measured operational definition for the concept time could be found in the report. It must be inferred that time was measured by a record that the investigator kept for each study participant.

RELATIONAL PROPOSITIONS. Relational propositions can be extracted from the list of research questions in the introductory section of the report, the description of the instruments, and the results of inferential statistical tests in the results section (Table E–2, middle-range theory Propositions 17, 20, 22, 24, 26, 28, 30, and 32). These relational propositions assert the existence of a relation between time and the concepts that address spouses' CABG-related stress experience. The relational existence propositions are:

There is a relation between time and the life events dimension of hardships and demands.

There is a relation between time and the functional support dimension of social support.

There is a relation between time and perception of illness severity.

There is a relation between time and the active coping dimension of coping responses.

There is a relation between time and the avoidance coping dimension of coping responses.

There is a relation between time and the physical and psychologic dimensions of stress responses.

There is a relation between time and the role strain dimension of stress responses.

There is a relation between time and the marital quality dimension of stress responses.

Still another relational proposition, which asserts the existence of a relation between the social network dimension of social support and stress responses, can be extracted from the results of inferential statistical tests (Table E–2, middle-range theory Proposition 21). Formalized, the relational existence proposition is:

There is a relation between the social network dimension of social support and stress responses.

HYPOTHESES. The research questions listed in the introductory section of the research report and the inferential statistical tests that were done imply that hypotheses were tested. The first research question implies that Artinian expected some level of existence for hardships and demands, social support, perception of illness severity, coping responses, and stress responses. Artinian did not, however, specify an a priori level for each concept. Thus, falsifiable hypotheses asserting a specific level of existence for each concept (e.g., high stress response) cannot be formulated. Actual levels of existence is noted only in the results section of the report (Table E–2, middle-range theory Propositions 18, 19, 22, 23, 25, 27, 29, 31, 33, 36, 39, and 42).

Each relational existence proposition, however, can be restated as a hypothesis, using concept names. Inasmuch as no a priori information was given with regard to the direction of each relational proposition, the implicit hypotheses, which are listed in Table E–3, are stated in the null form.

HIERARCHY OF PROPOSITIONS

Hierarchies of propositions based on level of abstraction can be constructed for all of the middle-range theory concepts except time by using nonrelational constitutive definitional propositions from the conceptual model and the theory concepts, a nonrelational representational definitional proposition, and a nonrelational opera-

---

Table E–3 ■ **IMPLICIT HYPOHESIS FOR ARTINIAN'S RESEARCH**

Null Hypotheses	Results of Testing Null Hypotheses
1. There is no difference in the life events dimension of hardships and demands from hospitalization to 6 weeks after discharge.	Supported Table E-2, Proposition 17
2. There is no difference in the functional support dimension of social support from hospitalization to 6 weeks after discharge.	Supported Table E-2, Proposition 20
3. There is no difference in perception of illness severity from hospitalization to 6 weeks after discharge.	Rejected Table E-2, Proposition 22
4a. There is no difference in the active coping dimension of coping responses from hospitalization to 6 weeks after discharge.	Supported Table E-2, Proposition 24
4b. There is no difference in the avoidance coping dimension of coping responses from hospitalization to 6 weeks after discharge.	Supported Table E-2, Proposition 26
5a. There is no difference in the physical and psychologic dimensions of stress responses from hospitalization to 6 weeks after discharge.	Rejected Table E-2, Proposition 28
5b. There is no difference in the role strain dimension of stress responses from hospitalization to 6 weeks after discharge.	Supported Table E-2, Proposition 30
5c. There is no difference in the marital quality dimension of stress responses from hospitalization to 6 weeks after discharge.	Rejected Table E-2, Proposition 32
6. There is no relation between the social network dimension of social support and stress responses.	Rejected Table E-2, Proposition 21

tional definitional proposition. Two examples are given. The first hierarchy based on level of abstraction is for the theory concept coping responses:

Abstract proposition: Mediating internal processes is defined as having three dimensions: perception, adaptive responses, and ineffective responses.

Somewhat concrete proposition: Roy's Adaptation Model concept mediating internal processes is represented by middle-range theory concept coping responses.

More concrete proposition: Coping responses is defined as having two dimensions: active coping and avoidance coping. Active coping is defined as cognitive or behavioral attempts to manage one's appraisal of the stressfulness of the event or deal directly with the problem and its effects. Avoidance coping is defined as attempts to avoid actively confronting the problem.

Most concrete proposition: Active and avoidance coping were measured by the Indices of Coping Responses.

The second hierarchy is for the role strain dimension of the theory concept stress responses:

Abstract proposition: Behavioral output is defined as having one dimension and four subdimensions. The dimension is health state, and the subdimensions are physiological mode, self-concept mode, role function mode, and interdependence mode.

Somewhat concrete proposition: The role function mode subdimension of Roy's Adaptation Model concept behavioral output is represented by the role strain dimension of middle-range theory concept stress responses.

More concrete proposition: Role strain is defined as disrupted or dysfunctional behavior dealing with arranging time to do various role-related activities.

Most concrete proposition: Role strain was measured by the Role Strain Scale.

Inasmuch as the relational propositions and derived hypotheses developed for the analysis of the middle-range theory of spouses' CABG-related stress experiences were not stated explicitly in the original research report, hierarchies of axioms and hypotheses stated in the vocabulary of empirical indicators were not constructed for this analysis.

DIAGRAMS

The conceptual-theoretical-empirical structure for the research is illustrated in Figure E–1. The question mark indicates that the theory concept time is not linked

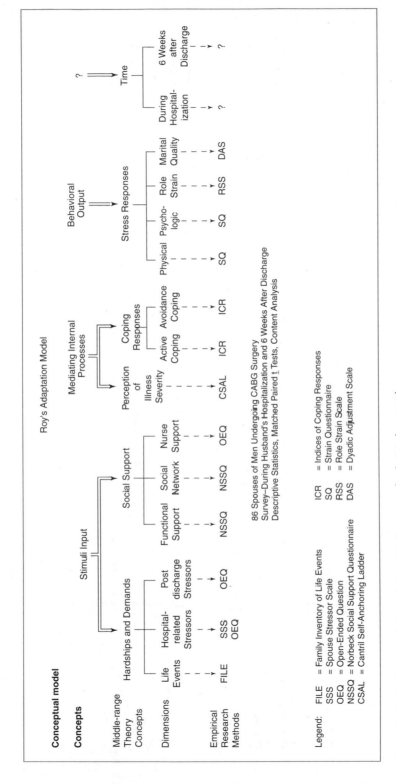

Figure E–1 ■ Conceptual-theoretical-empirical structure for Artinian's research.

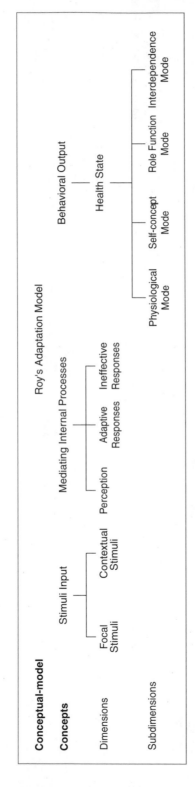

Figure E–2 ■ Diagram of conceptual model concepts and their dimensions for Artinian's research.

to any of Roy's model concepts. Another diagram was constructed to illustrate the concepts, dimensions, and subdimensions of Roy's Adaptation Model, as presented by Artinian for her research (Fig. E–2).

EVALUATION OF THE CONCEPTUAL-THEORETICAL-EMPIRICAL STRUCTURE

Analysis of Artinian's research report revealed that a middle-range descriptive classification theory of spouses' CABG-related stress experiences was tested. The theory is made up of six concepts, five of which are multidimensional (Table E–1 and Fig. E–1), and the propositions that describe and link the concepts.

EVALUATION OF THE CONCEPTUAL-THEORETICAL-EMPIRICAL LINKAGES

Specification Adequacy

The criterion of specification adequacy is met in part. The conceptual model that guided Artinian's theory-testing research is explicitly identified as Roy's Adaptation Model. However, the discussion of Roy's model is limited to one sentence. Consequently, only rudimentary constitutive definitions could be developed for the conceptual model concepts of interest through reference to a diagram that was included in the report. Moreover, the relation of the conceptual model to the middle-range theory was clear only by reference to the diagram and to Artinian's statement that "The Spouse Stress Theoretical Model that I deduced from Roy's conceptual model provided the overall framework for this study (Fig. 1)."

Linkage Adequacy

The criterion of linkage adequacy is met only in part. Artinian displayed the links between Roy's Adaptation Model concepts and the middle-range theory concepts in the diagram included in the report. However, the theory concept time was not linked to any conceptual model concept (Fig. E–1). Furthermore, with the exception of the theory concept role strain, the linkages between the particular dimensions and subdimensions of the conceptual model concepts and the theory concepts were not clear. For example, it might be inferred that the mediating internal process dimension of perception was linked to perception of illness severity, and that the dimensions of adaptive responses and ineffective responses were respectively linked to the active coping and avoidance coping dimensions of coping responses, but that inference is based only on the way in which the content of Figure 1 in the research report is displayed.

Conceptual Model Usage Rating Scale

Evaluation of the criteria of specification adequacy and linkage adequacy is summarized by application of the Conceptual Model Usage Rating Scale. Artinian's research report earned a score of 2, indicating minimal use of the conceptual model. The rating is based on the relative richness of information provided in Figure 1 of the report, contrasted with the paucity of explicit narrative about the relation of Roy's model to the research and the lack of a linkage between the conceptual model and the theory concept time.

EVALUATION OF THE THEORY

Significance

The middle-range theory of spouses' CABG-related stress experience meets the criterion of significance. Artinian addressed the social and theoretical significance of the research in the introductory section of the report. With regard to social significance, she identified the clinical problems in other family members that can result from the illness of one family member. More specifically, Artinian stated:

■ The family is the usual context in which illness occurs. Because the family is an interdependent system, illness or change in one member of the system is followed by change in other members. Not only does the patient's illness affect the family but also the family's ability to deal in an optimal manner with its ill member has a significant impact on the patient's physical and emotional adaptation to the illness.

Addressing the theoretical significance of the research, Artinian explained:

■ The stress of surgery may have a deleterious effect on the spouse's health, as well as impairing the spouse's ability to relate effectively with the patient. More research is needed to address the entire stress process of the spouse of the patient having CABG. Although problems and concerns of the spouse of the patient having CABG have been addressed, studies have not documented changes in stress process variables over time or investigated spouse perceptions of illness severity or of nurse support. In this study some of those gaps are addressed.

Internal Consistency

The middle-range theory of spouse's CABG-related stress experience meets the criterion of internal consistency in part. Semantic clarity is evident in that, with repeated reading of the research report, the dimensionality of the theory concepts could be identified and constitutive definitions could be developed. Moreover, although time is not identified explicitly as a concept, references to the two time periods for data collection are made throughout the report, and the acronym for each time period (T_1 for during hospitalization and T_2 for 6 weeks after discharge) is given in the introductory section. No concept redundancies are evident.

Semantic consistency is generally evident in that the same term is used for most theory concepts throughout the report. One exception and an area of potential confusion is introduced with the interchangeable use of the terms "mental" and "psychologic" when referring to one dimension of the theory concept stress responses.

Structural consistency is evident in that hierarchies based on level of abstraction could be constructed. There are no redundant propositions.

A. The Original Theory

Time ——————?—————— Life Events Dimension of Hardships and Demands

Time ——————?—————— Functional Support Dimension of Social Support

Time ——————?—————— Perception of Illness Severity

Time ——————?—————— Active Coping Dimension of Coping Responses

Time ——————?—————— Avoidance Coping Dimension of Coping Responses

Time ——————?—————— Physical and Psychologic Dimensions of Stress Responses

Time ——————?—————— Role Strain Dimension of Stress Responses

Time ——————?—————— Marital Quality Dimension of Stress Responses

Social Network Dimension of Social Support ——————?—————— Stress Responses

B. The Theory After Testing

Time ——————−—————— Perception of Illness Severity

Time ——————−—————— Physical and Psychologic Dimensions of Stress Responses

Time ——————−—————— Marital Quality Dimension of Stress Responses

Social Network Dimension of Social Support ——————+—————— Stress Responses

Figure E–3 ■ Diagram of the middle-range theory of spouses' CABG-related stress responses before (A) and after testing (B).

Parsimony

The middle-range theory of spouses' CABG-related stress experiences does not fully meet the criterion of parsimony. The analysis revealed that the theory is made up of six concepts and the propositions that describe or link those concepts. The theory is not excessively verbose. However, the theory that was tested is somewhat oversimplified, in that the analysis revealed that no nonrelational level of existence propositions and no explicit relational propositions are stated in the report.

The version of the theory that emerged from the testing is even more parsimonious. Indeed, just four of the original nine relational propositions that were extracted from the research report were retained (Table E–3; Fig. E–3). The question marks in this figure indicate that an a priori direction for each relation was not specified. The plus and minus signs give the direction of the relations obtained from the inferential statistical tests.

Testability

The middle-range theory of spouses' CABG-related stress experiences meets the criterion of testability. All concepts can be observed empirically. Implicit null hypotheses were tested, and some were falsified (Table E–3). Those hypotheses that were not falsified are potentially falsifiable in future studies (Table E–3).

More specifically, the findings of Artinian's study provide data on which to base falsifiable directional hypotheses in future research. For example, the research findings permit the development of an explicit falsifiable hypothesis stating that spouses' scores on a Cantril Self-Anchoring Ladder, which measures perception of illness severity, decrease from during hospitalization for CABG surgery to 6 weeks after discharge.

Furthermore, hypotheses based on nonrelational propositions asserting level of existence of the various stress experiences could be developed (Table E–2, Propositions 18, 19, 22, 23, 25, 27, 29, 31, 33, 36, 39, and 42). For example, the research findings permit the development of a falsifiable hypothesis stating that spouses' scores on the Role Strain Scale, which measures the role strain dimension of stress responses, indicate a low level of role strain during their husband's hospitalization for CABG surgery.

EVALUATION OF THE RESEARCH DESIGN

Operational Adequacy

The research design meets the criterion of operational adequacy in part. Artinian pointed out that the representativeness of the samples was limited by the use of a nonprobability sample, the method of sample selection, the female gender of all study participants, and the relatively high attrition rate from T_1 to T_2. The validity and reliability of most of the empirical indicators was reported, and reliability coefficients for the study sample were adequate. The data-collection procedure was explained in sufficient detail and was appropriate for a survey. Although the data-analysis techniques were appropriate, consideration might have been given to adjust the p value to take the number of statistical tests into account.

EVALUATION OF THE RESEARCH FINDINGS

Empirical Adequacy

Evaluation of the criterion of empirical adequacy is difficult in that Artinian did not specify a priori levels of existence for hardships and demands, social support, perception of illness severity, coping responses, or stress responses for each time period, or an a priori direction of change in level over time. Inasmuch as neither level nor direction was specified, empirical adequacy cannot be evaluated in terms of the support or rejection of hypotheses dealing with the level of existence of each concept or those dealing with the direction of change in the level over time. All that can be concluded from the research findings is that some level of each concept does exist at each time period and that the levels for perception of illness severity and the physical, psychologic, and marital quality dimensions of stress responses changed from during hospitalization to 6 weeks after discharge. Consequently, it can be concluded that the null form of implicit Hypotheses 1, 2, 4a, 4b, and 5b was supported, whereas the null form of implicit Hypotheses 3, 5a, and 5c was rejected (Table E–3; Fig. E–3). In addition, it can be concluded that the null form of implicit Hypothesis 6, which asserted no relation between the social network dimension of social support and a composite of all dimensions of stress responses was rejected (Table E–3; Fig. E–3). Artinian did not include alternative substantive or methodological explanations for the study findings.

EVALUATION OF THE UTILITY OF THE THEORY FOR PRACTICE

Pragmatic Adequacy

The findings of Artinian's theory-testing study meet the criterion of pragmatic adequacy. Indeed, Artinian explicitly addressed the implications of her findings for nursing practice. She pointed out that "nurses and other health professionals need to be attentive to the stress process experience of spouses after hospital discharge as well as during hospitalization."

To the extent that attention is limited to assessment of spouses' CABG-related stress experiences, the use of the instruments used by Artinian or similar assessment tools is feasible in clinical practice and clinicians have the legal ability to perform the assessment. Moreover, the study findings support the development of clinical practice guidelines that direct clinicians to perform such assessments. Although spouses of patients undergoing CABG surgery may be surprised that attention is being directed toward their experiences, it is anticipated that they would be receptive to such attention, at least during the time of the patient's hospitalization. The 22% attrition rate from hospitalization to 6 weeks postdischarge reported by Artinian suggests that some spouses may not be interested in continuing attention from clinicians.

Artinian noted that her research findings indicate that provisions for planned informational and emotional support should be targeted especially to women with large social networks. In addition, Artinian offered suggestions for specific nursing interventions, such as including spouses in cardiac preoperative and postoperative teaching, and preparing spouses for the uncertainty they might experience and for the symptoms that might be experienced by the patient during and after hospitalization. These suggestions go beyond the findings of the Artinian's study. Indeed, additional research is required to test the efficacy of planned support and other nursing interventions prior to their use in clinical practice.

EVALUATION OF THE CONCEPTUAL MODEL

Credibility

The credibility of Roy's Adaptation Model, which Artinian used to guide her research, is not addressed in the report. Based on the narrative and the diagram included in the report, it can be concluded only that the components of Roy's model provided a useful framework for the selection and organization of the middle-range theory concepts.

References

Artinian, N.T. (1991). Stress experiences of spouses of patients having coronary bypass during hospitalization and 6 weeks after discharge. *Heart and Lung, 20,* 52–59.

Roy, C. (1984). *Introduction to nursing: An adaptation model* (2nd ed.). Englewood Cliffs, NJ: Prentice-Hall.

Analysis and Evaluation of an Explanatory Theory-Testing Study:
Correlational Research

Correlates of Pain-Related Responses to Venipunctures in School-Age Children

Marie-Christine Bournaki

Guided by the Roy Adaptation Model of Nursing, the relationship of children's age, gender, exposure to past painful experiences, temperament, fears, and child-rearing practices to their pain responses to a venipuncture was examined. A sample of 94 children aged 8 to 12 years and their female caregivers were recruited from three outpatient clinics. During the venipuncture, children's behavioral and heart rate responses were monitored; immediately after, their subjective responses were recorded. Canonical correlation revealed two variates. In the first, age and threshold (temperamental dimension) correlated with pain quality, behavioral responses, and heart rate responses, explaining 12% of the variance. In the second, age, the temperamental dimensions of distractibility and threshold, and medical fears explained only 5.7% of the variance in pain quality and heart rate magnitude. Significant correlations between pain intensity, quality, behavioral responses, and heart rate responses support the multidimensionality of pain.

Venipunctures are described as painful procedures by hospitalized children (Van Cleve, Johnson, & Pothier, 1996; Wong & Baker, 1988) and the most difficult to deal with by adolescent oncology survivors (Fowler-Kerry, 1990). However, not all children respond similarly to venipunctures. Between 4% and 17% of school-age children rated their pain intensity to a venipuncture as severe (Fradet, McGrath, Kay, Adams, & Luke, 1990; Harrison, 1991), and 38% of children ages 3 to 10 had to be physically restrained during a venipuncture (Jacobsen et al., 1990). Manne,

Reprinted from *Nursing Research 46*(43), 147–154, 1997, with permission.

Jacobsen, and Redd (1992) reported that the pain intensity and behavioral responses of 3- to 10-year-old children were moderate. In a recent study by Van Cleve et al., hospitalized school-age children were found to rate venipuncture or intravenous cannulation as moderately painful.

Factors that account for variability in children's responses to venipunctures have not been fully identified. The purpose of this study, therefore, was to examine the relationship of a set of correlates, including age, gender, past painful experiences, temperament, general and medical fears, and child-rearing practices, on school-age children's subjective, behavioral, and heart rate responses to a venipuncture.

BACKGROUND

CONCEPTUAL FRAMEWORK: The Roy Adaptation Model of Nursing (RAM) (Roy and Andrews, 1991) and the research literature on children's responses to painful procedures guided this study. According to the RAM, the goal of nursing is to facilitate adaptation between the person and the environment through the management of stimuli (Roy & Corliss 1993). One of the assumptions of adaptation-level theory is that the person's "adaptive behavior is a function of the stimulus and adaptation level, that is, the pooled effects of the focal, contextual, and residual stimuli" (Roy & Corliss, 1993, p. 217). The focal stimulus immediately confronts the person; the contextual stimuli contribute to the effect of the focal stimulus; and residual stimuli are factors whose effects on the person's adaptation have not been clearly determined.

The focal and contextual stimuli are processed through coping mechanisms, such as the regulator and cognator subsystems. The regulator subsystem induces physiological responses through neural, chemical, and endocrine processes. The cognator subsystem elicits responses through perceptual/information processing, learning, judgment, and emotion processes (Andrews & Roy, 1991a). Outcomes of these coping mechanisms are the person's responses in four modes: self-concept, role function, interdependence, and physiological. The self-concept mode relates to feelings about one's personal and physical self. The role-function mode is associated with the need for social integrity based on roles assumed within society. The interdependence mode focuses on interactions that fulfill the need for affectional adequacy and support. The physiological mode is described as the person's physical responses to stimuli from the environment. In accordance with the proposition that stimuli serve as inputs to the person to elicit a response, children's pain-related responses were tested as a function of the pooled effects of the focal stimulus, the venipuncture, and the contributory effects of the contextual stimuli congruent with the RAM and the empiric pediatric pain literature. Contextual stimuli relate to culture, family, developmental stage, and cognator effectiveness, as well as those factors that have an effect on the person's adaptive responses in any of the modes (Andrews & Roy, 1991b). The pooled effects of a venipuncture, children's age, gender, exposure to past painful experiences, temperament, fears, and child-rearing practices were studied in relation to children's pain-related responses to the venipuncture.

Roy (1991) defined pain within the physiological mode, as a sensory experience of acute or chronic nature, coded into the somatosensory pathways. Acute pain refers to "discomfort which is intense but relatively short lived and reversible" (p. 166). Using principles from neurophysiology, Roy stated that a sensory experience such as pain involves the transmission of neural activity through specialized receptors, and transmission of information from sensory pathways to the cerebral cortex. A sensation results from receptors' activity and is converted into perceptual activity involving mental representations and interpretations (Roy). Thus, pain can be understood to be both a sensory and perceptual experience.

As a manifestation of the regulator subsystem activity, the sensory dimension was represented in this study by children's behavioral and heart rate responses. The perceptual dimension of pain, which is the response to the cognator subsystem activity, was portrayed by children's subjective responses about the location, intensity, and quality of pain.

REVIEW OF THE LITERATURE: Empirical evidence supports a negative relationship between the contextual stimulus of children's chronological age and pain intensity (Fradet et at. 1990; Lander & Fowler-Kerry, 1991; Manne et al., 1992) and behavioral responses to venipunctures (Fradet et al., 1990; Humphrey, Boon, van Linden van den Heuvell, van de Wiel, 1992; Jacobsen et al., 1990). Mean pain intensity responses to a venipuncture or intravenous cannulation were found to be greater in preschoolers than in school-age children; however, it is not clear whether this difference was statistically significant (Van Cleve et al., 1996). Gender has been believed to be a mediator in pain experiences (Katz, Kellerman, & Siegel, 1980). However, researchers have shown that gender has no effect on pain intensity responses (Fowler-Kerry & Lander, 1991; Fradet et al., 1990; Manne et al., 1992) and behavioral responses to venipunctures (Fradet et al.; Humphrey et al.; Jacobsen et al.). In view of the influence of socialization on school-age children's sex-role stereotypes, it was relevant to reexamine the effects of gender on pain responses.

Several researchers have reported that children's exposure to past painful procedures is inversely related to their behavioral responses to a venipuncture (Fradet et al., 1990; Jacobsen et al., 1990). However, in another study, this relationship did not reach statistical significance (Manne et al., 1992). The effects of past exposure to venipunctures on children's subjective, behavioral, and heart rate responses to a venipuncture remain unclear.

The contextual stimulus of temperament may explain the individual variability of responses across situations. According to Thomas and Chess (1977), temperament is the result of an interactive process between child and parent and consists of nine temperamental dimensions: activity, rhythmicity, approach/withdrawal, sensory threshold, intensity of reaction, quality of mood, distractibility, and attention span/persistence, and adaptability. Although the predictive effects of temperament have been studied in children's adaptation to chronic illness (Garrison, Biggs, & Williams, 1990; Wallander, Hubert, & Varni, 1988), the relationship between temperament and pain related to invasive procedures has only been examined in preschool children. Young and Fu (1988) found that a child's rhythmicity had a small effect on pain intensity and that approach accounted for 7% of children's behavioral responses to venipunctures. In view of the brevity of the venipuncture, the theoretical relevancy of each temperamental dimension, and school-age children's increased behavioral mastery, only sensory threshold, intensity, and distractibility were judged important in this study. Sensory threshold reflects sensitivity to stimulation and may be important in self-regulation and defense mechanisms (Rothbart & Derryberry, 1981). Intensity is the energy level of a response irrespective of the direction (Thomas & Chess, 1977). Distractibility, a measure of how sensitive one's attention is to environmental stimulation, may be relevant in children's coping mechanisms and adaptive responses.

Children fearful of medical procedures report higher pain intensity to venipunctures (Broome, Bates, Lillis, Wilson, & McGahee, 1990) and display more behavioral responses (Jacobsen et al., 1990). Nevertheless, investigators have not examined the contextual stimulus of children's medical fears in relation to a multidimensional view of the pain experience or accounted for another contextual stimulus, children's general fears. While fear is an immediate response to a threatening situation, general fears may serve as a context for the development of medical fears.

The family's influence on children's behaviors through the provision of structure and discipline is relevant in the study of children's responses to painful situations (Melamed & Bush, 1985). Parental restrictiveness and nurturance toward a child's behavioral expressiveness may help in understanding children's responses to pain. The contextual stimulus of child-rearing practices was examined in the situation of immunizations (Broome & Endsley, 1989). Children of authoritative (high-control, high-warmth) parents exhibited significantly fewer behavioral responses than those of authoritarian (high-control, low-warmth), permissive (low-control, high-warmth), and unresponsive (low-control, low-warmth) parents. This study extended examination of the influence of child-rearing practices to children's pain responses to venipunctures.

Previous studies of the effects of multiple variables on children's pain intensity and behavioral responses to venipunctures have been informative. However, children's pain has not been measured in a comprehensive fashion. The relationship between children's behavioral display and reported pain intensity has been found to be moderate in school-age children during venipunctures (Fradet et al., 1990; Humphrey et al., 1992; Manne et al., 1992) and during bone marrow aspirations (Jay & Elliott, 1984; Jay, Ozolins, Elliot, & Caldwell, 1983). Inasmuch as pain intensity represents one aspect of the pain experience, children's behavioral responses needed to be examined in relation to a global assessment of pain. Though not specific to pain, physiological responses have been described in acute pain experiences. However, studies involving cardiac rate during painful procedures have yielded equivocal results. Broome and Endsley (1987) found no relationship between preschoolers' behavioral responses and heart rate during a finger stick procedure, whereas Jay and Elliott (1984) reported a moderate correlation between behaviors and heart rate of school-age children and adolescents during bone marrow aspirations. These findings support the need to reexamine the role of sympathetic responses of heart rate combined with other pain measures during an invasive procedure. Based on the RAM and the empirical pediatric pain literature, the hypothesis tested was that there is a relationship between the set of independent variables age, gender, past painful experiences, temperament, medical fears, general fears, and child-rearing practices and the set of school-age children's responses to venipuncture: pain location, pain intensity, pain quality, observed behaviors, and heart rate.

METHOD

SAMPLE: The sample consisted of 94 children and their female caregivers recruited from three outpatient clinics (gastroenterology, nephrology, and preoperative) at a large pediatric hospital in a mid-Atlantic state. An initial power analysis for multiple regression with 9 independent variables, a power of .80, a medium effect size, and an alpha level of .05 revealed that 119 subjects were necessary (Cohen, 1988). However, the actual obtained power of the main analysis performed to test the study hypothesis was so low that an increase in sample size would not have yielded more meaningful results. Consequently, the study sample was judged sufficient.

Children between 8 and 12 years of age, cognitively normal for their school grade, accompanied by a female caregiver, and expected to receive a venipuncture during their clinic visit were asked to participate. Of the 121 subjects who were approached, 10 refused (8%) for lack of time or personal reasons. Of those who agreed, 17 (15%) were excluded for various reasons; 4 children had cognitive deficits, 2 were not accompanied by a female caregiver, 7 did not require a venipuncture, and 4 caregivers did not have time to complete the questionnaires. Children's mean age was 10.3 (SD = 1.4). The majority of the children were female (54.3%) and white (86.2%).

INSTRUMENTS: The Child Information Sheet (CHILDIS) was used to record information about the child's gender, age, school grade, number of past hospitalizations, and number of past venipunctures and other painful procedures. The Caregiver Information Sheet (CIS) was used to record demographic information about the caregiver, including age, gender, ethnicity, marital status, education level, employment status, and family income. Caregivers' perceptions about the child's experiences with past hospitalizations and painful procedures were also requested.

The Middle Childhood Temperament Questionnaire (MCTQ) (Hegvik, McDevitt, & Carey, 1982) was used to measure temperament of children 8 to 12 years old. The MCTQ is a 99-item parent report using a 6-point scale from 1 (almost always) to 6 (almost never) for each of nine temperamental dimensions. Three dimensions, distractibility, intensity, and threshold, were included in this study. Higher scores are indicative of higher distractibility and intensity but lower sensory threshold. Satisfactory criterion-related validity was evidenced in comparisons of children's temperament at ages 7 and 12 (Maziade, Câté, Boudreault, Thivierge, & Boutin, 1986). For this study, the Cronbach's alpha internal consistency reliability coefficients were threshold, .68, distractibility, .75, and intensity, .81.

The Child Medical Fears Scale (CMFS) (Broome, Hellier, Wilson, Dale, & Glanville, 1988) is used to measure children's levels of reported fears related to medical personnel and diagnostic or therapeutic procedures. Children rate their level of fear for 17 items on a scale of 1 (not at all), 2 (a little), and 3 = (a lot afraid), with higher scores indicating greater fear. Total scores range from 17 to 51. The content validity index for the CMFS is 78% (Broome et al.). Criterion validity was established with the original Fear Survey Schedule (Scherer & Nakamura, 1968), with a correlation of .71 (Broome et al.). The Cronbach's alpha internal consistency reliability coefficient was .87 for this study sample.

The Revised Fear Survey Schedule for Children (RFSSC) (Ollendick, 1983) is an 80-item questionnaire used to measure children's general fears. Children rate their level of fear to the unknown, supernatural events, bodily injury, small animals, and death on a 3-point scale of 1 (none), 2 (some), and 3 (a lot). Total scores range from 80 to 240, with higher scores indicating greater fear. Construct validity was established by discriminating fears of phobic and normal children (Ollendick) and by supporting a decline in children's fears with age (King, Gullone, & Ollendick, 1991). The generalizability of a five-factor structure has been shown across cultures (Ollendick & Yule, 1990). The Cronbach's alpha internal consistency coefficient for the present study was .95.

The Modified Child-Rearing Practices Report (M-CRPR) (Dekovic, Janssens, & Gerris, 1991; Rickel & Biasatti, 1982) was used to measure two parental attitudes toward child rearing: parental restrictiveness, characterized by a high degree of control and endorsement of strict rules and restrictions, and parental nurturance, characterized by the willingness of parents to share feelings with their children and to show responsiveness to the child's needs. The M-CRPR consists of 40 statements with a 6-point response format, from 1 (not at all descriptive of me) to 6 (highly descriptive of me). Two scores are obtained, with lower scores indicative of low restrictiveness (range 0 to 22) and low nurturance (range 0 to 18). The validity of the M-CRPR was supported by discriminating the child-rearing practices of parents of rejected and highly sociable children (Dekovic et al.) and by factor-structuring the scale (Dekovic et al.; Rickel & Biasatti). In this study, the Cronbach's alphas for the restrictiveness and nurturance subscales were .90 and .92, respectively.

The Adolescent Pediatric Pain Tool (APPT) (Savedra, Tesler, Holzemer, & Ward, 1992) is a self-report measure of location, intensity, and quality of pain in children aged 8 to 17 years. Pain location is measured using a body outline figure on which children are instructed to mark the location(s) of their current pain. The number of locations is summed, with scores ranging from 0 to 43 (Savedra, Tesler, Holzemer, Wilkie, & Ward, 1989). Criterion-related validity of the pain location scale was documented when children's markings and investigators' observations reached an agreement of at least 80% (Savedra, Tesler, Holzemer, Wilkie, & Ward, 1990). A postoperative decrease in pediatric surgical patients' pain sites was found, thus supporting construct validity (Savedra et al., 1990). Intrarater reliability estimates of the agreement between subjects' markings and pointings ranged from 83% to 94% (Savedra et al., 1989).

Pain intensity was measured using a 100-mm word-graphic rating scale, with scores ranging from 0 to 100. A decline in postoperative pain intensity scores supported construct validity (Savedra et al., 1990). Criterion-related validity was established through correlations with four other pain intensity scales (Tesler et al., 1991). Test-retest reliability was .91 (Tesler et al., 1991).

Pain quality was measured using a list of 67 words that relate to the sensory, affective, evaluative, and temporal experiences of pain (Tesler, Savedra, Ward, Holzemer, & Wilkie, 1988). Based on a factor analysis that confirmed only three factors (Wilkie et al., 1990), scores, which range from 0 to 56, are reported only for sensory, affective, and evaluative subscales. Criterion-related validity was evidenced by correlations with pain intensity scores (Savedra et al., 1990). A significant decrease in the number of words used by recovering pediatric surgical patients (Savedra et al., 1990; Savedra, Holzemer, Tesler, & Wilkie, 1993) supported construct validity. Test-retest reliability of total, sensory, affective, and evaluative scores of surgical patients revealed high correlations, .95, .91, .97, and .78, respectively (Tesler et al., 1991).

The Observed Child Distress (OCDS) (Jacobsen et al., 1990; Manne et al., 1992) was used to measure six behavioral responses to venipunctures: pain verbalizations, cry/scream, request for termination of procedure, refusing to assume body position, muscular rigidity, and requiring physical restraint. These behaviors are observed during three phases of the venipuncture (phase 1, from sitting in the chair until the tourniquet is applied; phase 2, from tourniquet application until needle is to be inserted; and phase 3, from piercing the skin to bandage application). They are rated for their presence (1) or absence (0), for a total score ranging from 0 to 18. Construct validity of the OCDS was supported by a positive correlation between behavioral scores and self-reports of pain intensity (Manne et al., 1992). Cronbach's alpha internal consistency coefficient for the study sample was .83.

A Nellcor electronic pulse oximeter (N-10; Haywood, CA) was used to measure heart rate during the venipuncture through a taped sensor to a finger. Heart rate was measured at rest and monitored every 10 seconds throughout the venipuncture. The magnitude of heart rate change (highest heart rate during phase 3 relative to baseline heart rate) was calculated for each child.

PROCEDURE: All subjects were recurited before their clinic appointments. Participation in the study was voluntary, and informed consents from female caregivers and children's assents were obtained in accordance with the institution's Committee for Protection of Human Subjects.

During waiting periods, caregivers completed the CIS, the MCTQ, and the M-CRPR. In the presence of their caregivers, children were asked to answer verbally to the CHILDIS, R-FSSC, and the CMFS. A baseline heart rate was obtained after each child had rested for 15 minutes in a sitting position. Throughout all phases of the procedure, children's behavioral responses were measured using the OCDS, and heart rate was monitored with a pulse oximeter. Data obtained during the third phase of the venipuncture, which is associated with the experience of pain, is reported in this study. Only one caregiver was absent during the venipuncture. Within 10 minutes following the procedure, children completed the APPT.

RESULTS

Examination of the distribution of the pain-related variables (Table 1) led to the exclusion of pain location scores from further statistical analyses due to limited variability. Since the distributions of pain intensity and quality scores were skewed, square root transformations were performed. Though the majority of children reported minimal pain intensity, 20% of the children regarded venipunctures as very painful procedures. Most children (98%) described their pain experiences using sensory descriptors, 75% chose evaluative words, and 40% selected affective qualitites. Children's behavioral responses associated with the insertion of the needle were minimal; however, heart rate changes were of greater magnitude. For most children (96.7%), magnitude in heart rate change was within two standard deviations. For 3.3% of the sample, important changes in heart rate were recorded (< or > 3 SD).

As presented in Table 1, data about children's past experiences with venipunctures were not normally distributed. Following transformation, the majority of children (64%) were found to have prior experience with venipunctures. The distributions for the temperamental dimensions of distractibility, intensity, and threshold were found to be normal. Children's scores on general fears were normally distributed; however, medical fear scores required square root transformation. Parental restrictiveness and nurturance scores were not normally distributed and were dichotomized into high and low groups. About half of the caregivers (43.6%) scored low on parental restrictiveness and 46.8% scored low on nurturance.

Correlations were computed between all independent and dependent variables. Threshold was correlated with pain quality ($r(94) = .25$, $p < .05$), that is, low sensory threshold was associated with more pain descriptors. Age, $r(93) = -.48$, $p < .001$, and threshold, $r(93) = .24$, $p < .05$, were correlated with behavioral responses, suggesting that with age, children manifest fewer behavioral responses, and that low sensory threshold is associated with more behavioral responses. Distractibility, $r(90) = .33$, $p < .05$, threshold, $r(90) = .23$, $p = .03$, general fears, $r(87) = .27$, $p < .05$, and medical fears, $r(86) = .26$, $p < .02$, were correlated with magnitude in heart rate change. Children with high distractibility, low threshold, and high general and medical fears had greater changes in heart rate. None of the

Table 1 ■ **SUMMARY OF CHILDREN'S SCORES ON DEPENDENT AND INDEPENDENT VARIABLES**

	n	M	(SD)	Range
Pain location	94	1.2	0.5	0–3
Pain intensity	94	29.4	24.0	0–100
Pain quality	94	8.0	6.3	0–41
Behavioral responses	93	1.7	1.4	0–6
Magnitude in heart rate change (%)	90	18.9	28.7	−40 to 101.3
Age	94	10.3	1.4	8–12
Past experiences with venipunctures	84	5.1	8.9	0–40
Temperament				
Distractability	94	4.07	0.9	1.5–6
Intensity	94	3.69	0.9	1.6–6
Threshold	94	3.85	0.8	2–5.5
General fears	90	137.9	24.3	94–212
Medical fears	90	27.6	6.8	17–49
Child-rearing practices				
Restrictiveness	84	64.2	19.2	32–130
Nurturance	86	93.3	11.9	21–107

independent variables were related to pain intensity. Consequently, pain intensity was excluded from the main analysis.

Examination of the correlations between the independent variables revealed multicollinearity for general and medical fears, $r(87) = .83, p < .001$. Consequently, general fears were excluded from the main analysis.

The correlation matrix for the dependent variables revealed low to moderate correlations between pain quality, intensity, behavioral responses, and magnitude in heart rate change. Specifically, pain quality correlated with pain intensity ($r(94) = 0.59, p < 0.001$), behavioral responses ($r(93) = 0.41, p < 0.001$), and magnitude in heart rate change ($r(90) = 32, p < 0.05$). Lower correlations were found between pain intensity and behavioral responses ($r(93) = 0.26, p < 0.05$) and magnitude in heart rate change ($r(90) = 0.22, p < 0.05$). As expected, behavioral responses were correlated with magnitude in heart rate change ($r(90) = 0.31, p < 0.01$). Together, these findings suggest that as children select more pain descriptors, they report higher pain intensity and exhibit more behavioral responses and greater heart rate responses.

Of the initial variables, only the independent and dependent variables that correlated significantly were retained for the canonical analysis. They were age, distractibility, threshold, medical fears, pain quality, behavioral responses, and magnitude of heart rate change. As can be seen in Table 2, two canonical variates were found to be significant. The first canonical variate (.526) was found for age and threshold, and correlated with pain quality, behavioral responses, and magnitude of heart rate change, explaining 12% of the variance. The second canonical variate (.411) revealed that age, medical fears, distractibility, and threshold correlated with pain quality and magnitude of heart rate change, explaining 5.7% of the variance. Overall, 17.7% of the variance was accounted for. Inasmuch as all variables did not enter the analysis, the study hypothesis was not supported.

A closer examination of the first variate in the set of independent variables supported an association between age and threshold. That is, with age, children learn to become less sensitive to environmental stimuli. In the set of dependent

---

Table 2 ■ **CANONICAL CORRELATION ANALYSIS SUMMARY TABLE BETWEEN AGE, DISTRACTIBILITY, THRESHOLD, AND MEDICAL FEARS (SET 1) AND PAIN QUALITY, BEHAVIORAL RESPONSES, AND HEART RATE MAGNITUDE (SET 2)**

Variables Sets	Canonical Variates	
	1	2
Set 1: independent variables		
Age of child	0.884[a]	−0.328[a]
Medical fears	−0.146	−0.582[a]
Distractibility	−0.251	−0.793[a]
Threshold	−0.572[a]	−0.504[a]
Set 2: dependent variables		
Pain quality	−0.463[a]	0.414[a]
Behavioral responses	−0.994[a]	0.055
Magnitude in heart rate change	−0.308[a]	0.912[a]
Canonical correlations	0.526	0.411
	$p < 0.001$	$p = 0.014$
Variance explained	12.0%	5.7%
Total variance explained	17.7%	

[a]Structure coefficients ≥ 0.30.

variables, pain quality was found to be associated with behavioral and heart rate responses. The second variate of the canonical analysis suggested that younger and fearful child tend to be more distractible and have low sensory thresholds.

Additional findings from t-test and chi-square analyses showed no differences on most independent and dependent variables between subjects from the preoperative clinic and those from the gastroenterology and nephrology clinics. However, children from the preoperative group had less experience with past venipunctures, χ^2 (1, $N = 84$) $= 4.24$, $p < .05$, and reported higher pain quality, $M = 2.7$, $SD = 1.1$, $T(93) = -2.1$, $p < .05$. In the total sample, girls had higher general fears than boys, $T(90) = -2.0$, $p < .001$, but no difference was found with regard to medical fears. Finally, girls had higher temperamental intensity than boys (girls, $M = 3.9$, $SD = 0.8$ vs. boys, $M = 3.5$, $SD = 0.9$; $T(94) = -2.05$, $p < .05$).

On all dependent variables, children were found to be homogeneous except that girls cried significantly more than boys during the venipuncture, χ^2 (1, $N = 93$) $= 4.22$, $p < .05$. No differences were noted in children experienced and inexperienced with venipunctures with regard to temperament, general and medical fears, pain intensity and pain quality scores, behavioral responses, and heart rate magnitude. Regardless of children's health problems, family income, and race, there were no differences in children's responses to pain.

DISCUSSION

Although the study hypothesis was not supported, the results from the canonical correlation revealed several important relationships. Data from the first variate showed that with increasing age and in children with high sensory threshold, fewer words are used to describe pain, fewer behavioral responses are manifested, and lower magnitude of change in heart rate is observed. With increasing age, children are more emotionally and behaviorally organized (Maccoby, 1983). Moreover, school-age children's greater understanding of the procedure, increasing awareness of socially acceptable behaviors, and competency in controlling behaviors may account for the restricted body movements. Finally, children less sensitive to sensory stimuli were less upset by the venipuncture and showed fewer behavioral responses and changes in heart rate.

Findings from the second variate suggest that younger, highly fearful, distractible, and sensitive children report higher pain quality and have higher heart rate reactivity. Lack of familiarity combined with a limited repertoire of coping skills may account for the younger child's increased vulnerability to stressful events. These findings support the need for the implementation of interventions for young children before and even during such relatively brief and simple medical procedures as venipunctures.

Correlations between the dependent variables as shown in the correlational matrix and in the first canonical variate support a relationship between the perceptual and sensory dimensions of pain. However, the relationship is low in magnitude. Gross motor responses may be less relevant in school-age children, suggesting that a focus on muscular rigidity and/or facial activity might be more appropriate for this group. In this study, no relationship was found between the independent variables and pain intensity. It may be that the venipuncture did not evoke enough variability in children's pain intensity or that no relationship can be established with pain intensity since it is essentially a subjective and unpredictable characteristic of pain.

The study results provided limited support for the Roy Adaptation Model. Based on the proposition that focal and contextual stimuli influence responses, empirical support was found for the contextual stimuli of age, medical fears, and the temperamental dimensions of distractibility and threshold. Only the contextual stimuli that affect developmental stage (age), self-concept (medical fears), and interdependence between parent and child (temperamental dimensions of distractibility and sensory threshold) were supported. The lack of a relationship between gender and subjective pain responses, though unexpected, is consistent with prior work on gender and pain intensity (Fowler-Kerry & Lander, 1991; Fradet et al., 1990; Manne et al., 1992). Limited support was found for the relationship between gender and behavioral responses, in that girls cried more than boys. The influence of parental child-rearing styles on responses to venipunctures was not noted in this study.

Contrary to prior research (Fradet et al., 1990; Jacobsen et al., 1990) but consistent with the work of Manne et al. (1992), the findings showed no relationship between experience with venipunctures and children's pain-related responses. This suggests that experienced children did not habituate to the procedure. It may also be that frequency of exposure is not sufficient information for understanding children's responses to pain. Rather, as the RAM suggests, children's coping abilities with procedures need to be taken into account.

Most importantly, findings from the correlational and canonical analyses support the multidimensionality of pain as conceptualized by the RAM. This empirical evidence is consistent with the need for clinicians and researchers to use a comprehensive approach to assess pain by integrating valid and reliable subjective, behavioral, and physiological measures. Such a global approach to understanding pain is in accordance with the RAM.

Several imstruments used in the study need further evaluation. The Revised Fear Survey Schedule for Children should be revised to be more sociohistorically appropriate for children. Low scores obtained by the Child Medical Fears Scale suggest a need to reexamine the relevancy of several items with a school-age population. In view of the fact that there was no relationship between behavioral responses and pain intensity, more attention needs to be paid to the meaning of behavioral responses. For example, it is important to understand which behavioral responses are reflective of the pain experience in different age groups. This information is particularly critical in the care of children unable to express their needs verbally.

This study supports the need to assess children's pain and to identify the factors that may aggravate the pain experience. Research on helping children cope with aversive medical procedures has produced somewhat equivocal results (Dahlquist, 1992). While certain strategies may be helpful to some children, others may have no or negative effects. In order to individualize the care of children undergoing procedures, future research may be directed toward matching interventions with children's age, fears, and temperament. The findings of this research have contributed to the extension of the knowledge base on school-age children's pain to venipunctures. ■

References

Andrews, H. A., & Roy, C. (1991a). Essentials of the Roy adaptation model. In C. Roy & H. A. Andrews (Eds.), *The Roy Adaptation Model: The definitive statement* (pp. 3–25). Norwalk, CT: Appleton & Lange.

Andrews, H. A., & Roy, C. (1991b). The nursing process according to the Roy adaptation model. In C. Roy & H. A. Andrews (Eds.), *The Roy Adaptation Model: The definitive statement* (pp. 27–54). Norwalk, CT: Appleton & Lange.

Broome, M. E., Bates, T. A., Lillis, P. P., & Wilson McGahee, T. (1990). Children's medical fears, coping behaviors, and pain perceptions during a lumbar puncture. *Oncology Nursing Forum, 17,* 361–367.

Broome, M. E., & Endsley, R. C. (1989). Maternal presence, childrearing practices, and children's response to an injection. *Research in Nursing and Health, 12,* 229–235.

Broome, M. E., Hellier, A., Wilson, T., Dale, S., & Glanville, C. (1988). Measuring children's fears of medical experiences. In C. F. Waltz & O. L. Strickland (Eds.), *Measurement of Nursing Outcomes* (Vol. 1, pp. 201–214). New York: Springer.

Cohen, J. (1988). *Statistical power analysis for the behavioral sciences* (2nd ed.). Hillsdale, NJ: Erlbaum.

Dahlquist, L. M. (1992). Coping with aversive medical treatments. In A. M. La Greca, L. J. Siegel, J. L. Wallander, & C. E. Walker (Eds.), *In stress and coping with child health* (pp. 345–376). New York: Guilford Press.

Dekovic, M., Janssens, J. M. A. M., & Gerris, J. R. M. (1991). Factor structure validity of the Block child rearing practices report (CRPR). *Psychological Assessment: A Journal of Consulting and Clinical Psychology, 3*, 182–187.

Fowler-Kerry, S. (1990). Adolescent oncology survivors' recollection of pain. In D. C. Tyler & E. J. Krane (Eds.), *Advances in pain research therapy* (Vol. 15, pp. 365–371). New York: Raven Press.

Fowler-Kerry, S., & Lander, J. (1991). Assessment of sex differences in children's and adolescents self-reported from venipunctures. *Journal of Pediatric Psychology, 16*, 783–793.

Fradet, C., McGrath, P. J., Kay, J., Adams, S., & Luke, B. (1990). A prospective survey of reactions to blood tests by children and adolescents. *Pain, 40*, 53–60.

Garrison, W. T., Biggs, D., & Williams, K. (1990). Temperament characteristics and clinical outcomes in young children with diabetes mellitus. *Child Psychology and Psychiatry, 31*, 1079–1088.

Harrison, A. (1991). Preparing children for venous sampling. *Pain, 45*, 299–306.

Hegvik, R. L., McDevitt, S. C., & Carey, W. B. (1982). The middle childhood temperament questionnaire. *Developmental and Behavioral Pediatrics, 3*, 197–200.

Humphrey, G. B., Boon, C. M. J., Van Linden van den Heuvell, G. F. E. C., & Van de Wiel, H. B. M. (1992). The occurrence of high levels of acute behavioral distress in children and adolescents undergoing routine venipunctures. *Pediatrics, 90*, 87–91.

Jacobsen, P. B., Manne, S. L., Gorfinkle, K., Schorr, O., Rapkin, B., & Redd, W. H. (1990). Analysis of child and parent behavior during painful medical procedures. *Health Psychology, 9*, 559–576.

Jay, S.M., & Elliot, C. (1984). Behavioral observation scale for measuring children's distress: The effects of increased methodological rigor. *Journal of Consulting and Clinical Psychology, 52*, 1106–1107.

Jay, S.M., Ozolins, M., Elliot, C.H., & Caldwell, S. (1983). Assessment of children's distress during painful medical procedures. *Health Psychology, 2*, 133–147.

Katz, E. R., Kellerman, J., & Siegel, S. (1980). Behavioral distress in children with cancer undergoing medical procedures: Developmental considerations. *Journal of Consulting and Clinical Psychology, 48*, 356–365.

King, N. J., Gullone, E., & Ollendick, T. H. (1991). Manifest anxiety and fearfulness in children and adolescents. *The Journal of Genetic Psychology, 153*, 63–73.

Lander, J., & Fowler-Kerry, (1991). Age differences in children's pain. *Perceptual and Motor Skills, 73*, 415–418.

Maccoby, E. E. (1983). Social-emotional development and response to stressor. In N. Garmezy & M. Rutter (Eds.), *Stress, coping, and development in children* (pp. 217–234). New York: McGraw-Hill.

Manne, S. L., Jacobsen, P. B., & Redd, W. H. (1992). Assessment of acute pediatric pain: Do child self-report, parent ratings and nurse ratings measure the same phenomenon? *Pain, 48*, 45–52.

Maziade, M., Coté, R., Boudreault, M., Thivierge, J., & Boutin, P. (1986). Family correlates of temperament continuity and change across middle childhood. *American Journal of Orthopsychiatry, 56*, 195–203.

Melamed, B. G., & Bush, J. P. (1985). Family factors in children with acute illness. In D. Turk & R. Kerns (Eds.), *Heath, illness and families: A life-span perspective* (pp. 183–219). New York: Wiley.

Ollendick, T. H. (1983). Reliability and validity of the revised fear survey schedule for children (FSSC-R). *Behavior Research Therapy, 21*, 685–692.

Ollendick, T. H., & Yule, W. (1990). Depression in British and American children and its relation to anxiety and fear. *Journal of Consulting and Clinical Psychology, 58*, 126–129.

Rickel, A. U., & Biasatti, L. L. (1982). Modification of the Block child rearing practice report. *Journal of Clinical Psychology, 38*, 129–134.

Rothbart, M. K., & Derryberry, D. (1981). Development of individual differences in temperament. In M. E. Lamb & A. L. Brown (Eds.), *Advances in developmental psychology: Vol.* (pp. 37–86). Hillsdale, NJ: Erlbaum.

Roy, C. (1991). Senses. In C. Roy & H. A. Andrews (Eds.), *The Roy Adaptation Model: The definitive statement* (pp. 164–189). Norwalk, CT: Appleton & Lange.

Roy, C., & Andrews, H. A. (1991). *The Roy Adaptation Model: The definitive statement.* Norwalk, CT: Appleton & Lange.

Roy, C., & Corliss, C. P. (1993). The Roy Adaptation Model: Theoretical update and knowledge for practice. In M. E. Parker (Ed). *Patterns of nursing theories in practice* (pp. 215–229). New York: National League for Nursing.

Savedra, M. C., Holzemer, W. L., Tesler, M. D., & Wilkie, D. J. (1993). Assessment of postoperative pain in children and adolescents using the adolescent pediatric pain tool. *Nursing Research, 42*, 5–9.

Savedra, M. C., Tesler, M. D., Holzemer, W. L., & Ward, J. A. (1992). *Adolescent Pediatric Pain Tool (APPT): User's manual.* San Francisco: University of California, School of Nursing.

Savedra, M. C., Tesler, M. D., Holzemer, W. L., Wilkie, D. J., & Ward, J. A. (1989). Pain location: Validity and reliability of body outline markings by hospitalized children and adolescents. *Research in Nursing and Health, 12*, 307–314.

Savedra, M. C., Tesler, M. D., Holzemer, W. L., Wilkie, D. J., & Ward, J. A. (1990). Testing a tool to assess postoperative pediatric and adolescent pain. In D. C. Tyler & E. J. Krane (Eds.), *Advances in Pain Therapy* (Vol. 15, pp. 85–93), New York: Raven Press.

Scherer, M. W., & Nakamura, C. Y. (1968). A fear survey for children (FSS-FC): A factor analytic comparison with manifest anxiety (CMAS). *Behavior Research and Therapy, 6*, 173–182.

Tesler, M., Savedra, M., Ward, J. A., Holzemer, W. L., & Wilkie, D. (1988). Children's language of pain. In R. Dubner, G. F. Gebhart, & M. R. Bond (Eds.), *Pain research and clinical management, Proceedings of the 5th World Congress on Pain* (Vol. 3, pp. 348–352). Amsterdam: Elsevier

Tesler, M. D., Savedra, M. C., Holzemer, W. L., Wilkie, D. J., Ward, J. A., & Paul, S. M. (1991). The word-graphic rating scale as a measure of children's and adolescents' pain intensity. *Research in Nursing and Health, 14*, 361–371.

Thomas, A., & Chess, S. (1977). *Temperament and development.* New York: Brunner and Mazel.

Van Cleve, L., Johnson, L., & Pothier, P. (1996). Pain responses of hospitalized infants and children to venipuncture and intravenous cannulation. *Journal of Pediatric Nursing, 11*, 169–174.

Wallander, J. L., Hubert, N. C., & Varni, J. W. (1988). Child and maternal temperament characteristics, goodness of fit, and adjustment in physically handicapped children. *Journal of Clincal Child Psychology, 17*, 336–344.

Wilkie, D.J., Holzemer, W.L., Tesler, M.D., Ward, J.A., Paul, S.M., & Savedra, M.C. (1990). Measuring pain quality: Validity and reliability of children's and adolescents' pain language. *Pain, 41*, 151–159.

Wong, D. L., & Baker, C. M. (1988). Pain in children: Comparison of assessment scales. *Pediatric Nursing, 14*, 9–17.

Young, M. R., & Fu, V. R. (1988). Influence of play and temperament on the young child's response to pain. *Children's Health Care, 16*, 209–215.

ANALYSIS OF THE CONCEPTUAL-THEORETICAL-EMPIRICAL STRUCTURE

The stated purpose of Bournaki's (1997) research was to examine the relationship of a set of correlates, including age, gender, past painful experiences, temperament, general and medical fears, and child-rearing practices, on school-age children's subjective, behavioral, and heart-rate responses to a venipuncture. The research was designed to test an explanatory theory of correlates of school-age children's pain-related responses to venipunctures, by means of correlational research.

INDENTIFICATION OF CONCEPTS

Conceptual Model Concepts

Analysis of the research report revealed that the research was guided by Roy's Adaptation Model of Nursing (Roy and Andrews, 1991). The particular conceptual model concepts employed in the research are stimuli and response mode.

Stimuli is a multidimensional concept encompassing three dimensions: focal stimulus, contextual stimuli, and residual stimuli. Bournaki used only the focal stimulus and contextual stimuli dimensions to guide her research.

Response mode also is a multidimensional concept; it encompasses four dimensions: physiological mode, self-concept mode, role function mode, and interdependence mode. Bournaki used only the physiological mode dimension to guide her research.

Middle-Range Theory Concepts

Further analysis of the research report revealed that the middle-range explanatory theory of correlates of school-age children's pain-related responses to venipunctures emcompasses eight concepts, several of which have more than one dimension (Table F–1).

CLASSIFICATION OF MIDDLE-RANGE
THEORY CONCEPTS

The classification of each middle-range theory concept is given in Table F–1. The theory concept school-age children's pain-related responses is classified as a theoretical term in Kaplan's schema, as a construct in Willer and Webster's schema, and as a summative unit in Dubin's schema because it is a complex, global phenomenon.

The theory concepts venipuncture, age, gender, and past painful experiences are classified as observational terms in Kaplan's schema and as observables in Willer and Webster's schema. Venipuncture is so classified because the procedure can be seen. Age, gender, and past painful experiences are so classified because, in this study, they were observed through each child's report of his or her age, gender, and past painful experiences. Indeed, the more appropriate label for each of these concepts is "report of age/gender/past painful experiences."

Venipuncture, age, and gender are classified as enumerative units in Dubin's schema because they are always present in this study. Past painful experiences is classified as an associative unit because, in this study, some children reported that

---

Table F–1 ■ **THE THEORY OF CORRELATES OF SCHOOL-AGE CHILDREN'S PAIN-RELATED RESPONSES TO VENIPUNCTURES: CONCEPTS, THEIR DIMENSIONS, AND CLASSIFICATION**

Concept Dimensions Subdimensions	Kaplan	Willer and Webster	Nonvariable or Variable	Dubin

School-age Children's Pain-related Responses
  Sensory Experience
    Observed behaviors
    Heart rate change
  Perceptual Experience
    Pain location
    Pain intensity
    Pain quality
	Theoretical Term	Construct	Variable	Summative Unit

Venipuncture	Observational Term	Observable	Nonvariable	Enumerative Unit
Age	Observational Term	Observable	Variable	Enumerative Unit
Gender	Observational Term	Observable	Variable	Enumerative Unit
Past Painful Experiences	Observational Term	Observable	Variable	Associative Unit

Temperament
 	
  Sensory Threshold
  Intensity
  Distractibility
	Construct	Construct	Variable	Relational Unit

Fears
  General Fears
  Medical Fears
	Construct	Construct	Variable	Relational Unit

Child-Rearing Practices
 	
  Parenteral Restrictiveness
  Parental Nurturance
	Construct	Construct	Variable	Relational Unit

---

they had not experienced any painful procedures in the past; thus, there was a real zero or absent value.

The theory concepts temperament, fears, and child-rearing practices are classified as constructs in both Kaplan's and Willer and Webster's schemata because all three concepts were invented for research purposes and must be inferred through responses to questionnaires. Temperament and child-rearing practices are classified as relational units in Dubin's schema because both concepts represent an interaction between the child and his or her parent. Fears is classified as a relational unit in Dubin's schema because it represents an interaction between the child and some real or imagined object.

The theory concept venipuncture is classified as a nonvariable because no other procedure was of interest in this correlational study. All other theory concepts are variables because each one demonstrated some fluctuation in this study.

INDENTIFICATION AND CLASSIFICATION OF PROPOSITIONS

Conceptual Model Propositions

Nonrelational and relational propositions from Roy's Adaptation Model were used to guide the research. All of the relevant propositions are listed in Table F–2.

Conceptual model Propositions 2, 3, and 8, along with a portion of conceptual model Proposition 1, can be formalized as a nonrelational proposition asserting a constitutive definition for the conceptual model concept stimuli. Formalized, the constitutive definition is:

> Stimuli is defined for the purposes of this study as having two dimensions: focal stimulus and contextual stimuli. The dimension focal stimulus is defined as the stimulus immediately confronting the person. The dimension contextual stimuli is defined as those stimuli that contribute to the effect of the focal stimulus, and encompass the subdimensions culture, family, developmental stage, cognator effectiveness, and other factors that have an effect on the person's adaptive responses in any of the response modes.

Conceptual model Propositions 4 and 6, along with a portion of conceptual model Proposition 5, can be formalized as a nonrelational proposition asserting a constitutive definition for the conceptual model concept response mode dimension. Formalized, the constitutive definition is:

> Response mode is defined for the purposes of this study as the outcome of the regulator and cognator coping mechanisms in the physiological mode dimension, which is the person's physical responses to stimuli from the environment.

Table F–2 ■ **CONCEPTUAL MODEL PROPOSITIONS FROM BOURNAKI'S RESEARCH REPORT**

Proposition	Classification
1. The person's adaptive behavior is a function of the stimulus and adaptation level, that is, the pooled effects of the focal, contextual, and residual stimuli.	Relational, Existence Nonrelational, Constitutive Definition
2. The focal stimulus immediately confronts the person.	Nonrelational, Constitutive Definition
3. The contextual stimuli contribute to the effect of the focal stimulus.	Nonrelational, Constitutive Definition
4. The focal and contextual stimuli are processed through coping mechanisms, such as the regulator and cognator subsystems.	Nonrelational, Constitutive Definition
5. Outcomes of these coping mechanisms are the person's responses in four modes: self-concept, role-function, interdependence, and physiological.	Nonrelational, Constitutive Definition
6. The physiological mode is described as the person's physical responses to stimuli from the environment.	Nonrelational, Constitutive Definition
7. Stimuli serve as inputs to the person to elicit a response.	Relational, Existence
8. Contextual stimuli relate to culture, family, developmental stage, and cognator effectiveness, as well as those factors that have an effect on the person's adaptive responses in any of the modes.	Nonrelational, Constitutive Definition

Conceptual model Propositions 1 and 7 can be formalized as a relational proposition asserting the existence of a relation between stimuli and response mode. Formalized, the relational proposition is:

There is a relation between stimuli and response mode.

Middle-Range Theory Propositions

Nonrelational and relational propositions that are central to the middle-range explanatory theory of correlates of school-age children's pain-related responses to venipunctures are evident in the research report. These propositions are listed in Table F–3.

NONRELATIONAL PROPOSITIONS. Middle-range theory Propositions 2, 3, and 4 can be formalized as a nonrelational proposition asserting the level of existence for the theory concept school-age children's pain-related responses. Formalized, the nonrelational level of existence proposition is:

School-age children's pain-related responses to venipuncture range from moderate to severe.

Middle-range theory Propositions 8 and 9, along with portions of Propositions 28, 35, 36, and 37 can be combined as a nonrelational proposition asserting a constitutive definition for the theory concept school-age children's pain-related responses. Formalized, the constitutive definition is:

School-age children's pain-related responses is defined as discomfort that is intense but relatively short-lived and reversible and encompasses two dimensions: sensory experience and perceptual experience. The sensory experience dimension is made up of two subdimensions: observed behaviors and heart rate change. The subdimension observed behaviors is defined as the behavioral responses of pain verbalizations, cry/scream, request for termination of procedure, refusing to assume body position, muscular rigidity, and requiring physical restraint. The subdimension heart rate change is defined as the highest heart rate during phase 3 of data collection relative to baseline heart rate. The perceptual experience dimension is made up of three subdimensions: pain location, pain intensity, and pain quality. Pain location is defined as the location of pain on the body. Pain intensity is defined as a word-graphic expressing the intensity of the pain. Pain quality is defined as sensory, affective, and evaluative words about pain.

Middle-range theory Proposition 1, along with information extracted from the instrument section of the research report, can be formalized as a nonrelational proposition asserting a constitutive definition for the theory concept venipuncture. Formalized, the constitutive definition is:

Venipuncture is defined as a painful procedure that involves using a needle to pierce the skin and puncture the vein.

A portion of middle-range theory Proposition 12, along with information extracted from the sample section of the report, can be formalized as a nonrelational

text continues on page 354

Table F–3 ■ **MIDDLE-RANGE THEORY PROPOSITIONS FROM BOURNAKI'S RESEARCH REPORT**

Proposition	Classification
1. Venipunctures are described as painful procedures by hospitalized children.	Nonrelational, Constitutive Definition
2. Between 4% and 17% of school-age children rated their pain intensity to a venipuncture as severe, and 38% of children ages 3 to 10 had to be physically restrained during a venipuncture.	Nonrelational, Level of Existence
3. Manne, Jacobsen, and Redd reported that the pain intensity and behavioral responses of 3- to 10-year-old children were moderate.	Nonrelational, Level of Existence
4. In a recent study by Van Cleve et al., hospitalized school-age children were found to rate venipuncture or intravenous cannulation as moderately painful.	Nonrelational, Level of Existence
5. Children's pain-related responses were tested as a function of the pooled effects of the focal stimulus, the venipuncture.	Nonrelational, Representational Definition
6. Children's pain-related responses were tested as a function of the pooled effects of the . . . contributory effects of the contextual stimuli congruent with the RAM (Roy's Adaptation Model) and the empiric pediatric pain literature . . . The pooled effects of . . . children's age, gender, exposure to past painful experiences, temperament, fears, and child-rearing practices were studied.	Nonrelational, Representational Definition
7. Roy defined pain within the physiological mode, as a sensory experience of acute or chronic nature, coded into the somatosensory pathways.	Nonrelational, Representational Definition
8. Acute pain refers to discomfort which is intense but relatively short lived and reversible.	Nonrelational, Constitutive Definition
9. Pain can be understood to be both a sensory and perceptual experience.	Nonrelational, Constitutive Definition
10. As a manifestation of the regulatory subsystem activity, the sensory dimension of pain was represented in this study by children's behavioral and heart rate responses.	Nonrelational, Constitutive Definition Representational Definition
11. The perceptual dimension of pain, which is the response to the cognator subsystem activity, was portrayed by children's subjective responses about the location, intensity, and quality of pain.	Nonrelational, Constitutive Definition Representational Definition
12. Empirical evidence supports a negative relationship between the contextual stimulus of children's chronological age and pain intensity and behavioral responses to venipunctures.	Relational, Existence Direction Nonrelational, Constitutive Definition Representational Definition
13. Gender has been believed to be a mediator in pain experiences. However, researchers have shown that gender has no effect on pain intensity responses and behavioral responses to venipunctures. In view of the influence of socialization on school-age children's sex-role stereotypes, it was relevant to reexamine the effects of gender on pain responses.	Relational, Existence
14. Several researchers have reported that children's exposure to past painful procedures is inversely related to their behavioral responses to a venipuncture. However, in another study, this relationship did not reach significance. The effects of past exposure to venipunctures on children's subjective, behavioral, and heart rate responses to a venipuncture remain unclear.	Relational, Existence Nonrelational, Constitutive Definition
15. The contextual stimulus of temperament may explain the individual variability of responses across situations.	Nonrelational, Representational Definition

(continued on page 352)

Proposition	Classification
16. Temperament is the result of an interactive process between child and parent and consists of nine temperamental dimensions: activity, rhythmicity, approach/withdrawal, sensory threshold, intensity of reaction, quality of mood, distractibility, attention span/persistence, and adaptability . . . Only sensory threshold, intensity, and distractibility were judged important in this study.	Nonrelational, Constitutive Definition
17. Young and Fu found that a child's rhythmicity had a small effect on pain intensity and that approach accounted for 7% of children's behavioral responses to venipunctures.	Relational, Existence Strength
18. Sensory threshold reflects sensitivity to stimulation and may be important in self-regulation and defense mechanisms.	Nonrelational, Constitutive Definition
19. Intensity is the energy level of a response irrespective of the direction.	Nonrelational, Constitutive Definition
20. Distractibility, a measure of how sensitive one's attention is to environmental stimulation, may be relevant in children's coping mechanisms and adaptive responses.	Nonrelational, Constitutive Definition
21. Children fearful of medical procedures report higher pain intensity to venipunctures and display more behavioral responses.	Relational, Existence Direction
22. Investigators have not examined the contextual stimulus of children's medical fears . . . or accounted for another contextual stimulus, children's general fears.	Nonrelational, Representational Definition
23. Fear is an immediate response to a threatening situation.	Nonrelational, Constitutive Definition
24. Parental restrictiveness and nurturance toward a child's behavioral expressiveness may help in understanding children's responses to pain.	Relational, Existence
25. The contextual stimulus of child-rearing practices was examined.	Nonrelational, Representational Definition
26. Children of authoritative . . . parents exhibited significantly fewer behavioral responses than those of authoritarian . . . permissive, . . . and unresponsive . . . parents.	Relational, Existence Direction
27. The relationship between children's behavioral display and reported pain intensity has been found to be moderate in school-age children during venipunctures . . . Studies involving cardiac rate during painful procedures have yielded equivocal results. Broome and Endsley found no relationship between preschoolers' behavioral responses and heart rate during a finger stick procedure, whereas Jay and Elliott reported a moderate correlation between behaviors and heart rate of school-age children and adolescents during bone marrow aspirations.	Relational, Existence Implicit Hypothesis
28. The hypothesis tested was that there is a relationship between the set of independent variables age, gender, past painful experiences, temperament, medical fears, general fears, and child-rearing practices and the set of school-age children's responses to venipuncture: pain location, pain intensity, pain quality, observed behaviors, and heart rate.	Relational, Existence Hypothesis Nonrelational, Constitutive Definition
29. The Child Information Sheet (CHILDIS) was used to record information about the child's gender, age, . . . number of past venipunctures and other painful experiences.	Nonrelational, Measured Operational Definition
30. The Caregiver Information Sheet (CIS) was used to record . . . caregivers' perceptions about the child's experiences with past . . . painful procedures.	Nonrelational, Measured Operational Definition

Table F–3 ■ **MIDDLE-RANGE THEORY PROPOSITIONS FROM
BOURNAKI'S RESEARCH REPORT** *(Continued)*

Proposition	Classification
31. The Middle Childhood Temperament Questionnaire (MCTQ) was used to measure temperament.	Nonrelational, Measured Operational Definition
32. The Child Medical Fears Scale (CMFS) [was] used to measure children's level of reported fears related to medical personnel and diagnostic or therapeutic procedures.	Nonrelational, Measured Operational Definition Constitutive Definition
33. The Revised Fear Survey Schedule for Children (R-FSSC) [was] used to measure children's general fears. Children rate their level of fear to the unknown, supernatural events, bodily injury, small animals, and death.	Nonrelational, Measured Operational Definition Constitutive Definition
34. The Modified Child-Rearing Practices Report (M-CRPR) was used to measure two parental attitudes toward child rearing: parental restrictiveness, characterized by a high degree of control and endorsement of strict rules and restrictions, and parental nurturance, characterized by the willingness of parents to share feelings with their children and to show responsiveness to the child's needs.	Nonrelational, Measured Operational Definition Constitutive Definition
35. The Adolescent Pediatric Pain Tool (APPT) is a self-report measure of location, intensity, and quality of pain in children . . . Pain location is measured using a body outline figure on which children are instructed to mark the location(s) of their current pain. . . . Pain intensity was measured using a 100-mm word-graphic rating scale. . . . Pain quality was measured using a list of 67 words that relate to the sensory, affective, evaluative, and temporal experiences of pain . . . scores . . . are reported only for sensory, affective, and evaluative subscales.	Nonrelational, Measured Operational Definition Constitutive Definition
36. The Observed Child Distress [Scale] (OCDS) was used to measure six behavioral responses to venipunctures: pain verbalizations, cry/scream, request for termination of procedure, refusing to assume body position, muscular rigidity, and requiring physical restraint.	Nonrelational, Measured Operational Definition Constitutive Definition
37. A Nellcor electronic pulse oximeter (N-10) was used to measure heart rate. . . . The magnitude of heart rate change (highest heart rate during phase 3 relative to baseline heart rate) was calculated for each child.	Nonrelational, Measured Operational Definition Constitutive Definition
38. The correlation matrix for the dependent variables revealed low to moderate correlations between pain quality, [pain] intensity, behavioral responses, and magnitude in heart rate change. . . . Together, these findings suggest that as children select more pain descriptors, they report higher pain intensity and exhibit more behavioral reponses and greater heart rate responses.	Relational, Result of testing implicit hypothesis
39. Two canonical variates were found to be significant. The first canonical variate (.526) was found for age and threshold, and correlated with pain quality, behavioral responses, and magnitude of heart rate change, explaining 12% of the variance. The second canonical variate (.411) revealed that age, medical fears, distractibility, and threshold correlated with pain quality and magnitude of heart rate change, explaining 5.7% of the variance. Overall, 17.7% of the variance was accounted for. Inasmuch as all variables did not enter the analysis, the study hypothesis was not supported.	Relational, Result of testing main research hypothesis

proposition asserting a constitutive definition for the theory concept age. Formalized, the constitutive definition is:

Age is defined as chronological age from 8 to 12 years.

A nonrelational proposition asserting a constitutive definition for the theory concept gender can be extracted from the sample section of the report. Formalized, the constitutive definition is:

Gender is defined as being male or female.

A portion of middle-range theory Proposition 14 can be formalized as a nonrelational proposition asserting a constitutive definition for the theory concept past painful experiences. Formalized, the constitutive definition is:

Past painful experiences is defined as past exposure to venipunctures.

Middle-range theory Propositions 16, 18, 19, and 20 can be formalized as a nonrelational proposition asserting a constitutive definition for the theory concept temperament. Formalized, the constitutive definition is:

Temperament is defined as the result of an interactive process between child and parent and consists of nine dimensions: activity, rhythmicity, approach/withdrawal, sensory threshold, intensity of reaction, quality of mood, distractibility, attention span/persistence, and adaptability. The present study was limited to the sensory threshold, intensity, and distractibility dimensions. The sensory threshold dimension is defined as sensitivity to stimulation. The intensity dimension is defined as the energy level of a response, irrespective of the direction. The distractibility dimension is defined as how sensitive one's attention is to environmental stimulation.

Middle-range theory Proposition 23, along with portions of Propositions 28, 32, and 33, can be formalized as a nonrelational proposition asserting a constitutive definition for the theory concept fears. Formalized, the constitutive definition is:

Fear is defined as an immediate response to a threatening situation and has two dimensions: general fears and medical fears. The general fears dimension is defined as fear of the unknown, supernatural events, bodily injury, small animals, and death. The medical fears dimension is defined as fears related to medical personnel and diagnostic or therapeutic procedures.

A portion of middle-range theory Proposition 34 can be formalized as a nonrelational proposition asserting a constitutive definition for the theory concept child-rearing practice. Formalized, the constitutive definition is:

Child-rearing practices is defined as parental attitudes toward child rearing and has two dimensions: parental restrictiveness and parental nurturance. The parental restrictiveness dimension is defined as a high degree of control and endorsement of strict rules and restrictions. The parental nurturance dimension is defined as the willingness of parents to share feelings with their children and to show responsiveness to the child's needs.

Middle-range theory Propositions 5, 6, 7, 10, 11, 15, 22, and 25, along with a portion of Proposition 12, can be formalized as nonrelational propositions that assert representational definitions. Formalized, the representational definitions are:

> The physiological mode dimension of Roy's Adaptation Model concept response mode is represented by middle-range theory concept school-age children's pain-related responses.

> The focal stimulus dimension of Roy's Adaptation Model concept stimulus is represented by middle-range theory concept venipuncture.

> The contextual stimulus dimension of Roy's Adaptation Model concept stimulus is represented by middle-range theory concepts age, gender, past painful experiences, temperament, fears, and child-rearing practices.

These representational propositions clearly link the conceptual model concepts stimuli and response mode with the middle-range theory concepts.

Middle-range theory Propositions 29, 30, 31, 32, 33, 34, 35, 36, and 37 can be formalized as nonrelational propositions that assert measured operational definitions. These measured operational definitions clearly link the middle-range theory concepts with their respective empirical indicators. Formalized, the measured operational definitions are:

> The observed behaviors subdimension of school-age children's pain-related responses was measured by the Observed Child Distress Scale.

> The heart rate change subdimension of school-age children's pain-related responses was measured by a Nellcor electronic pulse oximeter (N-10).

> The pain location, pain intensity, and pain quality subdimensions of school-age children's pain-related responses were measured by the Adolescent Pediatric Pain Tool.

> Age was measured by an item on the Child Information Sheet.

> Gender was measured by an item on the Child Information Sheet.

> Past painful experiences was measured by an item on the Child Information Sheet and an item on the Caregiver Information Sheet.

> The sensory threshold, intensity, and distractibility dimensions of temperament were measured by the Middle Childhood Temperament Questionnaire.

> The general fears dimension of fears was measured by the Revised Fear Survey Schedule for Children.

> The medical fears dimension of fears was measured by the Child Medical Fears Scale.

> The parental restrictiveness and parental nurturance dimensions of child-rearing practices were measured by the Modified Child-Rearing Practices Report.

Although Bournaki conducted correlational rather than experimental research, the description for the theory concept venipuncture represents a nonrelational proposition that asserts an experimental operational definition. The experimental operational definition, which was formalized from information extracted from the instruments and procedure sections of the research report, is:

> Venipuncture consists of three phases. Phase 1 extends from sitting in the chair until the tourniquet is applied; phase 2, from tourniquet application until needle is to be inserted; and phase 3, from piercing the skin to bandage application. Only data obtained from phase 3 were used for the research.

RELATIONAL PROPOSITIONS. Middle-range theory Proposition 12 can be formalized as a relational proposition asserting the existence and direction of a relation between age and school-age children's pain-related responses:

> There is a negative relation between age and school-age children's pain-related responses.

Middle-range theory Proposition 13 can be formalized as a relational proposition asserting the existence of a relation between gender and school-age children's pain-related responses:

> There is a relation between gender and school-age children's pain-related responses.

Middle-range theory Proposition 14 can be formalized as a relational proposition asserting the existence of a relation between past painful experiences and school-age children's pain-related responses:

> There is a relation between past painful experiences and school-age children's pain-related responses.

Middle-range theory Proposition 17 can be formalized as a relational proposition asserting the existence and strength of a relation between temperament and school-age children's pain-related responses:

> There is a relation of small magnitude between temperament and school-age children's pain-related responses.

Middle-range theory Proposition 21 can be formalized as a relational proposition asserting the existence and direction of a relation between the medical fears dimension of the concept fears and school-age children's pain-related responses:

> There is a positive relation between medical fears and school-age children's pain-related responses.

Middle-range theory Propositions 24 and 26 can be formalized as a relational proposition asserting the existence of a relation between child-rearing practices and school-age children's pain-related responses:

> There is a relation between child-rearing practices and school-age children's pain-related responses.

Here, it should be noted that the direction of the relation was not specified in the formalized proposition because the correspondence of the dimensions of child-rearing practices mentioned in Proposition 26 (authoritative, authoritarian, permissive, unresponsive) and those used in Bournaki's research (parental restrictiveness and parental nurturance) could not be determined.

HYPOTHESES: Middle-range theory Proposition 28, which is a relational existence proposition, states the main research hypothesis that was tested, using the names of the middle-range theory concepts. Formalized, the hypothesis is:

> There is a relation between the set of concepts age, gender, past painful experiences, temperament (sensory threshold, intensity, and distractibility dimensions), fears (general fears and medical fears dimensions), and child-rearing practices (parental restrictiveness and parental nurturance dimensions), and the set of subdimensions of school-age children's pain-related responses to venipuncture: pain location, pain intensity, pain quality, observed behaviors, and heart rate.

Middle-range theory Proposition 27 is a relational proposition that asserts the existence of a relation between the various subdimensions of the theory concept school-age children's pain-related responses. Information presented in the results section of the research report indicates that this proposition represents an implicit hypothesis. Formalized, the implicit hypothesis is:

> There is a relation between the set of subdimensions of school-age children's pain-related responses: pain location, pain intensity, pain quality, observed behaviors, and heart rate.

HIERARCHY OF PROPOSITIONS

A hierarchy of propositions based on level of abstraction can be constructed by using the relational proposition for the conceptual model concepts, the nonrelational representational definitional propositions, and the hypothesis, using the names of the middle-range theory concepts. The hierarchy is:

Abstract proposition: There is a relation between stimuli and response mode.

Somewhat concrete propositions: The focal stimulus dimension of Roy's Adaptation Model concept stimulus is represented by middle-range theory concept venipuncture.

The contextual stimulus dimension of Roy's Adaptation Model concept stimulus is represented by middle-range theory concepts age, gender, past painful experiences, temperament, fears, and child-rearing practices.

The physiological mode dimension of Roy's Adaptation Model concept response mode is represented by middle-range theory concept school-age children's pain-related responses.

More concrete proposition: There is a relation between the set of concepts age, gender, past painful experiences, temperament (sensory threshold, intensity, and distractibility dimensions), fears (general fears and medical fears dimensions), and child-rearing practices (parental restrictiveness and parental nurturance dimensions), and the set of subdimensions of school-age children's pain-related responses to venipuncture: pain location, pain intensity, pain quality, observed behaviors, and heart rate.

A hierarchy of propositions based on deductive reasoning can be constructed for the main research hypothesis, by using the hypothesis stated in concept names and the measured operational definitions to deduce the hypothesis stated in the language of the empirical indicators. The deductive hierarchy is:

Axiom$_1$: If there is a relation between the set of concepts age, gender, past painful experiences, temperament (sensory threshold, intensity, and distractibility dimensions), fears (general fears and medical fears dimensions), and child-rearing practices (parental restrictiveness and parental nurturance dimensions), and the set of subdimensions of school-age children's pain-related responses to venipuncture: pain location, pain intensity, pain quality, observed behaviors, and heart rate, and

Axiom$_2$: if age was measured by an item on the Child Information Sheet, and

Axiom$_3$: if gender was measured by an item on the Child Information Sheet, and

Axiom$_4$: if past painful experiences was measured by an item on the Child Information Sheet and an item on the Caregiver Information Sheet, and

Axiom$_5$: if the sensory threshold, intensity, and distractibility dimensions of temperament were measured by the Middle Childhood Temperament Questionnaire, and

Axiom$_6$: if the general fears dimension of fears was measured by the Revised Fear Survey Schedule for Children, and

Axiom$_7$: if the medical fears dimension of fears was measured by the Child Medical Fears Scale, and

Axiom$_8$: if the parental restrictiveness and parental nurturance dimensions of child-rearing practices were measured by the Modified Child-Rearing Practices Report, and

Axiom$_9$: if the observed behaviors subdimension of school-age children's pain-related responses was measured by the Observed Child Distress Scale, and

Axiom$_{10}$: if the heart rate change subdimension of school-age children's pain-related responses was measured by a Nellcor electronic pulse oximeter, and

Axiom$_{11}$: if the pain location, pain intensity, and pain quality subdimensions of school-age children's pain-related re-

sponses were measured by the Adolescent Pediatric Pain
Tool, then

Hypothesis: there is a relation between the set of scores from
the Child Information Sheet items, the Caregiver
Information Sheet item, the Middle Childhood
Temperament Questionnaire, the Revised Fear Survey
Schedule for Children, the Child Medical Fears Scale, and
the Modified Child-Rearing Practices Report, and the set of
scores from the Adolescent Pediatric Pain Tool, the
Observed Child Distress Scale, and the Nellcor electronic
pulse oximeter.

DIAGRAMS

The conceptual-theoretical-empirical structure for the research is illustrated in
Figure F–1. Another diagram was constructed to illustrate the conceptual model relational proposition (Fig. F–2). Diagrams for the middle-range theory relational
propositions that are evident in the research report are given in Figure F–3. The
question marks in Figure F–3 indicate that the direction of the relation is not known.
A diagram for the main research hypothesis that was tested, stated in concept names,
is given in Figure F–4.

EVALUATION OF THE CONCEPTUAL-THEORETICAL-EMPIRICAL STRUCTURE

Analysis of Bournaki's research report revealed that a middle-range explanatory theory of correlates of school-age children's pain-related responses to venipunctures was tested. The concepts of the theory and their dimensions and subdimensions are listed in Table F–1 and illustrated in Figure F–1.

EVALUATION OF THE CONCEPTUAL-THEORETICAL-EMPIRICAL LINKAGES

Specification Adequacy

The criterion of specification adequacy is met. Bournaki provided a clear and
concise overview of Roy's Adaptation Model and explained the relation of the conceptual model to the middle-range theory that was tested.

Linkage Adequacy

The criterion of linkage adequacy is met. All conceptual model and middle-
range theory concepts are clearly and explicitly linked by nonrelational representational definitional propositions that are given in the introductory and instruments
sections of the research report. *text continues on page 362*

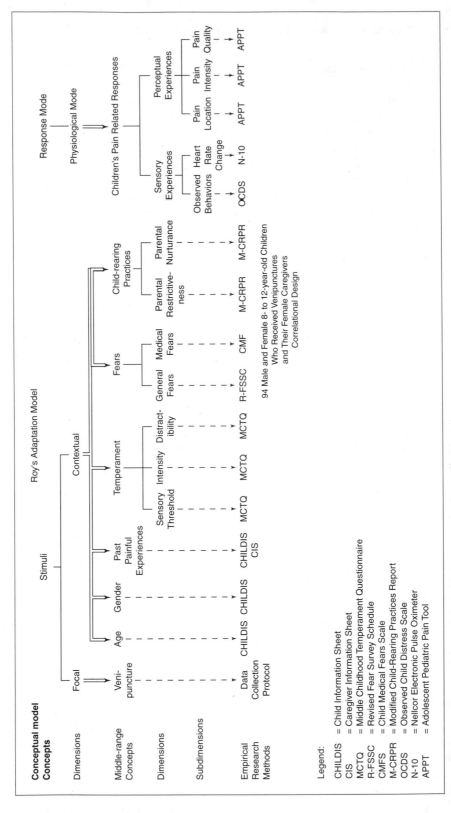

Figure F-1 ■ Conceptual-theoretical-empirical structure for Bournaki's research.

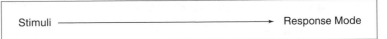

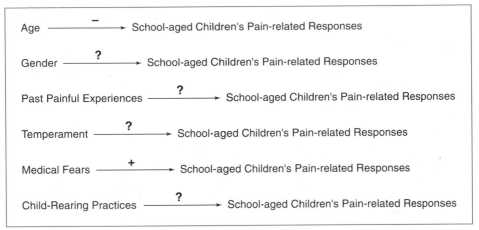

Figure F–2 ■ Diagram of the conceptual model relational proposition for Bournaki's research.

Figure F–3 ■ Diagrams of the relational propositions for the middle-range theory of correlates of school-aged children's pain-related responses to venipunctures.

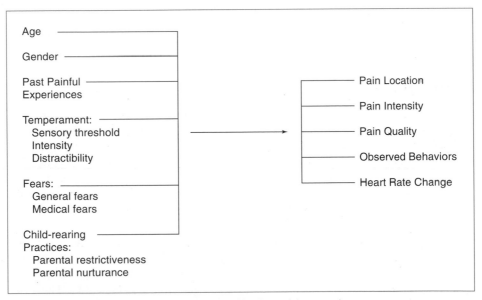

Figure F–4 ■ Diagram of the hypothesis tested by Bournaki's research.

Conceptual Model Usage Rating Scale

Evaluation of the criteria of specification adequacy and linkage adequacy is summarized by application of the Conceptual Model Usage Rating Scale. Bournaki's research report earned a score of 3, indicating adequate use of Roy's Adaptation Model.

EVALUATION OF THE THEORY

Significance

The middle-range theory of correlates of school-age children's pain-related responses to venipunctures meets the criterion of significance. Bournaki addressed the social significance of her study in the introductory section of the research report. She stated:

> ■ Venipunctures are described as painful procedures by hospitalized children and the most difficult to deal with by adolescent oncology survivors . . . Between 4% and 17% of school-age children rated their pain intensity to a venipuncture as severe, and 38% of children ages 3 to 10 had to be physically restrained during a venipuncture. Manne, Jacobsen, and Redd reported that the pain intensity and behavioral responses of 3- to 10-year-old children were moderate. In a recent study by Van Cleve et al., hospitalized school-age children were found to rate venipuncture or intravenous cannulation as moderately painful.

Bournaki also addressed the theoretical significance of her study in the introductory section and again later in the background section of the report. She explained: "Not all children respond similarly to venipunctures. . . . Factors that account for variability in children's responses to venipunctures have not been fully identified." Continuing, Bournaki pointed out that "Previous studies of the effects of multiple variables on children's pain intensity and behavioral responses to venipunctures have been informative. However, children's pain has not been measured in a comprehensive fashion."

Internal Consistency

The middle-range theory of correlates of school-age children's pain-related responses to venipunctures meets the criterion of internal consistency in part. Semantic clarity is evident, in that constitutive definitions are explicitly given or can be easily extracted from the report for all middle-range theory concepts. Semantic consistency is generally evident in that the same terms are used for the same concepts throughout the report. Although the terms "observed behaviors" and "behavioral responses" are used interchangeably throughout the research report, this does not create much confusion. There are no redundant concepts.

Structural consistency is evident, in that a hierarchy based on level of abstraction could be constructed. In addition, a hierarchy based on deductive reasoning could be constructed, leading from the main research hypothesis stated in concept names to the hypothesis stated in the names of the empirical indicators. However, a flaw in structural consistency was noted, in that no relational proposition is given for the relation between the general fears dimension of the theory concept fears and school-age children's pain-related responses. Furthermore, no propositions are given for the relation between the specific dimensions of the theory concept temperament and school-age children's pain-related responses, or for the relation between the specific dimensions of the theory concept child-rearing practices and school-age children's pain-related responses. In both cases, the relational proposition asserted a relation between only the theory concept (that is, temperament and child-rearing practices) and school-age children's pain-related responses. There are no redundant propositions.

Parsimony

The middle-range theory of correlates of school-age children's pain-related responses to venipunctures meets the criterion of parsimony. Although the original theory is made up of eight concepts, some of which are multidimensional, it is neither oversimplified nor excessively verbose (Table F-1). Moreover, the theory that emerged from the testing is even more parsimonious (Table F–3, middle-range theory Proposition 39; Fig. F-4; Fig. F–5).

Testability

The middle-range theory of correlates of school-age children's pain-related responses to venipunctures meets the criterion of testability. Measured operational definitions clearly link the middle-range theory concepts with their respective empirical indicators. An explicit, testable hypothesis is given in the research report, and it was falsified. Moreover, a falsifiable hypothesis based on the theory that

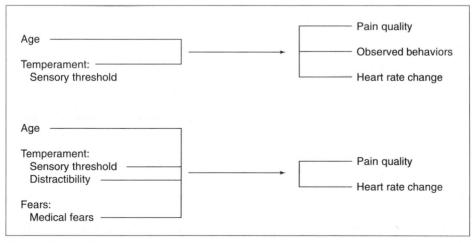

Figure F–5 ■ Diagram of the explanatory theory of correlates of school-aged children's pain-related responses to venipunctures after testing.

emerged from the theory-testing research could easily be developed (Table F–3, middle-range theory Proposition 39; Fig. F–5). In addition, an implicit, falsifiable hypothesis was extracted from the research report (Table F–3, middle-range theory Proposition 38).

EVALUATION OF THE RESEARCH DESIGN

Operational Adequacy

The research design meets the criterion of operational adequacy. The correlational design is clearly explained and was implemented appropriately. A power analysis for the size of the sample is reported and a rationale is given for using a smaller sample than was required by the original power analysis. Moreover, psychometirc data are reported for the empirical indicators. In addition, the statistical technique of canonical correlation was used appropriately. For example, data transformations were performed for concepts that were not normally distributed. Moreover, the pain location dimension of the concept school-age children's pain-related responses was eliminated from the analyses due to very limited variability, and the general fears dimension of the concept fears was excluded from the canonical correlation analysis because of multicollinarity with the medical fears dimension of fears.

EVALUATION OF THE RESEARCH FINDINGS

Empirical Adequacy

The middle-range theory of correlates of school-age children's pain-related responses to venipunctures does not meet the criterion of empirical adequacy. The main research hypothesis required that all concepts and dimensions of those concepts that were designated as the independent variables had to be related to all of the subdimensions of the concept school-age children's pain-related responses. Based on the results of the canonical correlation procedure, Bournaki explicitly concluded, "Inasmuch as all variables did not enter the analysis, the study hypothesis was not supported" (Table F–3, middle-range theory Proposition 39; Fig. F–5).

Furthermore, it was evident from middle-range theory Proposition 27 (Table F–3), which was formalized as an implicit hypothesis, that Bournaki expected the subdimensions of the concept school-age children's pain-related responses to be interrelated. The correlation matrix and the results of the canonical correlation procedure revealed some correlations between subdimensions. Bournaki concluded, "Correlations between the dependent variables as shown in the correlational matrix and in the first canonical variate support a relationship between the perceptual and sensory dimensions of pain. However, the relationship is low in magnitude" (Table F–3, middle-range theory Propositions 38 and 39).

Bournaki offered alternative substantive and methodological explanations for the research finding. For example, she addressed both substantive and methodological explanations when she stated:

■ Contrary to prior research but consistent with the work of Manne et al., the findings showed no relationship between experience with venipunctures [i.e., past painful procedures] and school-age children's pain-related responses. This suggests that experienced children did not habituate to the procedure. It may also be that frequency of exposure is not sufficient information for understanding children's responses to pain. Rather, as [Roy's Adaptation Model] suggests, children's coping abilities with procedures need to be taken into account.

EVALUATION OF THE UTILITY OF THE THEORY FOR PRACTICE

Pragmatic Adequacy

The findings of Bournaki's theory-testing research meet the criterion of pragmatic adequacy. Bournaki pointed out that:

■ This empirical evidence is consistent with the need for clinicians . . . to use a comprehensive approach to assess pain by integrating valid and reliable subjective, behavioral, and physiological measures. . . . This study supports the need to assess children's pain and to identify the factors that may aggravate the pain experience.

Comprehensive assessment of school-age children's responses to venipuncture, employing the instruments used by Bournaki or other clinical tools, is feasible, and clinicians have the legal ability to perform such assessments. Moreover, inasmuch as children and their families expect that attention will be given to pain, comprehensive assessments should be congruent with their expectations. Furthermore, the theory that emerged from testing highlights the areas of assessment that should be incorporated into clinical practice guidelines. To her credit, Bournaki went on to recommend additional research before adopting a particular strategy for helping children to cope with aversive medical procedures.

EVALUATION OF THE CONCEPTUAL MODEL

Credibility

The credibility of Roy's Adaptation Model, which Bournaki used to guide the development of her research, is addressed explicitly in the report. Bournaki commented:

■ The study results provided limited support for the Roy Adaptation Model. Based on the proposition that focal and contextual stimuli influence responses, empirical support was found for the contextual stimuli of age, medical fears, and the temperamental dimensions of distractibility and [sensory] threshold. Only the contextual stimuli that affect developmental stage (age), self-concept (medical fears) and interdependence between parent and child (temperamental dimensions of distractibility and sensory threshold) were supported. . . . Most importantly, findings from the correlational and canonical analyses support the multidimensionality of pain as conceptualized by [Roy's Adaptation Model].

References

Bournaki, M-C. (1997). Correlates of pain-related responses to venipunctures in school-age children. *Nursing Research, 46,* 147–154.

Roy, C., & Andrews, H.A. (1991). *The Roy adaptation model: The definitive statement.* Norwalk, CT: Appleton and Lange.

Analysis and Evaluation of a Predictive Theory-Testing Study: Experimental Research

Boomerang Pillows and Respiratory Capacity

KATHYRN L. ROBERTS
MAUREEN BRITTIN
MARGARET-ANN COOK
JUNE deCLIFFORD

An experimental study was done to determine whether subjects placed on boomerang pillows would have lower vital capacities than subjects placed on straight pillows after 30 minutes. A sample of 42 subjects took part in the study in a nursing laboratory. A crossover design was used in which subjects were measured in both conditions. The findings indicated that there was no significant difference in the vital capacities of subjects in the two conditions. An associated finding was that the vital capacities were significantly lower in a semi-Fowler's position than in a straight chair. It was concluded that boomerang pillows are safe to use for persons without respiratory problems. Further research is needed into the effect of boomerang pillows on persons with respiratory deficits.

Hospitalized patients are now using "boomerang" pillows that are shaped like an inverted letter U or V to increase comfort while in bed.[1] This pillow is designed to fit behind the head and down the shoulders. One pillow replaces the three pillows (one behind the head and one behind each arm and shoulder) that have traditionally been used to achieve the "armchair" position. Figure 1 illustrates this pillow, which is approximately 90 cm across its widest dimension. The pillows are promoted by manufacturers as preventing aching backs, promoting comfort and

Reprinted from *Clinical Nursing Research*, 3(2), 157–165, 1994, with permission.

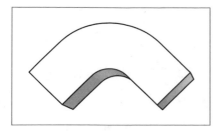

Figure I ■ A boomerang pillow.

support, and as being especially beneficial to the elderly and bedridden. This study was stimulated by the observation of one of the researchers that some patients being supported by boomerang pillows in the semi-Fowler's position were inclined to slump into the pillow because the fixed shape of the pillow prevented the patient from moving the pillow away from the sides of the body. It was hypothesized that this would create posterior convexity of the lumbar curvature and an anterior flexion of the shoulders that could lead to restricted chest expansion during inspiration and resultant lowering of lung capacity. The purpose of this study was to determine whether the use of boomerang pillows as compared with conventional or straight pillows decreased the respiratory capacity.

Levine's Conservation Model (Levine, 1991) provided the theoretical framework for this study. Specifically, the study was based on the principle of conservation on energy, which involves the appropriate use of energy and the prevention of energy depletion (Schaeffer, 1991a). Any factor that limits the individual's ability to expand the lungs fully will limit the lung capacity, thereby decreasing the oxygen transfer, cellular oxygen levels, and thus available energy for metabolism in the body. Levine (1991) stated that respiration is a quantifiable measure of energy use. She had previously noted that proper positioning for maximum respiratory benefit is a major nursing responsibility and that to maintain a straight airway with no interference in the flow of air and to accommodate the muscular activity that controls the size and shape of the thorax are two nursing concerns (Levine, 1973). It has also been suggested that an adequate supply of oxygen as well as rest will help to develop energy reserve to promote structural, personal, and social integrity (Schaeffer, 1991b).

An extensive search of the literature did not reveal any other research studies that investigated the relationship between patient positioning on pillows and lung capacity. Because the boomerang pillows are fairly new there has not been much research carried out as yet. However, one study linking posture and vital capacity was found. Peacock, Westers, Enright, Thomas, and Houlston (1982) compared vital capacities in the fetal position (sitting with hips, knees, and ankles fully flexed, hands clasping ankles), the Trendelenberg position, the supine position, and the lean-standing (standing, arms leaning on a table) and high-grasp position (standing, arms raised grasping bars above head level, with arms spread). Subjects had a higher vital capacity in the latter two positions in which they were upright with the arms away from the body and the abdominal contents were not compressed. The authors concluded that the fixation of the shoulder girdle and the relaxation of pressure on the diaphragm that occurs in both postures would account for the findings. Their study was a pilot study and was done on a small sample; however, a conservative statistical analysis was done.

Because Peacock et al. (1982) showed that a posture in which there was more pressure on the chest from the arms resulted in a lower vital capacity, the hypothesis for the current study was that, because of increased compression of the chest from the boomerang pillow, subjects positioned on boomerang pillows would have lower vital capacities than those positioned on straight pillows.

METHOD

Design
The design of the study was an experimental crossover design in which the vital capacity of well persons was compared at rest in a semi-Fowler's position. Subjects were measured before and after a period of resting on a boomerang pillow and before and after a period of resting on straight pillows. Each subject was measured both in the control (straight pillows) and treatment (boomerang pillows) position and subjects therefore served as their own controls. This design minimized the possibility of differences between groups. Subjects were commenced alternately on boomerang and straight pillows to control for fatigue effects. Random allocation to the first condition was not considered necessary because each subject was tested in both conditions and there was a 50% likelihood of the subject entering each commencing condition.

Sample
The minimum sample size for this study was calculated, using a formula to calculate sample size for a single mean with a 95% level of confidence and a 90% probability of detecting a true difference (Dawson-Saunders & Trapp, 1990). According to figures provided by the Work Health Authority in Darwin, the normal mean vital capacity for a female of average height (165 cm) is 3.6 liters. A standard deviation of 20% was considered to be reasonable. It was considered that a difference of 360 mls would detect a 10% difference in the means. The minimum sample size was calculated at 42 in each condition. Because subjects served as their own controls and were measured twice, the sample size needed was 42.

A convenience sample of 42 volunteer subjects took part in the study. They were persons who were generally healthy and without any condition that would affect their respiratory system. It was decided to carry out the study on well persons initially to establish baseline data because no previous similar research had been done. The subjects were adult females in order to eliminate any difference between male and female breathing patterns such as differences in diaphragmatic and costal breathing. Smokers were not excluded because the measurements were comparing pre- and posttreatment readings in the same individuals. It was expected that the vital capacity of subjects measured after 30 minutes on boomerang pillows would be lower than that of subjects measured after the same time on straight pillows.

Equipment
The study used the beds in the Nursing Laboratory at the Northern Territory University, Darwin, Australia. New boomerang and straight pillows were used to make sure that each pillow was the same as the others of its type. The vital capacity was measured at rest using a Vitallograph, an electronically controlled spirometer with an accuracy of $\pm 3\%$. A mouthpiece is connected by a tube to the Vitallograph that measures the vital capacity and gives a digital reading. Disposable mouthpieces were used for reasons of hygiene.

Procedure
The subjects were informed about the project and asked to fill in a consent form. The procedure for measuring the vital capacity was explained to the subjects. The vital capacity was measured in a sitting position on a chair at the beginning of the experiment to accustom the subject to the procedure and at a 5-minute interval

to record baseline data in a sitting position. The subject was asked to take as deep a breath as possible and then to breathe out into the mouthpiece as deeply as possible. Following the initial readings, the subjects were asked to lie on a bed raised to an angle of 45°, or in the semi-Fowler's position. They were positioned on either two straight pillows or one boomerang pillow on top of a straight pillow, which provided the same angle of elevation for both conditions. Subjects were requested to lie quietly and not to talk during the procedure. An initial reading was taken at 2 minutes and another at 30 minutes, while the subjects were still in position on the pillows. Then the subjects were switched over to the other type of pillow and another set of readings was done at 2 and 30 minutes. Data were recorded on specially prepared data rosters, using code numbers to protect the anonymity of the subjects.

Data Analysis

Data were analyzed using the StatView program on a Macintosh computer. The data for all means were normally distributed with 66% of measurements falling within one standard deviation of the mean. Paired t tests were therefore used to determine significant differences in the means, because different measurements from the same subjects were compared. A 95% level of confidence was set.

FINDINGS

The mean vital capacity of all subjects at the initial sitting measurement was 3.9 liters with an SD of 1.1 liters, and after 5 minutes the mean was 4.3 liters with an SD of 1.0 liters. Table 1 shows the comparison of results for the two types of pillows.

There was no significant difference between the vital capacities on the two types of pillows at 30 minutes (paired one-tailed t test, $p \geq .05$). In addition, there was no significant difference in the 2-minute and 30-minute readings on either type of pillow or between pillows at 2 minutes. Thus the hypothesis that the vital capacity of subjects on boomerang pillows would be lower than that of those on straight pillows after 30 minutes was not supported. An interesting finding was that the mean vital capacity sitting at 5 minutes was higher than that taken in bed for the straight pillows ($p = .06$) and significantly higher than that taken in bed for the boomerang pillows ($p = .0001$), indicating that there is slightly greater lung capacity (300 mls to 400 mls) in a sitting position upright on a chair than at rest in a semi-Fowler's position in bed.

DISCUSSION

This study has shown that in well persons the use of boomerang pillows does not inhibit the respiratory capacity any more than the use of straight pillows does. Although it was not specifically planned to investigate the differences between chair and bed, the results of the study also indicate that positioning in an upright chair does appear to provide slightly better lung capacity than in a bed in a semi-Fowler's position. This finding supports the finding of Peacock et al. (1982) that a more upright posture increases vital capacity, a finding that is explained by the lower position of the diaphragm in the sitting position. These results suggest that the use of

Table 1 ■ **VITAL CAPACITY ON TWO TYPES OF PILLOW (IN LITERS)**

Type of Pillow	2 minutes		30 minutes	
	X	**SD**	**X**	**SD**
Straight	4.1	1.2	3.9	1.1
Boomerang	3.9	1.1	3.9	1.0

boomerang pillows does not interfere with the conservation of energy as proposed by Levine's model and that positioning patients out of bed in a comfortable, upright chair may improve the lung capacity and therefore assist conservation of energy as proposed by Levine (1991) and supported by Schaeffer (1991a, 1991b).

The study was limited in that it used only well persons and a convenience sample so that the results cannot be generalized to all patients. Further research using elderly and/or ill persons who may have respiratory problems is indicated. A future study on this topic could improve the design of the experiment by using a longer measurement such as minute volume rather than vital capacity to diminish the individual variation effects. Further research comparing lung expansion of persons in semi-Fowler's position in a bed, high Fowler's position in bed, and sitting up in a chair could also be useful. Such studies can improve nursing practice by adding to the knowledge about safe measurements to assure patient comfort while maintaining conservation of energy.

IMPLICATIONS FOR PRACTICE

On the basis of this study, boomerang pillows appear to be just as safe as straight pillows for use in the home or in the hospital as long as the person does not have an acute illness or impaired breathing. However, because this study used a convenience sample and was the first to investigate these pillows, a replication study using a larger sample that is more representative and includes males would be a more convincing demonstration of their safety. Until further research demonstrates whether boomerang pillows are indicated for persons with decreased respiratory capacity, they should be used with caution on any patient with a breathing problem and the patient's respirations should be monitored.

In this study, there was an improvement of approximately 10% in vital capacity when subjects sat upright compared with leaning back at an angle of 45°. Thus having patients sit up out of bed where possible will result in an improved lung capacity.

In summary, clinicians may have confidence in using boomerang pillows for persons who are relatively well, but should monitor their use with patients until further research demonstrates their safety. ■

NOTE

1. *Boomerang pillow* is a generic term for these pillows in Australia. They are marketed under various trade names.

REFERENCES

Dawson-Saunders, B., & Trapp, R. (1990). *Basic and clinical biostatistics.* East Norwalk, CT: Appleton-Lange.

Levine, M. (1973). *Introduction to clinical nursing.* Philadelphia: F.A. Davis.

Levine, M. (1991). The conservation principles, a model for health. In K. Schaefer & J. Pond (Eds.), *Levine's conservation model* (pp. 1–11). Philadelphia: F. A. Davis.

Peacock, J., Westers, T., Enright, M., Thomas, A., & Houlston, C. (1982). Posture and vital capacity. *Physiotherapy Canada, 34*(6), 337–340.

Schaeffer, K. (1991a). Levine's conservation principles and research. In K. Schaefer & J. Pond (Eds.), *Levine's conservation model* (pp. 45–59). Philadelphia: F. A. Davis.

Schaeffer, K. (1991b). Care of the patient with congestive heart failure. In K. Schaefer & J. Pond (Eds.), *Levine's conservation model* (pp. 119–131). Philadelphia: F. A. Davis.

ANALYSIS OF THE CONCEPTUAL-THEORETICAL-EMPIRICAL STRUCTURE

The stated purpose of Roberts, Brittin, Cook, and deClifford's (1994) research was to determine whether the use of boomerang pillows decreased the vital capacity as compared with conventional or straight pillows. The research was designed to test a middle-range predictive theory of the effect of position on vital capacity, by means of experimental research.

IDENTIFICATION OF CONCEPTS

Conceptual Model Concepts

Analysis of the research report revealed that the research was guided by Levine's (1991) Conservation Model. The conceptual model concept of interest for the research is conservation of energy.

Middle-Range Theory Concepts

Further analysis of the research report revealed that the middle-range predictive theory of the effect of position on vital capacity encompasses two concepts: position and vital capacity. Vital capacity is a unidimensional concept. Position has three dimensions: boomerang pillow, straight pillow, and sitting upright. The decision to include the dimension sitting upright was made when this position emerged as central to the theory in the results section of the research report.

CLASSIFICATION OF MIDDLE-RANGE THEORY CONCEPTS

The middle-range theory concept position is classified as an observational term in Kaplan's schema and as an observable in Willer and Webster's schema because each position can be seen. The concept is classified as a variable because it has three forms—boomerang pillow, straight pillow, or sitting upright. It is classified as an enumerative unit in Dubin's schema because the subjects were always in some kind of position.

The middle-range theory concept vital capacity is classified as a construct in Kaplan's and Willer and Webster's schemata because it was invented for research and clinical purposes and can be observed only by reference to measurements on a calibrated instrument. The concept is classified as a variable because its measurement reflected a range of values in this study. It is classified as an enumerative unit in Dubin's schema because all study participants had some level of vital capacity.

IDENTIFICATION AND CLASSIFICATION OF PROPOSITIONS

Conceptual Model Propositions

Nonrelational and relational propositions from Levine's Conservation Model were used to guide the research. The relevant propositions are listed in Table G–1.

Conceptual model Proposition 1 can be formalized as a nonrelational proposition asserting the constitutive definition for conservation of energy:

> Conservation of energy is defined as the appropriate use of energy and the prevention of energy depletion.

Conceptual model Proposition 2 can be formalized as a relational proposition asserting the existence, direction, and contingent nature of the relation between certain factors and energy. The formalized proposition is:

> Certain factors are negatively related to the ability to extend the lungs fully, which in turn is positively related to lung capacity, which in turn is positively related to oxygen transfer and cellular oxygen, which in turn are positively related to energy.

It should be noted that this proposition includes concepts that are not relevant to Roberts et al.'s research. In particular, Roberts et al. limited their research to the examination of one factor (position) and lung (vital) capacity; they did not include any middle-range theory concepts derived from the conceptual model concepts oxygen transfer, cellular oxygen, and energy.

Middle-Range Theory Propositions

Nonrelational and relational propositions that are central to the middle-range predictive theory of the effect of position on vital capacity are evident in the research report. These propositions are listed in Table G–2.

NONRELATIONAL PROPOSITIONS. Middle-range theory Proposition 1, combined with the stated purpose of the study and information extracted from the procedure

---

Table G–I ▓ **CONCEPTUAL MODEL PROPOSITIONS FROM ROBERTS, BRITTIN, COOK, AND DECLIFFORD'S RESEARCH REPORT**

Proposition	Classification
I. The principle of conservation of energy . . . involves the appropriate use of energy and the prevention of energy depletion.	Nonrelational, Constitutive Definition
2. Any factor that limits the individual's ability to expand the lungs fully will limit the lung capacity, thereby decreasing the oxygen transfer, cellular oxygen levels, and thus available energy for metabolism in the body.	Relational, Existence Direction Contingent

---

Table G–2 ■ **MIDDLE-RANGE THEORY PROPOSITIONS FROM ROBERTS, BRITTIN, COOK, AND DECLIFFORD'S RESEARCH REPORT**

Proposition	Classification
1. Boomerang pillows . . . are shaped like an inverted letter U or V . . . This pillow is designed to fit behind the head and down the shoulders. One pillow replaces the three pillows (one behind the head and one behind each arm and shoulder) that have traditionally been used to achieve the "armchair" position. . . . this pillow . . . is approximately 90 cm across its widest dimension.	Nonrelational, Constitutive Definition
2. Levine's Conservation Model provided the [conceptual] framework for this study. Specifically, the study was based on the principle of conservation of energy.	Nonrelational, Representational Definition
3. Levine stated that respiration is a quantifiable measure of energy use. She had previously noted that proper positioning for maximum respiratory benefit is a major nursing responsibility and that to maintain a straight airway with no interference in the flow of air and to accommodate the muscular activity that controls the size and shape of the thorax are two nursing concerns.	Nonrelational, Representational Definition
4. One study [linked] posture and vital capacity . . . Peacock et al. showed that a posture in which there was more pressure on the chest from the arms resulted in a lower vital capacity.	Relational, Existence Direction
5. The hypothesis for the current study was that, because of increased compression of the chest from the boomerang pillow, subjects positioned on boomerang pillows would have lower vital capacities than those positioned on straight pillows.	Relational, Existence Direction Hypothesis
6. The vital capacity of well persons was compared at rest in a semi-Fowler's position. Subjects were measured before and after a period of resting on a boomerang pillow and before and after a period of resting on straight pillows.	Nonrelational, Experimental Operational Definition
7. Each subject was measured in both the control (straight pillows) and treatment (boomerang) position.	Nonrelational, Experimental Operational Definition
8. It was expected that the vital capacity of subjects measured after 30 minutes on boomerang pillows would be lower than that of subjects measured after the same time on straight pillows.	Relational, Existence Direction Hypothesis
9. New boomerang and straight pillows were used.	Nonrelational, Experimental Operational Definition
10. The vital capacity was measured at rest using a Vitallograph.	Nonrelational, Measured Operational Definition
11. A mouthpiece is connected by a tube to the Vitallograph that measures the vital capacity and gives a digital reading. Disposable mouthpieces were used.	Nonrelational, Experimental Operational Definition
12. The vital capacity was measured in a sitting position on a chair at the beginning of the experiment to accustom the subject to the procedure and at a 5-minute interval to record baseline data in a sitting position. The subject was asked to take as deep a breath as possible and then to breathe out into the mouthpiece as deeply as possible. Following the initial readings, the subjects were asked to lie on a bed raised to an angle of 45°, or in the semi-Fowler's position. They were positioned on either two straight pillows or one boomerang pillow on top of a straight	Nonrelational, Experimental Operational Definition Constitutive Definition

(continued on page 375)

Table G–2 ■ MIDDLE-RANGE THEORY PROPOSITIONS FROM ROBERTS, BRITTIN, COOK, AND DECLIFFORD'S RESEARCH REPORT (*Continued*)

Proposition	Classification
pillow, which provided the same angle of elevation for both conditions. Subjects were requested to lie quietly and not to talk during the procedure. An initial reading was taken at 2 minutes and another at 30 minutes, while the subjects were still in position on the pillows. Then the subjects were switched over to the other type of pillow and another set of readings was done at 2 and 30 minutes.	
13. There was no significant difference between the vital capacities on the two types of pillows at 30 minutes (paired one-tailed *t* test, $p \geq .05$). In addition, there was no significant difference in the 2-minute and 30-minute readings on either type of pillow or between pillows at 2 minutes. Thus the hypothesis that the vital capacity of subjects on boomerang pillows would be lower than that of those on straight pillows after 30 minutes was not supported.	Relational, Result of testing main research hypothesis
14. An interesting finding was that the mean vital capacity sitting [upright] at 5 minutes was higher than that taken in bed for the straight pillows ($p = .06$) and significantly higher than that taken in bed for the boomerang pillows ($p = .0001$), indicating that there is slightly greater lung capacity (300 mls to 400 mls) in a sitting position upright in a chair than at rest in a semi-Fowler's position in bed.	Relational, Result of testing implicit hypothesis Nonrelational, Constitutive Definition

section of the report, can be formalized as a nonrelational proposition asserting a constitutive definition for the theory concept position. The constitutive definition is:

> Position is defined as having three dimensions: boomerang pillow, straight pillow, and sitting upright. The dimension boomerang pillow is defined as a pillow that is shaped like an inverted letter U or V and is approximately 90 cm at its widest part. This pillow is designed to fit behind the head and down the shoulders. The dimension straight pillow is defined as a conventional pillow. The dimension sitting upright is defined as a sitting position on a chair.

A portion of middle-range theory Proposition 12 can be formalized as a nonrelational proposition asserting a constitutive definition for the theory concept vital capacity. The constitutive definition is:

> Vital capacity is defined as the maximum amount of air expelled after taking as deep a breath as possible.

Middle-range theory Propositions 2 and 3 can be formalized as a nonrelational proposition that asserts a representational definition. Formalized, the representational definition, which links the conceptual model concept with the middle-range theory concepts, is:

> Levine's Conservation Model concept conservation of energy was represented by the middle-range theory concepts position and vital capacity.

It should be noted that the development of this representational definition requires the inference that Roberts et al. equated respiration with vital capacity.

The experimental nature of Roberts et al.'s research led to the search for an experimental operational definition for each theory concept. Such a definition for the theory concept position is evident in middle-range theory Propositions 7, 9, and 12. Analysis of these propositions, combined with the stated purpose of the research, revealed that the dimension boomerang pillow is the experimental condition, and that the dimensions straight pillow and sitting upright are the control conditions. Formalized, the experimental operational definition for the experimental boomerang pillow condition is:

> The subject was asked to lie on a bed raised to an angle of 45°, or in the semi-Fowler's position. She was positioned on one new boomerang pillow on top of one new straight pillow. The subject was requested to lie quietly and not to talk during the procedure. The subject was switched over to the other type of pillow after 30 minutes.

Formalized, the experimental operational definition for the control straight pillow condition is:

> The subject was asked to lie on a bed raised to an angle of 45°, or in the semi-Fowler's position. She was positioned on two straight pillows. The subject was requested to lie quietly and not to talk during the procedure. The subject was switched over to the other type of pillow after 30 minutes.

Formalized, the experimental operational definition for the control sitting upright condition is:

> The subject was placed in a sitting position on a chair for 5 minutes at the beginning of the experiment.

The experimental operational definition describes the empirical indicators for the three dimensions of the concept position, that is, the experimental condition protocol for the dimension boomerang pillow, and the control condition protocols for the dimensions straight pillow and sitting upright.

Middle-range theory Proposition 10 can be formalized as a nonrelational proposition that asserts a measured operational definition for vital capacity. Formalized, the measured operational definition, is:

> Vital capacity was measured by a Vitallograph.

This operational definition clearly links the theory concept vital capacity to its empirical indicator, that is, the Vitallograph.

Middle-range theory Propositions 6, 7, 11, and 12 can be formalized as a nonrelational proposition that asserts an experimental operational definition for the theory concept vital capacity. Formalized, the experimental operational definition is:

> Vital capacity was measured with the subject in a sitting position on a chair at the beginning of the experiment to accustom her to the procedure and at a 5-minute interval to record baseline data in a sitting position. The subject was asked to take as deep a breath as possible and then to breathe out as deeply as possible into a disposable mouthpiece connected by a tube to the Vitallograph. Another

Vitallograph reading was taken 2 minutes after the subject had been positioned on either the boomerang pillow or straight pillows and again 30 minutes later, while the subject was still in position on the pillows. Then the subject was switched over to the other type of pillow and another set of readings was done at 2 and 30 minutes.

This experimental operational definition clearly describes the protocol used to record the data from the empirical indicator (the Vitallograph) for the theory concept vital capacity.

RELATIONAL PROPOSITION. Middle-range theory Propositions 4 and 5 can be formalized as a relational proposition that asserts the existence, direction, and contingent nature of the relation between position and vital capacity. The relational proposition is:

Position is negatively related to chest compression, which in turn is positively related to vital capacity, such that use of a boomerang pillow results in greater chest compression than use of straight pillows, which in turn results in lower vital capacity.

This proposition provides the explanation for the hypothesized effect of position on vital capacity. More specifically, the proposition asserts that chest compression is the factor responsible for the differential effects of the dimensions of the theory concept position on vital capacity.

HYPOTHESES. Middle-range theory Propositions 5 and 8, along with information extracted from the sample and data-analysis sections of the report, can be combined and formalized as a relational proposition that asserts the main research hypothesis. The hypothesis asserts the existence, direction, and magnitude of the relation, as well as the required level of probability for acceptance. Stated in concept names, the hypothesis is:

Position is negatively related to vital capacity, such that 30 minutes of being at rest in a semi-Fowler's position in bed using a boomerang pillow will result in a vital capacity of at least 360 mls lower than vital capacity after 30 minutes of being at rest in a semi-Fowler's position in bed using straight pillows, at the 95% level of confidence.

Middle-range theory Proposition 14, which was extracted from the results section of the report, can be formalized as two implicit hypotheses that extend the main research hypothesis. Inasmuch as these hypotheses are implicit, they are stated in the null form. Formalized and stated in concept names, the implicit hypotheses are:

There is no relation between position and vital capacity, such that there is no difference in the vital capacity of subjects when they are sitting upright and when they are at rest in a semi-Fowler's position in bed using a boomerang pillow.

There is no relation between position and vital capacity, such that there is no difference in the vital capacity of subjects when they are sitting upright and when they are at rest in a semi-Fowler's position in bed using straight pillows.

HIERARCHY OF PROPOSITIONS

A hierarchy of propositions based on level of abstraction can be constructed from the conceptual model nonrelational constitutive definitional proposition, the conceptual model relational proposition, the middle-range theory nonrelational representational definitional proposition, and the middle-range theory relational proposition. The hierarchy is:

Abstract propositions: Conservation of energy is defined as the appropriate use of energy and the prevention of energy depletion.

Certain factors are negatively related to the ability to extend the lungs fully, which in turn is positively related to lung capacity, which in turn is positively related to oxygen transfer and cellular oxygen, which in turn are positively related to energy.

Somewhat concrete proposition: Levine's Conservation Model concept conservation of energy was represented by the middle-range theory concepts position and vital capacity.

More concrete proposition: Position is negatively related to chest compression, which in turn is positively related to vital capacity, such that use of a boomerang pillow results in greater chest compression than use of straight pillows, which in turn results in lower vital capacity.

In addition, a hierarchy of propositions based on deductive reasoning can be constructed for the main research hypothesis, by using the hypothesis stated in concept names and the operational definitions to deduce the hypothesis stated in terms of the empirical indicators. That hierarchy is:

Axiom$_1$: If position is negatively related to vital capacity, such that 30 minutes of being at rest in a semi-Fowler's position in bed using a boomerang pillow will result in a vital capacity of at least 360 mls lower than vital capacity after 30 minutes of being at rest in a semi-Fowler's position in bed using straight pillows, at the 95% level of confidence, and

Axiom$_2$: if use of a boomerang pillow is the experimental condition protocol, and

Axiom$_3$: if use of straight pillows is a control condition protocol, and

Axiom$_4$: if vital capacity is measured by the Vitallograph, then

Hypothesis: study participants will have a Vitallograph reading of at least 360 mls lower when under the experimental boomerang pillow condition protocol for 30 minutes than

when under the control straight pillow condition protocol
for 30 minutes, at the 95% level of confidence.

DIAGRAMS

The conceptual-theoretical-empirical structure for the research is illustrated in
Figure G–1. Another diagram was constructed to illustrate the relational proposition from the conceptual model (Fig. G–2). This diagram illustrates the contingent
relation between certain factors and energy as an inventory of antecedents and consequences. Still another diagram was constructed to illustrate the middle-range theory proposition that position is related to vital capacity (Fig. G–3). The negative
sign of this relational proposition indicates that use of the boomerang pillow (the
experimental condition) would result in lower vital capacity than use of the straight
pillows (one of the control conditions).

EVALUATION OF THE CONCEPTUAL-THEORETICAL-EMPIRICAL STRUCTURE

Analysis of Roberts et al.'s research report revealed that a middle-range predictive theory of the effect of position on vital capacity was tested. The concepts

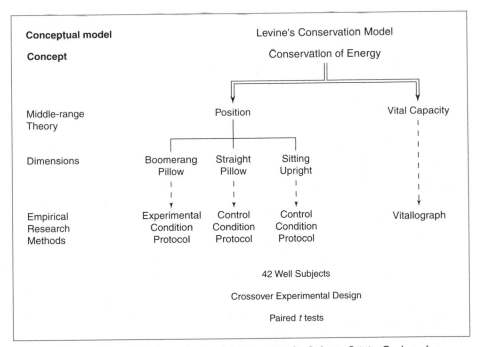

Figure G–I ■ Conceptual-theoretical-empirical structure for Roberts, Brittin, Cook, and deClifford's research.

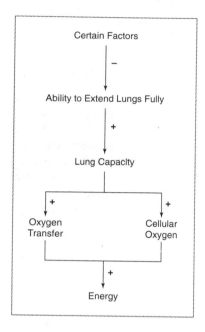

Figure G–2 ■ An inventory of antecedents and consequences: the conceptual model relational proposition guiding Roberts, Brittin, Cook, and deClifford's research.

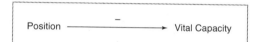

Figure G–3 ■ Diagram of the middle-range theory relational proposition for Roberts, Brittin, Cook, and deClifford's research.

are position, which has the three dimensions of boomerang pillow, straight pillow, and sitting upright, and vital capacity.

EVALUATION OF THE CONCEPTUAL-THEORETICAL-EMPIRICAL LINKAGES

Specification Adequacy

The criterion of specification adequacy is met. The conceptual model that guided Roberts et al.'s theory-testing research is explicitly identified as Levine's Conservation Model. Levine's model concept principle of the conversation of energy was discussed in sufficient breadth and depth so that its relation to the middle-range theory and the empirical research methods is clear.

Linkage Adequacy

The criterion of linkage adequacy is met. The linkage between the conceptual model concept conservation of energy and the middle-range theory concepts position and vital capacity is evident in the research report. It should be noted, however, that the linkage requires the inference that Roberts et al. equated respiration with vital capacity. Taken together, the conceptual model and middle-range theory relational propositions support that inference.

Conceptual Model Usage Rating Scale

Evaluation of the criteria of specification adequacy and linkage adequacy is summarized by application of the Conceptual Model Usage Rating Scale. Roberts et al.'s research report earned a score of 3, indicating adequate use of Levine's Conservation Model.

EVALUATION OF THE THEORY

Significance

The middle-range theory of the effect of position on vital capacity meets the criterion of significance. Roberts et al. addressed the social significance of their research in the very first sentence of their report: "Hospitalized patients are now using 'boomerang' pillows . . . to increase comfort while in bed." A few sentences later, they claimed that "The pillows are promoted by manufacturers as preventing aching backs, promoting comfort and support, and as being especially beneficial to the elderly and bedridden."

Continuing, Roberts et al. addressed the theoretical significance of the research:

▨ This study was stimulated by the observation of one of the researchers that some patients being supported by boomerang pillows in the semi-Fowler's position were inclined to slump into the pillow because the fixed shape of the pillow prevented the patient from moving the pillow away from the sides of the body. It was hypothesized that this would create posterior convexity of the lumbar curvature and an anterior flexion of the shoulders that could lead to restricted chest expansion during inspiration and resultant lowering of lung capacity. . . . An extensive search of the literature did not reveal any other . . . studies that investigated the relationship between patient positioning and lung capacity. Because boomerang pillows are fairly new there has not been much research carried out as yet.

Internal Consistency

The middle-range theory of the effect of position on vital capacity meets the criterion of internal consistency in part. Semantic clarity is evident, in that two of the dimensions for the theory concept position are clearly identified as boomerang pillow and straight pillow, and the dimension boomerang pillow is explicitly defined. Although an explicit constitutive definition for the dimension straight pillow is not given, Roberts et al. refer it as a "conventional or straight pillow" in the introductory section of the report. In contrast, the dimension sitting upright had to be extracted from the results section of the research report, and its constitutive definition had to be extracted from the procedure section. Furthermore, the constitutive definition for the theory concept vital capacity is embedded in an experimental operational definition and is recognized as such only if the reader has sufficient clinical knowledge of this concept or has access to a medical dictionary (Thomas, 1997, p. 300). Semantic consistency is evident for the concept position; Roberts et al. consistently use the terms "boomerang pillow" and "straight pillow." Semantic consistency is not evident, however, for the concept vital capacity; indeed, Roberts et al. use the terms "respiratory capacity," "lung capacity," and "vital capacity" interchangeably throughout the report. The theory contained no redundant concepts.

Structural consistency is evident, in that hierarchies of propositions based on level of abstraction and on deductive reasoning could be constructed. The theory contained no redundant propositions.

Parsimony

The middle-range theory of the effect of position on vital capacity meets the criterion of parsimony. The theory is neither oversimplified nor excessively verbose.

Testability

The middle-range theory of the effect of position on vital capacity meets the criterion of testability. Experimental operational definitions clearly link position and vital capacity with their respective empirical indicators. Moreover, the main research hypothesis proposed by Roberts et al. was falsified. In addition, Roberts et al. used an unanticipated study finding from their study (i.e., the result of testing the implicit hypothesis) to propose an alternative hypothesis, also derived from Levine's model concept conservation of energy. They proposed that: "Positioning patients out of bed in a comfortable, upright chair may improve the lung capacity and therefore assist conservation of energy as proposed by Levine." If another dimension of position (e.g., sitting in bed) is added, this hypothesis is falsifiable.

EVALUATION OF THE RESEARCH DESIGN

Operational Adequacy

The research design meets the criterion of operational adequacy. The crossover experimental design is clearly explained, rationale are given for each aspect of the design and data-collection procedure, and the design was implemented appropriately. Sample size calculations support the actual number of participants in the study, and a rationale is given for limiting the sample to well female adults. In addition, rationale are given for the use of new pillows and disposable mouthpieces. Moreover, the reliability of the Vitallograph is noted.

EVALUATION OF THE RESEARCH FINDINGS

Empirical Adequacy

The middle-range theory of the effect of position on vital capacity does not meet the criterion of empirical adequacy. Roberts et al. explicitly stated, "The hypothesis that the vital capacity of subjects on boomerang pillows would be lower than that of those on straight pillows after 30 minutes was not supported" (Table G–2, middle-range theory Proposition 13). In particular, no evidence of a difference in vital capacity for the experimental boomerang pillow condition and the control straight pillow condition was found at the a priori 95% level of confidence for a one-tailed paired *t* test.

Although Roberts et al. did not offer alternative substantive or methodological explanations for the lack of empirical adequacy of their theory, they did offer a substantive explanation for the unanticipated finding of higher vital capacity when subjects were sitting upright in a chair then when they were in bed with boomerang or straight pillows (Table G–2, middle-range theory Proposition 14). They stated, "This finding supports the findings of Peacock et al. that a more upright posture increased vital capacity, a finding that is explained by the lower position of the diaphragm in the sitting position."

EVALUATION OF THE UTILITY OF THE THEORY FOR PRACTICE

Pragmatic Adequacy

The findings of Roberts et al.'s theory-testing research meets the criterion of pragmatic adequacy. Roberts et al. carefully pointed out that, on the basis of their research, the use of boomerang pillows should be limited to persons who are well. The use of boomerang pillows certainly is feasible, and clinicians have the legal ability to monitor individuals' vital capacity when they are using these pillows. The cost of the pillows and the monitoring equipment, however, may not be supported by administrators.

To their credit, Roberts et al. recommended further research and careful monitoring of any patient who is placed on a boomerang pillow. In particular, they proposed the following clinical practice guideline:

■ Until further research demonstrates whether boomerang pillows are indicated for persons with decreased respiratory capacity, they should be used with caution on any patient with a breathing problem and the patient's respirations should be monitored. . . . Clinicians may have confidence in using boomerang pillows for persons who are relatively well, but should monitor their use with patients until further research demonstrates their safety.

EVALUATION OF THE CONCEPTUAL MODEL

Credibility

The credibility of Levine's Conservation Model, which Roberts et al. used to guide the development of their research, is addressed explicitly in the report. Roberts et al. stated:

▓ The results [of the study] suggest that the use of boomerang pillows does not interfere with the conservation of energy as proposed by Levine's model and that positioning patients out of bed in a comfortable, upright chair may improve the lung capacity and therefore assist conservation of energy.

Roberts et al. did, however, recommend that further research on the effects of position be guided by Levine's model concept conservation of energy. They stated:

▓ Further research comparing lung expansion of persons in semi-Fowler's position in a bed, high Fowler's position in bed, and sitting up in a chair could also be useful. Such studies can improve nursing practice by adding to the knowledge about safe measures to assure patient comfort while maintaining conservation of energy.

Given the unanticipated finding of the study with regard to higher vital capacity when study participants were sitting upright in a chair than when they were in bed with boomerang or straight pillows, the recommendation for further research that is guided by Levine's Conservation Model is warranted.

References

Levine, M. (1991). The conservation principles: A model for health. In K. Schaefer & J. Pond (Eds.), *Levine's conservation model* (pp. 1–11). Philadelphia: F.A. Davis.

Roberts, K.L., Brittin, M., Cook, M-A., & deClifford, J. (1994). Boomerang pillows and respiratory capacity. *Clinical Nursing Research, 3,* 157–165.

Thomas, C.L. (Ed.). (1997). *Taber's cyclopedic medical dictionary* (18th ed.). Philadelphia: F.A. Davis.

Index

Page numbers followed by an f indicate figures; those followed by a t indicate tables.